PRACTICAL OSSEOUS SURGERY IN PERIODONTICS AND IMPLANT DENTISTRY

PRACTICAL OSSEOUS SURGERY IN PERIODONTICS AND IMPLANT DENTISTRY

Edited by

Serge Dibart, DMD
Jean-Pierre Dibart, MD

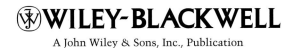

A John Wiley & Sons, Inc., Publication

Library of Congress Cataloging-in-Publication Data

Practical osseous surgery in periodontics and implant dentistry / edited by Serge Dibart, Jean-Pierre Dibart.
   p. ; cm.
  Includes bibliographical references and index.
  ISBN 978-0-8138-1812-2 (hardcover : alk. paper)
  1. Osseointegrated dental implants. 2. Dental implants.
3. Periodontal disease. I. Dibart, Serge. II. Dibart, Jean-Pierre.
[DNLM: 1. Oral Surgical Procedures, Preprosthetic–methods. 2. Alveolar Process–surgery. 3. Dental Implantation, Endosseous–methods. 4. Guided Tissue Regeneration, Periodontal–methods. 5. Periodontal Diseases–surgery. WU 500]
  RK667.I45P73 2011
  617.4'710592–dc22

2011009940

A catalogue record for this book is available from the British Library.

This book is published in the following electronic formats: ePDF 9780470960561; ePub 9780470960578; Mobi 9780470960585

Set in 9.5/12 pt HelveticaNeue-Light by Toppan Best-set Premedia Limited
Printed and bound in Singapore by Fabulous Printers Pte Ltd

Disclaimer

Table of Contents

Foreword

I am delighted to be asked to write the forward for this new book on practical osseous surgery. This book is greatly needed in dentistry and, quite frankly, is overdue. I am especially glad that Serge Dibart and Jean-Pierre Dibart decided to undertake this work and to provide the dental profession with a much-needed resource in the management of intraoral bone.

I cannot help but smile when I see the words "bone" or "alveolar bone" or "osseous." I am reminded of long ago at the start of my graduate training program in periodontology at Harvard under the mentorship of Paul Goldhaber. I did not realize until I arrived in Boston that Paul was a world authority on bone and that he would begin to teach my fellow residents and me all of the intricacies and exciting mysteries of bone. Quite frankly, I thought I was at Harvard to study "periodontal pockets." I remember that in the first month of the residency program, my classmates and I rotated through orthopedic surgery at Massachusetts General Hospital. Paul wanted us to see the management of bone up close and firsthand. And so we watched as hips, knees, and elbows were repaired or replaced or tumors removed from legs and arms and subsequent osseous defects grafted. It was an amazing introduction to osseous surgery. And soon thereafter, upon returning to the dental school, we were given new Ochsenbein chisels and Schluger files and shown how to remove and contour the alveolar bony defects associated with periodontitis. We were also taught the initial steps in bone regeneration using allograft material and later, tissue-guiding membranes. It was a phenomenal time of being "immersed" in the training of the surgical management of bone.

Osseous surgery has clearly come a very long way since I was a resident in periodontics. It is extraordinary what has been introduced to dentistry in the last 30 years, and quite frankly, there is no looking back. Resective osseous surgery, while not as popular as it once was, is nonetheless an essential part of managing bony defects in the treatment of periodontitis and placing dental implants. Sophisticated instruments such as the Piezotome have been introduced to make bone cutting and resection easier and with much fewer complications. Bone regeneration for both periodontal disease management and implant placement management has come a very long way. We now have at our disposal signaling molecules such as growth and differentiation factors that can greatly enhance our ability to regenerate bone. Even as we are adopting specific signaling molecules into our practice, new molecules are being developed that may prove to be more efficacious.

The subsequent introduction of guided bone regeneration principles and techniques has taught us that we can in fact regenerate bone where it is critically needed prior to implant placement. And this new ability to regenerate bone where needed ushered in the era of "prosthetically driven" implant placement. Guided bone regeneration, coupled with bone grafts, signaling molecules, and tissue excluding/guiding membranes have allowed the clinician to dictate where bone will be regenerated. No longer does the mere presence of bone dictate where an implant will be placed. Moreover, extraction sockets are now carefully managed during tooth removal, using a combination of atraumatic techniques, bone grafts, and membranes to ensure maximal preservation of the site.

And now, with no end in sight, osseous surgery has also advanced orthodontic tooth movement. Several years ago the Wilcko brothers brought periodontally accelerated osteogenic orthodontics to the forefront through a series of intriguing cases presented in publications and at meetings. It became clear that the manipulation of bone through osseous surgery, combined with bone regeneration techniques, could foster quicker tooth movement. A more minimally invasive surgical technique introduced will likely make this approach to tooth movement even more acceptable to orthodontists and patients.

All told, I say "lucky us". Serge and Jean-Pierre Dibart have provided us with a first-rate book that provides current concepts and techniques for managing "bone" in periodontics, orthodontics, and implant dentistry. Realizing how far and how quickly dentistry's management of osseous conditions has advanced, I look forward to the future and the continual development of this aspect of patient management in dentistry, knowing that clinicians such as the Dibarts will help advance this very exciting area of dentistry.

Ray C. Williams, DMD
Professor and Dean
School of Dental Medicine
Stony Brook University
Stony Brook, NY 11794

Contributors

Editors

Serge Dibart, DMD
Professor and Director
Graduate Periodontology and Oral Biology
Henry M. Goldman School of Dental Medicine
Boston University
Boston MA
USA

Jean-Pierre Dibart, MD
Rheumatology and Sport Medicine
Private Practice
Marseille, France

Contributors

Rima Abdallah BDS, CAGS, DSc
Department of Periodontology and Oral Biology
Henry M. Goldman School of Dental Medicine
Boston University
Boston, MA
USA

Fahad Al-Harbi, BDS, MSD, FACP, DScD
Dean
College of Dentistry
University of Dammam
Dammam
Saudi Arabia

Obadah H. Attar, BDS
Certificate in Endodontics, Post Doctoral Fellowship in Implantology
DScD in Endodonitcs
Resident
Endodontic Department
Boston University Goldman School of Dental Medicine
Boston, MA
USA

Rayyan Kayal, BDS, DSc
Diplomate, American Board of Periodontology
Assistant Professor and Consultant of Periodontology
King Abdulaziz University—Faculty of Dentistry
Jeddah
Saudi Arabia

Mohamad Koutrach, DDS
Assistant Professor of Prosthodontics
Boston University Institute for Dental Research & Education—Dubai
Dubai, United Arab Emirates

Francis Louise, DDS
Professor and Director
Department of Periodontology
School of Dental Medicine
Université de la Méditerranée
Marseille
France

Yves Macia, DDS, MS (anthropology)
Associate Professor
Department of Periodontology
Université de la Méditerranée
Marseille
France

Luigi Montesani, MD, DMD
Specialist in Periodontology and Prosthetic Dentistry
Private Practice
Rome, Italy

Steven M. Morgano, DMD
Professor and Director
Division of Postdoctoral Prosthodontics
Department of Restorative Sciences and Biomaterials
Henry M. Goldman School of Dental Medicine
Boston University
Boston, MA
USA

Albert M. Price, DMD, DSc
Associate Clinical Professor
Department of Periodontology and Oral Biology
Henry M. Goldman School of Dental Medicine
Boston University
Boston MA
USA

Ulrike Schulze-Späte, DMD, PhD
Assistant Professor of Dental Medicine
Division of Periodontics
Section of Oral and Diagnostics Sciences
College of Dental Medicine
Columbia University
New York, NY
USA

**Saynur Vardar Sengul, DDS, PhD, CAGS
in Periodontology**
Department of Periodontology and Oral Biology
Henry M. Goldman School of Dental Medicine
Boston University
Boston, MA
USA

Mingfang Su, DMD, MSc
Associate Clinical Professor
Department of Periodontology and Oral Biology
Henry M. Goldman School of Dental Medicine
Boston University
Boston, MA
USA

Ray Williams, DMD
Professor and Dean
School of Dental Medicine
Stony Brook University
Stony Brook, NY
USA

Oreste D. Zanni, DDS
Assistant Clinical Professor
Department of Periodontology and Oral Biology
Henry M. Goldman School of Dental Medicine
Boston University
Boston, MA
USA

Yun Po Zhang, PhD, DDS (hon)
Director
Clinical Dental Research
Colgate-Palmolive Company
Piscataway, New Jersey
USA

Acknowledgments

The authors would like to thank Mary O. Taber for her considerable help and expertise in editing and formatting this manuscript. And special thanks to Dr. George Gallagher for providing the histological picture for the book's cover.

The authors would also like to thank Dr. Gurkan Goktug for his contribution to Chapter 16 and Dr. Anuradha Deshmukh and Anastasios Moschidis for their contribution to Chapter 7.

Section 1

Body-Mouth Connection: Relevant Pathologies Affecting Dental Treatment, Guidelines, Prevention, and Necessary Precautions

Chapter 1 Body Weight, Diet, and Periodontitis

Jean-Pierre Dibart, MD

BODY WEIGHT

Introduction

The body mass index relates body weight to height. Body mass index, or BMI, is defined as the weight in kilograms divided by the height in meters squared. Obesity is defined as a body mass index greater than $30 \, kg/m^2$; BMI between $25 \, kg/m^2$ and $30 \, kg/m^2$ defines overweight people, the normal weight being between $19 \, kg/m^2$ and $25 \, kg/m^2$. Obesity is a chronic disease with many important medical complications. The main cause of obesity is an imbalance between energy intake and energy expenditure.

The necessary treatment includes

- a calorie-restricted diet,

- increased physical activity, and

- nutritional modifications, with reduction of fat and sugar intake

The prevalence of obesity has increased in Western countries. It is a metabolic disease that predisposes to many medical complications such as cardiovascular disease, cancer, arthrosis, and diabetes, and it has also been implicated as a risk factor for chronic health conditions such as periodontitis. Obesity is associated with periodontal disease because the adipose tissues secrete some cytokines and hormones that are involved in inflammatory process. A high body mass index is associated with a systemic low-grade inflammatory state. Tumor necrosis factor-α, a proinflammatory cytokine, is produced in adipose tissues and is responsible for lowered insulin sensitivity, called insulin resistance which is responsible for elevated plasma glucose levels.

Periodontitis is characterized by alveolar bone loss, which is the consequence of bone resorption by the osteoclasts. Bone-forming cells (osteoblasts) and bone-resorbing cells (osteoclasts) are under hormonal control; the bone formation is negatively regulated by the hormone leptin, produced from adipocytes.

Health education should encourage better nutritional habits to reach normal weight and prevent obesity, and also to promote better oral hygiene to prevent periodontal disease (Alabdulkarim et al. 2005; Dalla Vecchia et al. 2005; Ekuni et al. 2008; Khader et al. 2009; Lalla et al. 2006; Linden et al. 2007; Nishida et al. 2005; Reeves et al. 2006; Saito et al. 2001; Saito et al. 2005; Wood, Johnson, and Streckfus 2003; Ylostalo et al. 2008).

Body Mass Index

High body mass index is a risk factor for periodontitis. There is a 16% increased risk for periodontitis per $1 \, kg/m^2$ of increased body mass index. Body mass index is also significantly associated with the community periodontal index score (Ekuni et al. 2008). Total body weight is associated with periodontitis. Adolescents aged 17 to 21 years old have a 1.06 times increased risk for periodontal disease per 1 kg increase in body weight (Reeves et al. 2006). There is a significant correlation between body mass index and periodontitis, with a dose-response relationship (Nishida et al. 2005). Obesity is a risk factor for periodontitis; there is an association between high body weight and periodontal infection (Ylostalo et al. 2008). High body mass index is significantly associated with periodontitis, with an odds ratio of 2.9 (Khader et al. 2009). Obesity with a body mass index greater than $30 \, kg/m^2$ is significantly associated with periodontitis, with an odds ratio of 1.77 (Linden et al. 2007).

Obese patients are 1.86 times more likely to present periodontitis according to the following groups:

- For patients older than 40 years of age, the odds ratio is 2.67.

- For females, the odds ratio is 3.14.

- For nonsmokers, the odds ratio is 3.36 (Alabdulkarim et al. 2005).

There is a positive correlation between body mass index and periodontitis, with a significantly higher prevalence in females. Obese females are significantly (2.1 times) more likely to have

Practical Osseous Surgery in Periodontics and Implant Dentistry, First Edition. Edited by Serge Dibart, Jean-Pierre Dibart.

periodontitis (Dalla Vecchia et al. 2005). Obesity is also associated with deep probing pockets. High body mass index and body fat are significantly associated with the highest quintile of mean probing pocket depth (Saito 2005). There is a positive and significant association between high body mass index and the number of teeth with periodontal disease; this may be explained by obesity being responsible for a systemic low-grade inflammatory state (Lalla et al. 2006). People with higher categories of body mass index and upper body abdominal fat have a significantly increased risk of presenting with periodontitis (Saito et al. 2001).

There are significant correlations between body composition and periodontal disease. Body mass index and abdominal visceral fat are significantly associated with periodontitis (Wood, Johnson, and Streckfus 2003). Only 14% of normal-weight people have periodontitis; although 29.6% of overweight people and 51.9% of obese people present with periodontitis. High percentage of body fat, which is a person's total fat divided by that person's weight, is significantly associated with periodontal disease, with an odds ratio of 1.8 (Khader et al. 2009).

Physical Activity

There is an inverse linear association between sustained physical activity and periodontal disease: increased physical activity induces an improvement in insulin sensitivity and glucose metabolism. Periodontitis risk decreases with increased average physical activity. Compared with men in the lowest quintile for physical activity, those in the highest quintile have a significant 13% lower risk of periodontitis. Physically active patients present with significantly less average radiographic alveolar bone loss (Merchant et al. 2003).

Waist-to-Hip Ratio and Waist Circumference

High waist-to-hip ratio is a significant risk factor for periodontitis. Upper-body obesity as measured by the waist-to-hip ratio or the waist circumference is related to visceral abdominal adiposity. Because of induced systemic inflammation and insulin resistance by adipose tissue, it represents a risk factor for type 2 diabetes and cardiovascular diseases. Patients with a high waist-to-hip ratio present a significantly increased risk for periodontitis (Saito et al. 2001). Periodontitis is more frequent among patients with high waist circumference and high waist-to-hip ratio; high waist circumference is significantly associated with periodontitis with an odds ratio of 2.1 (Khader et al. 2009). Adolescents aged 17 to 21 years old have an 1.05 times increased risk of periodontal disease per 1-cm increase in waist circumference (Reeves et al. 2006). Waist-to-hip ratio, which characterizes abdominal visceral fat, is statistically significantly associated with periodontitis. There

are significant correlations between body composition and periodontal disease, waist-to-hip ratio being the most significant element associated with periodontitis (Wood, Johnson, and Streckfus 2003). High waist-to-hip ratio is also significantly associated with the highest quintile of mean probing pocket depth (Saito et al. 2005).

Adipokines

Adipocytes produce cytokines, or adipokines, which are responsible for the association between obesity and other disease. Adipocytes in the adipose tissues of obese people produce large quantities of leptin, which regulates energy expenditure and body weight (Nishimura et al. 2003). Adiponectin and resistin are adipokines, which are responsible for systemic inflammation and insulin resistance in obese people. Serum resistin levels are higher in patients with periodontitis than in healthy subjects. Periodontitis patients with at least one tooth with a probing pocket depth greater than 6 mm have two times higher serum resistin levels than subjects without periodontitis (Furugen et al. 2008). Periodontitis is significantly associated with increased resistin levels. Resistin and adiponectin are secreted from adipocytes, and resistin plays an important role in inflammation (Saito et al. 2008).

Experimentation

Experimental calorie-restriction diet may have anti-inflammatory effects. A low-calorie diet results in a significant reduction in ligature-induced gingival index, bleeding on probing, probing depth, and attachment level. Periodontal destruction is significantly reduced in low-calorie-diet animals (Branch-Mays et al. 2008). After oral infection with *Porphyromonas gingivalis*, mice with diet-induced obesity present a significantly higher level of alveolar bone loss, with 40% increase in bone loss 10 days after inoculation. Accompanying the increase in bone loss, obese mice show an altered immune response with elevated bacterial counts for *P. gingivalis* (Amar et al. 2007).

The Metabolic Syndrome

Metabolic syndrome is characterized by the following:

- Central visceral obesity
- Hypertriglyceridemia and low levels of high-density lipoprotein cholesterol
- Hypertension
- Insulin resistance

Abdominal visceral obesity is characterized by an increased waist circumference.

Atherogenic dyslipidemia is defined by raised triglycerides and low concentrations of high-density lipoprotein cholesterol, elevated apolipoprotein B, small high-density lipoprotein cholesterol particles, and small low-density lipoprotein cholesterol particles.

Hypertension is characterized by chronic elevated blood pressure.

Insulin resistance or lowered insulin sensitivity is associated with high risk for cardiovascular disease and diabetes.

A proinflammatory state is generally present with the elevation of serum C-reactive protein because adipose tissues release inflammatory cytokines, inducing the elevation of C-reactive protein.

Prothrombotic state is characterized by raised serum plasminogen activator inhibitor and high fibrinogen (Grundy et al. 2004). The metabolic syndrome is associated with severe periodontitis; these patients are 2.31 times more likely to present with the metabolic syndrome. The prevalence of the metabolic syndrome is

- 18% among patients with no or mild periodontitis,

- 34% among patients with moderate periodontitis, and

- 37% among patients with severe periodontitis (D'Aiuto et al. 2008).

NUTRITION

Omega-3 Polyunsaturated Fatty Acids

Sources of omega-3 polyunsaturated fatty acids (eicosapentaenoic acid and docosahexaenoic acid) can be found in animals and especially in fish such as salmon, tuna, and mackerel. They are also present in many vegetables and nuts (alphalinolenic acid), such as walnuts and almonds. They are capable of reducing proinflammatory cytokine levels (Enwonwu and Ritchie 2007).

Fish oil rich in omega-3 polyunsaturated fatty acids, especially eicosapentaenoic acid and docosahexaenoic acid, may protect from bone loss in chronic inflammatory diseases, such as rheumatoid arthritis or periodontitis.

A fish oil-enriched diet inhibit alveolar bone resorption after experimental *P. gingivalis* infection. *P. gingivalis* infected rats fed omega-3 polyunsaturated fatty acids have the same alveolar bone levels as do the healthy animals. Omega-3 polyunsaturated fatty acid dietary supplementation can modulate inflammatory reactions leading to periodontitis, with reduction of the alveolar bone resorption (Kesavalu et al. 2006).

Free Radicals, Reactive Oxygen Species, and Antioxidants

Free radical-induced tissue damage and antioxidant defense mechanisms are important factors present in inflammatory diseases. High levels of reactive oxygen species activity combined with low antioxidant defense can lead to inflammatory diseases such as periodontitis.

Oxidative stress is an imbalance between excess production of reactive oxygen species and low antioxidant defense. The reactive oxygen species are

- superoxide anions,

- hydroxyl radicals, and

- peroxyl radicals (Nassar, Kantarci, and van Dyke 2007).

P. gingivalis induces the release of inflammatory cytokines such as interleukin-8 and tumor necrosis factor-α, leading to an increased activity of polymorphonucleocytes. After the stimulation by bacterial antigens, activated polymorphonucleocytes produce the reactive oxygen species (Sculley and Langley 2002).

Systemic inflammation accelerates the consumption of antioxidants such as vitamins and minerals. Increased production of reactive oxygen species necessitates more antioxidant elements such as zinc, copper, and selenium. Selenium has oxidation-reduction functions, and selenium-dependent glutathione enzymes are necessary for reduction of damaging lipids (Enwonwu and Ritchie 2007). In periodontitis, oxidative stress is present either locally and in the serum. Low serum antioxidant concentrations are associated with higher relative risk for periodontitis. Low serum total antioxidant concentrations are inversely associated with severe periodontitis (Chapple et al. 2007).

Lycopene is an antioxidant carotenoid contained in vegetables, particularly in tomatoes. In periodontitis patients, there is a significant inverse relationship between serum lycopene levels and C-reactive protein, and between monthly tomato consumption and white blood cell count. There is also an inverse relationship between monthly tomato consumption and congestive heart failure risk. For moderate monthly tomato consumption, the risk ratio for congestive heart failure is 3.15; for low monthly tomato consumption, the risk ratio is 3.31; and for very low monthly tomato consumption, the risk ratio is 5.1. For people without periodontitis and with moderate serum lycopene level, the risk ratio for congestive heart failure is 0.25 (Wood and Johnson 2004). Peri-implant disease is caused by bacteria infection associated with inflammation and tissue destruction, which is induced by free radicals and reactive oxygen species. In saliva of patients with peri-implant disease, the total antioxidant status and the concentrations of antioxidants such as uric acid and ascorbate are significantly decreased. On the contrary, total antioxidant status and concentrations of uric acid and ascorbate are higher in healthy people (Liskmann et al. 2007). The total antioxidant capacity of the gingival crevicular fluid and plasma is significantly lower in chronic periodontitis. Successful periodontal therapy increases significantly the total antioxidant capacity of gingival crevicular fluid (Chapple et al. 2007). Gingival crevicular fluid antioxidant concentration is significantly lower in periodontitis. Total antioxidant capacity of plasma is also lower in periodontitis, which can result from excessive systemic inflammation or may induce the periodontal destruction (Brock et al. 2004).

Fusobacterium-stimulated polymorphonucleocytes induce the release of reactive oxygen species, which are responsible for a high degree of lipid peroxidation (Sheikhi et al. 2001). Imbalance between oxidative stress and antioxidant capacity may be responsible for periodontal disease. Lipid peroxidation is significantly higher in periodontitis patients. On the contrary, total antioxidant capacity in saliva is significantly lower in periodontitis patients (Guentsch et al. 2008). Reactive oxygen species are responsible for the destruction of periodontal tissues because of the imbalance between oxidant and antioxidant activity.

In periodontitis, gingival crevicular fluid presents a significantly higher lipid peroxidation level. Saliva shows lower antioxidant glutathione concentration and higher lipid peroxidation level. Periodontal therapy induces a significant decrease of lipid peroxidation and a significant increase in glutathione concentrations (Tsai et al. 2005). Gingival crevicular fluid total antioxidant capacity is significantly decreased in periodontitis patients, presenting lower mean plasma antioxidant capacity. Concentrations of glutathione, which has antioxidant activity, are lower in gingival crevicular fluid because of decreased glutathione synthesis and increased local degradation. In periodontitis plasma and gingival crevicular fluid contain a lower mean total antioxidant capacity (Chapple et al. 2002). Total salivary antioxidant concentrations are significantly lower in periodontitis because of the enhanced action of the reactive oxygen species, which may also predispose to increased effects of reactive oxygen species on periodontal tissues (Chapple et al. 1997).

Superoxide dismutases are antioxidant enzymes that neutralize superoxide radicals. Copper, zinc, and superoxide dismutase are antioxidants that play a protective role against oxidation caused by infections (Balashova et al. 2007).

After stimulation by bacterial antigens, polymorphonucleocytes produce superoxide radicals. The increased number and activity of leukocytes induce an important reactive oxygen species release, with damage to periodontal tissues and to alveolar bone. Ascorbate, albumin, and urate are antioxidant elements of plasma; although urate is the main antioxidant of saliva (Sculley and Langley-Evans 2002). Reactive oxygen species are produced by leukocytes during an inflammatory response. Periodontal destruction is secondary to the imbalance in the antioxidant and oxidant activity in periodontal pockets. Reactive oxygen species are responsible for extracellular matrix proteoglycan degradation because of their oxidant action (Waddington, Moseley, and Embery 2000).

Nutritional Status

Nutrition

Malnutrition impairs phagocytic function, cell-mediated immunity, complement system, and antibody and cytokine production. Protein energy malnutrition is responsible for impaired immunity and multiplication of oral anaerobic pathogens.

Inflammation necessitates the use of increased quantities of vitamins and minerals. Adequate energy and nutrients are necessary for the production of acute phase proteins, inflammatory mediators, and antioxidants.

Calcium and Vitamin D

Calcium and vitamin D are two important elements for bone metabolism. Women with hip osteoporosis have more than three times the alveolar bone loss around posterior teeth than do women without hip osteoporosis. Calcium and phosphorus are major minerals in hydroxyapatite crystals, and vitamin D regulates calcium and phosphorus metabolism and intestinal absorption. Calcium and vitamin D dietary intake is essential for bone health in periodontitis. Calcium and vitamin D medical supplementation is always necessary for osteoporosis treatment and prevention (Kaye 2007).

Whole Grain

Periodontitis may decrease with higher dietary whole-grain intake; four whole-grain servings per day may decrease the risk. Men in the highest quintile of whole-grain intake are 23% less likely to have periodontitis than are those in the lowest (Merchant et al. 2006).

Diet

Patients with metabolic syndrome who undergo 1 year of a nutritional program show the following significant changes in gingival crevicular fluid:

- Reduction of clinical probing depth
- Reduction of gingival inflammation
- Reduced levels of interleukin-1β
- Reduced levels of interleukin-6 (Jenzsch et al. 2009)

Cranberry

A treatment with a cranberry antioxidant fraction prepared from cranberry juice inhibits *Aggregatibacter actinomycetemcomitans*-induced interleukin-6, interleukin-8, and prostaglandin E2 inflammatory mediators production, as well as cycloxygenase-2 inflammatory enzyme expression (Bodet, Chandad, and Grenier 2007).

Green Tea

Catechins are antioxidants derived from green tea; they are able to reduce collagenase activity and tissue destruction. Collagenase activity in gingival crevicular fluid of highly progressive periodontitis patients is inhibited by green tea catechins. Among green tea catechins, epicatechin gallate and epigallocatechin gallate have the most important inhibitory effect (Makimura et al. 1993). Green tea catechins may help in the treatment of periodontal disease. Green tea catechins show a bactericidal effect against Gram-negative anaerobic bacteria such as *P. gingivalis* and *Prevotella* spp. After a mechanical treatment and the local application of green tea catechins, pocket depth and proportion of Gram-negative anaerobic rods are significantly reduced (Hirasawa et al. 2002).

Garlic

Garlic has antimicrobial properties against periodontal pathogens and their enzymes. Periodontal pathogens present among the lowest minimal inhibitory concentrations and the lowest minimum bactericidal concentrations of garlic. Garlic inhibits trypsin-like and total protease activity of *P. gingivalis* (Bakri and Douglas 2005).

Onion

Onion extracts may possess a bactericidal effect on some oral pathogens such as *Streptococcus mutans*, *Streptococcus sobrinus*, *P. gingivalis,* and *Prevotella intermedia* (Kim 1997).

Vitamins

Vitamin C

There is a significant association between low vitamin C levels and periodontal attachment loss. Patients with vitamin C deficiency show more attachment loss than subjects with normal serum vitamin C levels (Amaliya et al. 2007). Serum vitamin C level is inversely correlated to attachment loss; clinical attachment loss is 4% greater in patients with lower serum vitamin C level (Amarasena et al. 2005). Low serum vitamin C is inversely associated with periodontitis, especially in severe disease. Higher serum vitamin C concentrations are associated with less-severe periodontitis, with an odds ratio of 0.5 (Chapple, Miward, and Dietrich 2007). Chronic peri-

odontitis patients present significantly reduced plasma vitamin C levels; after 2 weeks of dietary vitamin C intake as grapefruit consumption, the plasma levels rise significantly and the sulcus bleeding index is reduced (Staudte, Sigush and Glockmann 2005). *P. gingivalis* infection is associated with low levels of serum vitamin C; there is a highly significant inverse association between plasma vitamin C and *P. gingivalis* antibody levels. High antibody titers to *A. actinomycetemcomitans* and *P. gingivalis* are inversely correlated with low levels of vitamin C, especially for vitamin C concentrations lower than 4 mg/L (Pussinen et al. 2003).

Vitamin B

Chronic periodontitis patients supplemented with multiple vitamin B medications, show significantly lower mean clinical attachment levels (Neiva et al. 2005).

Alcohol Consumption

There is a significant positive linear relationship between high alcohol consumption and periodontal parameters such as mean clinical attachment loss and mean probing depth (Amaral, Luiz, and Leao 2008).

Deep probing depth is significantly associated with high alcohol consumption with an odds ratio of 7.72 (Negishi et al. 2004). Alcohol consumption is significantly associated with increased severity of clinical attachment loss, with the following odds ratios:

- 1.22 for 5 drinks per week
- 1.39 for 10 drinks per week
- 1.54 for 15 drinks per week
- 1.67 for 20 drinks per week (Tezal et al. 2004)

Alcohol consumption is significantly associated with probing depth and attachment loss. For 15–29.9 g alcohol per day, patients have a significantly higher odds ratio (2.7) of having more than 35% of their teeth with probing depth greater than 4 mm (Shimazaki et al. 2005). People who drink alcohol have a higher risk of getting periodontal disease: it is an independent risk factor for periodontitis.

- For 0.1–4.9 g per day, the relative risk is 1.24.
- For 5–29.9 g per day, the relative risk is 1.18.
- For more than 30 g per day, the relative risk is 1.27 (Pitiphat et al. 2003).

Gamma-glutamyl transpeptidase enzyme serum levels are elevated in case of liver damage by chronic alcohol intake. Severe alcohol use with plasma gamma-glutamyl transpeptidase level greater than 51 IU/L is significantly associated with periodontal parameters such as plaque index, gingival margin level, gingival index, probing depth, and attachment loss (Khocht et al. 2003).

Elevated levels of reactive oxygen species following chronic alcohol consumption induce an increased periodontal inflammation, high oxidative damage, and elevated tumor necrosis factor-α concentrations. In rats with ligature-induced periodontitis, ethanol feeding decreases the ratio of reduced oxidized glutathione. Alcohol intake increases polymorphonuclear leukocyte infiltration, tumor necrosis factor-α production, and gingival oxidative damage (Irie et al. 2008).

REFERENCES

Alabdulkarim M, Bissada N, Al-Zahrani M, et al. 2005. *J Int Acad Periodontol*. 7(2):34–38.

Amaliya, Timmerman MF, Abbas F, et al. 2007. *J Clin Periodontol*. 34(4):299–304.

Amar S, Zhou Q, Shaik-Dasthargirisaheb Y, et al. 2007. *Proc Natl Acad Sci USA*. 104(51):20466–71.

Amaral Cda S, Luiz RR, Leao AT. 2008. *J Periodontol*. 79(6):993–98.

Amarasena N, Ogawa H, Yoshihara A, et al. 2005. *J Clin Periodontol*. 32(1):93–97.

Balashova NV, Park DH, Patel JK, et al. 2007. *Infect Immun*. 75(9):4490–97.

Bakri IM, Douglas CW. 2005. *Arch Oral Biol*. 50(7):645–51.

Bodet C, Chandad F, Grenier D. 2007. *Eur J Oral Sci*. 115(1):64–70.

Branch-Mays GL, Dawson DR, Gunsolley JC, et al. 2008. *J Periodntol*. 79(7):1184–91.

Brock GR, Butterworth CJ, Matthews JB, et al. 2004. *J Clin Periodontol*. 31(7):515–21.

Chapple IL, Brock G, Eftimiadi C, et al. 2002. *Mol Pathol*. 55(6):367–73.

Chapple IL, Brock GR, Milward MR, et al. 2007. *J Clin Periodontol*. 34(2):103–10.

Chapple IL, Mason GI, Garner I, et al. 1997. *Ann Clin Biochem*. 34(Pt 4):412–21.

Chapple IL, Miward MR, Dietrich T. 2007. *J Nutr*. 137(3):657664.

D'Aiuto F, Sabbah W, Netuveli G, et al. 2008. *J Clin Endocrinol Metab*. 93(10):3989–94.

Dalla Vecchia CF, Susin C, Rosing CK, et al. 2005. *J Periodontol*. 76(10):1721–28.

Ekuni D, Yamamoto T, Koyama R, et al. 2008. *J Periodontal Res*. 43(4):417–21.

Enwonwu CO, Ritchie CS. 2007. *J Am Dent Assoc*. 138(1):70–73.

Furugen R, Hayashida H, Yamaguchi N, et al. 2008. *J Periodontal Res*. 43(5):556–62.

Grundy SM, Brewer B, Cleeman JI, et al. 2004. *Circulation*. 109:433–38.

Guentsch A, Preshaw PM, Bremer-Streck S, et al. 2008. *Clin Oral Investig*. 12(4):345–52.

Hirasawa M, Takada K, Makimura M, et al. 2002. *J Periodontal Res*. 37(6):433–38.

Irie K, Tomofuji T, Tamaki N, et al. 2008. *J Dent Res*. 87(5):456–60.

Jenzsch A, Eick S, Rassoul F, et al. 2009. *Br J Nutr*. 101(6):879–85.

Kaye EK. 2007. *J Am Dent Assoc*. 138(5):616–19.

Kesavalu L, Vasudevan B, Raghu B, et al. 2006. *J Dent Res*. 85(7):648–52

Khader YS, Bawadi HA, Haroun TF, et al. 2009. *J Clin Periodontol*. 36(1):18–24.

Kim JH. 1997. *J Nihon Univ Sch Dent*. 39(3):136–41.

Khocht A, Janal M, Schleifer S, et al. 2003. *J Periodontol*. 74(4):485–93.

Lalla E, Cheng B, Lal S, et al. 2006. *Diabetes Care*. 29(2):295–99.

Linden G, Patterson C, Evans A, et al. 2007. *J Clin Periodontol*. 34(6):461–66.

Liskmann S, Vihalemm T, Salum O, et al. 2007. *Clin Oral Implants Res*. 18(1):27–33.

Makimura M, Hirasawa M, Kobayashi K, et al. 1993. *J Periodontol*. 64(7):630–36.

Merchant AT, Pitiphat W, Franz M, et al. 2006. *Am J Clin Nutr*. 83(6):1395–1400.

Merchant AT, Pitiphat W, Rimm EB, et al. 2003. *Eur J Epidemiol*. 18(9):891–98.

Nassar H, Kantarci A, van Dyke TE. 2007. *Periodontol 2000*. 43:233–44.

Negishi J, Kawanami M, Terada Y, et al. 2004. *J Int Acad Periodontol*. 6(4):120–24.

Neiva RF, Al Shammari K, Nociti FH Jr, et al. 2005. *J Periodontol*. 76(7):1084–91.

Nishida N, Tanaka M, Hayashi N, et al. 2005. *J Periodontol*. 76(6):923–28.

Nishimura F, Iwamoto Y, Mineshiba J, et al. 2003. *J Periodontol*. 74(1):97–102.

Pitiphat W, Merchant AT, Rimm EB, et al. 2003. *J Dent Res*. 82(7):509–13.

Pussinen PJ, Laatikainen T, Alfthan G, et al. 2003. *Clin Diagn Lab Immunol*. 10(5):897–902.

Reeves AF, Rees JM, Schiff M, et al. 2006. *Arch Pediatr Adolesc Med*. 160(9):894–99.

Saito T, Shimazaki Y, Kiyohara Y, et al. 2005. *J Periodontal Res*. 40(4):346–53.

Saito T, Shimazaki Y, Koga T, et al. 2001. *J Dent Res*. 80(7):1631–36.

Saito T, Yamaguchi N, Shimazaki Y, et al. 2008. *J Dent Res*. 87(4):319–22.

Sculley DV, Langley-Evans SC. 2002. *Proc Nutr Soc*. 61(1):137–43.

Sheikhi M, Bouhafs RK, Hammarstrom KJ, et al. 2001. *Oral Dis*. 7(1):41–46.

Shimazaki Y, Saito T, Kiyohara Y, et al. 2005. *J Periodontol*. 76(9):1534–41.

Staudte H, Sigush BW, Glockmann E. 2005. *Br Dent J*. 199(4):213–17.

Tezal M, Grossi SG, Ho AW, et al. 2004. *J Clin Periodontol*. 31(7):484–88.

Tsai CC, Chen HS, Chen SL, et al. 2005. *J Periodontal Res*. 40(5):378–84.

Waddington RJ, Moseley R, Embery G. 2000. *Oral Dis*. 6(3):138–51.

Wood N, Johnson RB. 2004. *J Clin Periodontol*. 31(7):574–80

Ylostalo P, Suominen-Taipale L, Reunanen A, et al. 2008. *J Clin Periodontol*. 35(4):297–304.

Wood N, Johnson RB, Streckfus CF. 2003. *J Clin Periodontol*. 30(4):321–27.

Chapter 2 Diabetes and Periodontitis

Jean-Pierre Dibart, MD

INTRODUCTION

Definitions

The characteristic metabolic disorder in diabetes is hyperglycemia. Diabetes mellitus is characterized by chronic elevated levels of glucose in the blood. The diagnosis of diabetes is made with fasting plasma glucose levels of 126 mg/dL or greater. Diabetes mellitus results from a dysregulation of glucose metabolism due to the decreased production of insulin by the β cells of islets of Langerhans in the pancreas.

Diabetes is a chronic disease of adults and children and is of two types:

1. diabetes mellitus type 1, which occurs predominantly in youth, although it can occur at any age, and

2. diabetes mellitus type 2, which is the most prevalent type of diabetes and which occurs predominantly in overweight people.

High levels of glycosylated hemoglobin (HbA1c) are the result of elevated blood glucose levels over a period of a few months before the day of blood analysis. HbA1c is a good measure of long-term glucose levels. The normal serum levels of glycosylated hemoglobin are between 4% and 6% (Ship 2003). Severely elevated levels are greater than 9%, and mildly elevated levels are between 7% and 9% (Madden et al. 2008).

Glycemic control is based on following factors:

- better nutrition
- weight loss
- self-monitoring of blood glucose levels
- prevention and treatment of infections (Madden et al. 2008)

Complications

Poorly controlled blood glucose level is the principal cause of vascular complications. There are two types of cardiovascular complications in diabetes:

1. Macrovascular pathology or macroangiopathy, with increased risk of myocardial infarction, peripheral arterial disease, and stroke.

2. Microvascular pathology or microangiopathy, with

   - retinopathy and vascular damage of the retina;
   - nephropathy, with renal failure, renal insufficiency, and end-stage renal disease;
   - neuropathy of peripheral nerves;
   - poor wound healing;
   - enhanced risk of infection; and
   - periodontal disease.

Diabetic microangiopathy is responsible for compromised delivery of nutrients to tissues and poor elimination of metabolic products. Diabetes induces most of its complications on blood vessels, on large vessels with macroangiopathy, and on small vessels with microangiopathy.

Uncontrolled diabetes with poor glycemic control is a risk factor for severe periodontitis. The treatment of periodontitis improves glycemic control (Boehm and Scannapieco 2007). Mean advanced alveolar bone loss is significantly associated with eye vascular complication or retinopathy, with an odds ratio of 8.86 (Negishi et al. 2004). *Porphyromonas gingivalis* is capable of invading endothelial cells causing vascular damage; infection worsens glycemic control inducing hyperglycemia and increases the severity of microvascular and macrovascular pathology (Grossi et al. 2001).

Patient Management

Periodontitis may influence the severity of diabetes because of inflammation and uncontrolled glucose levels, and treatment of periodontal disease may be beneficial to diabetes control. Health education to encourage better oral care is necessary to reduce the prevalence of the diabetic disease and its complications.

Practical Osseous Surgery in Periodontics and Implant Dentistry, First Edition. Edited by Serge Dibart, Jean-Pierre Dibart.
© 2011 John Wiley & Sons, Inc. Published 2011 by John Wiley & Sons, Inc.

For dentists, knowledge of the general and oral signs of diabetes are necessary. Dentists must be prepared to manage diabetic emergencies:

- low blood glucose levels or hypoglycemia (the most frequent complication)
- high blood glucose levels or hyperglycemia, with possible ketoacidosis or coma.

Dentists should be aware of circumstances that can induce hyperglycemia, such as infections, corticosteroids, surgery, stress, and medications, or circumstances that can induce hypoglycemia, such as an inappropriate diet or treatment and associated medications (Ship 2003).

Diabetes care should include personal glucose monitoring with blood tests. Regular care should also include laboratory information regarding levels of blood glucose, glycosylated hemoglobin for glycemic control, leukocyte count for infections, C-reactive protein for inflammation, and creatinine for renal failure. Before any oral procedure, fasting glucose and glycosylated hemoglobin must be checked (Taylor 2003).

In case of surgery, antibiotic therapy may be used to prevent or treat oral infections, because opportunistic infections are more frequent with uncontrolled diabetes.

Endodontic and periodontic lesions of teeth are associated with hyperglycemia and may necessitate a sudden increase in insulin demand in order to normalize glucose levels. But after dental and periodontal treatment, the insulin need returns to baseline (Schulze, Schonauer, and Busse 2007).

Diabetes and Periodontitis

Periodontitis is twice as prevalent in diabetic patients than in healthy subjects (Grossi et al. 2001). Diabetes is a modifying and aggravating factor in the severity of periodontal disease. Periodontitis results from an interplay of bacterial infection and host response. Severe periodontitis often coexists with diabetes mellitus; periodontitis increases the severity of diabetes and complicates metabolic control. Infection and advanced glycation end products–mediated cytokine response is responsible for periodontal tissue destruction. The host response to infection is an important factor in extension and severity of periodontal disease; periodontitis severity and prevalence are increased in diabetes. Diabetes and periodontitis can both stimulate chronic production of inflammatory cytokines. These cytokines are elevated in periodontitis and may in turn predispose to diabetes. Cytokines can promote insulin resistance and cause the destruction of pancreatic beta cells, inducing diabetes (Duarte et al. 2007; Grossi 2001; Iacopino 2001; Kuroe et al. 2006; Nassar, Kantarci, and van Dyke 2000; Nibali et al. 2007; Nishimura et al. 2003; Novak et al. 2008). Oral diseases are associated with diabetes. Periodontitis is a risk factor for poor glycemic control and complications of diabetes. Sometimes periodontitis may be the first clinical manifestation of diabetes (Lamster, Lalla, and Borgnakke 2008). Periodontal indices, such as probing depth, attachment loss, and tooth loss, are significantly higher in diabetes family members (Meng 2007). There is a significant association between diabetes and deep probing depths and severe alveolar bone loss (Negishi et al. 2004). Periodontal infection is responsible for chronic inflammation, periodontal tissue destruction, and impaired tissue repair (Iacopino 2001).

Periodontal Therapy

Successful anti-infectious periodontal therapy has a beneficial effect on metabolic control of type 2 diabetes and glucose regulation. Proinflammatory cytokines, such as tumor necrosis factor-α (TNF-α), produced from excess amount of adipocytes, are responsible for lowered insulin sensitivity, called *insulin resistance*, and hyperglycemia. Diabetes can affect the periodontal tissues and the treatment of periodontal disease. Successful antimicrobial periodontal therapy may then result in improved insulin resistance and better glycemic control (Grossi et al. 1997; Katz 2005; Lalla, Kaplan et al. 2007; Madden 2008; Navarro-Sanchez, Faria-Almeida, and Bascones-Martinez 2007; O Connell 2008). Diabetes and periodontitis are secondary to chronic inflammation, altered host response, or insulin resistance. Periodontitis is associated with an elevated systemic inflammatory state and increased risk of hyperglycemia. Periodontal therapy that causes the decrease of oral bacterial load and reduction of periodontal and systemic inflammation can improve blood glucose control (Mealey and Rose 2008).

TYPE 2 DIABETES MELLITUS

Periodontal Treatment

Preventive periodontal therapy should be intense enough to reduce periodontal inflammation and glycosylated hemoglobin levels. Periodontitis treatment should include scaling, root planing, oral hygiene instruction, and chlorexidine rinse treatment (Madden et al. 2008). After nonsurgical periodontal therapy, significant probing depth reduction is observed after full-mouth scaling and root planing, with improvement in glycemic control and reduction in glycated hemoglobin levels (Rodrigues, Taba, and Novaes 2003). After full-mouth subgingival debridement in diabetic patients, many subgingival bacterial species are reduced, such as *P. gingivalis*, *Tannerella forsythensis*, *Treponema denticola*, and *Prevotella intermedia*. *P. gingivalis* is detected more frequently in patients with increased glycosylated hemoglobin levels and worse glycemic control (Makiura et al. 2008). After periodontal therapy, including scaling, root planing, and doxycycline, there is a significant reduction of 1.1 mm in probing depth, a reduction of 1.5% in glycosylated hemoglobin levels, and reduction in serum inflammatory mediators such interleukin-6 (IL-6) and granulocyte colony-stimulating factor (O'Connell et al. 2008). After subgingival scaling and root planing, patients show significant reduction in total gingival crevicular fluid volume and levels of IL-1β and TNF-α. There is an improvement in metabolic glycemic control, with significant reduction in glycosylated hemoglobin, at 3 and 6 months after treatment (Navarro-Sanchez, Faria-Almeida, and Bascones-Martinez 2007). Periodontitis can contribute for poorer glycemic control in diabetes. IL-6, IL-1β, and TNF-α are produced in response to periodontopathic bacteria and can modify glucose metabolism. Periodontal therapy has a beneficial effect on glycemic control. Diabetic patients should receive regular oral examination for periodontitis prevention and periodontal treatment (Taylor 2003). After full-mouth subgingival debridement, the percentage of macrophages releasing TNF-α decreases significantly by 78%, high-sensitivity C-reactive protein decreases significantly by 37%, and soluble E selectin decreases by 16.6% (Lalla, Kaplan, et al. 2007). After periodontal therapy including doxycycline, there is great reduction in probing depth and subgingival *P. gingivalis* concentrations. Treatment can improve glycemic control. Patients receiving periodontal treatment show a reduction of periodontal inflammation and significant reduction in mean glycosylated hemoglobin levels about 10% (Grossi et al. 1997). In diabetics local minocycline administration in every periodontal pocket once a week for a month significantly reduces the serum TNF-α levels, with an average reduction of 0.49 pg/mL (Iwamoto et al. 2001).

Advanced Glycation End Products

Nonenzymatic reaction of glucose with amino acids in proteins leads to accumulation of irreversible molecules called *advanced glycation end products*. They promote inflammatory response and the production of reactive oxygen species. Tissue destruction is associated with oxidative stress due to the imbalance between reactive oxygen species and antioxidant defense. Oxidative stress can damage proteins, lipids, and DNA. Glycation end products can interact directly or indirectly by reacting with receptors for advanced glycation end products. Hyperglycemia causes the production of advanced glycation end products and reactive oxygen species, which are responsible for oxidative damage leading to vascular complications. Inflammatory response is secondary to the action of advanced glycation end products, which induce production of reactive oxygen species and inflammatory mediators (Nassar, Kantarci, and van Dyke 2007). In diabetes, glycation and oxidation of proteins and lipids lead to the formation of advanced glycation end products and promotion of oxidative stress in periodontal tissues. There is an increased immunoreactivity for advanced glycation end products in the gingiva of diabetics, with increased oxidant stress in periodontal tissues (Schmidt et al. 1996). Elevated levels of blood glucose lead to the production of irreversible advanced glycation end products, which are partly respon-

sible for development of diabetic vascular complications. They induce the production of inflammatory mediators and tissue-destructive enzymes. Activation of receptors for advanced glycation end products causes enhanced inflammation and tissue destruction. Chronic accumulation of advanced glycation end products is responsible for the destruction and inflammation in diabetic periodontium (Lalla et al. 2000). Diabetes promotes degenerative vascular changes in gingival tissues. Vascular degeneration worsens with poor glycemic control and duration of diabetes. Hyperglycemia induces alteration of gingival collagen by amino-acid nonenzymatic glycation and formation of advanced glycation end products, with production of modified collagen and poor wound healing. Advanced glycation end products induce oxidant stress and interact with receptors for advanced glycation end products, with production of enzymes, cytokines, and inflammatory mediators (Ryan et al. 2003). Serum advanced glycation end products are significantly associated with aggravation of periodontitis (Takedo et al. 2006). Advanced glycation end products and their receptors are involved in the pathogenesis of periodontitis. Receptors for advanced glycation end products are expressed in gingival tissues from diabetic patients with periodontitis. The expression of receptors for advanced glycation end products is positively correlated with TNF-α levels (Meng 2007). Receptors for advanced glycation end products are present in human periodontium. Advanced glycation end products, through interaction with their receptors, have destructive effects on gingival tissues in patients with periodontitis and diabetes (Katz et al. 2005).

Impaired Glucose Tolerance

Impaired glucose tolerance after an oral glucose tolerance test may be the symptom of a prediabetic state. Impaired glucose tolerance is significantly associated with periodontitis and alveolar bone loss. Having deep pockets is significantly associated with past glucose intolerance. The proportion of subjects with impaired glucose tolerance increases significantly in patients in the higher tertiles of alveolar bone loss (Saito et al. 2006). A significant 3.28 times increase of alveolar bone loss is present among patients with newly diagnosed diabetes, compared with people with normal glucose tolerance (Marugame et al. 2003). Experimentally high-fat-fed periodontitis rats develop more severe insulin resistance, and they present earlier impaired glucose tolerance (Watanabe et al. 2008). Prediabetic rats with periodontitis present increased impaired glucose tolerance. Periodontitis in prediabetic rats is associated with increased fasting glucose and increased insulin resistance (Pontes Andersen et al. 2007).

Glycated Hemoglobin

Periodontitis patients with diabetes present significantly higher glycated hemoglobin levels (Jansson et al. 2006).

Periodontitis is associated with high values of glycated hemoglobin (greater than 9%), with an odds ratio of 6.1. Mean advanced alveolar bone loss is also significantly associated with high glycated hemoglobin levels, with an odds ratio of 4.94. High values of glycated hemoglobin are significantly associated with advanced periodontitis, presenting more than 50% mean alveolar bone loss and two or more teeth with probing depth greater than 6 mm (Negishi et al. 2004). Hyperglycemia induces inflammatory cytokine production and periodontal inflammation. Glycated hemoglobin level greater than 8% is significantly associated with gingival crevicular fluid IL-1β levels. Probing depth, attachment levels, bleeding on probing, and random glucose are significantly associated with gingival crevicular fluid IL-1β levels (Engebretson et al. 2004). Patients with glycated hemoglobin levels greater than 9 percent have a significantly higher prevalence of severe periodontitis, with an odds ratio of 2.9 (Tsai, Hayes, and Taylor 2002). Periodontal therapy may improve HbA1c levels. After full mouth scaling and root planing, there is a significant reduction in glycated hemoglobin levels (Rodrigues et al. 2003). Local minocycline administration in every periodontal pocket significantly reduces serum glycated hemoglobin levels, with an average reduction of 0.8% (Iwamoto et al. 2001).

Systemic Inflammation

In periodontal inflammation, IL-1β, IL-6, IL-8, and interferon gamma levels are higher in gingival tissues. IL-1β and IL-6 are elevated in cases of diabetes and periodontitis (Duarte et al. 2007). In diabetes hyperglycemia is associated with higher levels of inflammatory cytokines, TNF-α, IL-1β, and IL-6. They are responsible for initiation and progression of inflammation and periodontal disease severity (Nassar, Kantarci, and van Dyke 2007). Circulating TNF-α is produced by adipocytes in adipose tissue of obese patients and is responsible for insulin resistance. TNF-α concentrations are significantly correlated with periodontitis severity, attachment loss, and gingival crevicular fluid IL-1β levels (Engebretson et al. 2007). TNF-α is produced by adipocytes, macrophages, and monocytes. It is elevated in obese patients and decreases with weight loss. It is responsible for hyperglycemia due to insulin resistance (Nishimura et al. 2003). Persistent elevation of TNF-α, IL-1β, and IL-6 levels is responsible for damage to the liver cells, release of acute-phase proteins, dyslipidemia, and damage to pancreatic β cells (Grossi 2001). People with diabetes have dyslipidemia with elevated levels of low-density lipoprotein cholesterol and triglycerides. Periodontitis may also lead to increased low-density lipoprotein cholesterol and triglyceride levels. Periodontitis causes systemic bacteremia with elevated serum IL-1β and TNF-α levels, which are responsible for metabolic disorders and dyslipidemia (Iacopino 2001). TNF-α produced by periodontal inflammation is responsible for altered glucose regulation and insulin resistance (Iwamoto et al. 2001).

Clinical Parameters

Diabetes is associated with significantly more calculus formation, tooth loss, and increased severity of periodontitis. Patients have three times higher mean attachment levels and frequency of probing depth greater than 6 mm than non-diabetic patients. There is also a significantly higher frequency of sites with attachment levels greater than 3 mm (Novak et al. 2008). Diabetes patients show a

- significant increased prevalence of periodontitis
- significant lower number of teeth
- significant increase in probing depths greater than 4 mm and pocket depths greater than 4 mm
- significant association with bleeding on probing
- significant association with plaque
- significant association with the presence of *P. gingivalis* and *T. forsythensis* (Campus et al. 2005).

Severe generalized periodontitis is associated with low-grade systemic inflammation, and with significantly increased blood leukocyte counts.

The metabolic modifications include dyslipidemia with significantly lower high-density lipoprotein cholesterol and higher low-density lipoprotein cholesterol, and significantly increased non-fasting glucose levels (Nibali et al. 2007). Diabetic patients present a positive association between the severity of periodontal infection and serum lipids. Especially high low-density lipoprotein cholesterol levels are significantly associated with antibody titer to *P. gingivalis* (Kuroe et al. 2006).

TYPE 1 DIABETES MELLITUS

Clinical Parameters

Patients with type 1 diabetes mellitus are predisposed to periodontitis. Children and adolescents with type 1 diabetes mellitus present significantly more plaque and more gingival inflammation. Periodontitis is associated with type 1 diabetes, with an odds ratio of 2.78. The severity of periodontal destruction is significantly associated with mean glycated hemoglobin and duration of diabetes. Periodontal disease prevalence depends on duration of diabetes, glycemic control, and importance of gingival inflammation (Dakovic and Pavlovic 2008). From 6 to 11 years old, and more so after 12, periodontal destruction is increased in type 1 diabetes. Diabetes is a significant risk factor for periodontitis, especially for 12- to 18-year-old children. Children with type 1 diabetes present significantly more dental plaque, gingival inflammation, and attachment loss (Lalla, Cheng, et al. 2006). Periodontal destruction is related to the level of glycemic metabolic control. there is a significant positive association between mean glycated hemoglobin levels and periodontal disease, with an odds ratio of 1.31 (Lalla, Cheng, et al. 2007). Periodontal disease is significantly associated with mean duration of type 1 diabetes. Diabetes is significantly associated with a higher prevalence of *P. gingivalis* and *P. intermedia* presence in subgingival plaque samples. Serum immunoglobulin G antibody levels against *P. gingivalis* are significantly elevated in periodontitis patients with diabetes (Takahashi et al. 2001). Type 1 diabetic pregnant women present significantly higher plaque index, gingival inflammation, mean probing depth, and mean clinical attachment level (Guthmiller et al. 2001).

Chronic Inflammation

Hyperglycemia induces glycation of amino acids with production of advanced glycation end products, promoting inflammatory response with release of TNF-α and IL-6. People with diabetes have significantly higher gingival crevicular fluid, prostaglandin E2, and IL-1β levels. Type 1 diabetes patients have abnormal monocytic inflammatory secretion in response to lipopolysaccharide of *P. gingivalis*. Monocytes of diabetic patients secrete more prostaglandin E2, TNF-α, and IL-1β (Salvi, Beck, and Offenbacher 1998). Diabetic patients present a significantly higher TNF-α monocytic secretion in response to *P. gingivalis* lipopolysaccharide. These patients present an upregulated monocytic TNF-α secretion phenotype, which is associated with a more severe periodontal disease (Salvi et al. 1997).

Periodontal Therapy

Periodontal therapy has a beneficial effect on glycemic control in type 1 diabetes. Periodontitis treatment and prevention are necessary for a good metabolic control in type 1 diabetic patients (Taylor 2003). Young patients with diabetes should have regular periodontitis treatment and prevention in order to stop periodontitis progression and periodontal destruction (Lalla et al. 2006). Full-mouth disinfection applied every 3 months significantly improves periodontal status and glycemic control. After full-mouth disinfection, type 1 diabetes adult periodontitis patients present significantly lower plaque index, less bleeding on probing, less probing depth, and gain of clinical attachment (Schara, Medvesck, and Skaleric 2006).

REFERENCES

Boehm TK, Scannapieco FA. 2007. *J Am Dent Assoc*. 138(suppl):26S–33S.

Campus G, Salem A, Uzzau S, et al. 2005. *J Periodontol*. 76(3):418–25.

Dakovic D, Pavlovic MD. 2008. *J Periodontol*. 79(6):987–92.

Duarte PM, de Oliveira MC, Tambeli CH, et al. 2007. *J Periodontal Res*. 42(4):377–81.

Engebretson S, Chertog R, Nichols A, et al. 2007. *J Clin Periodontol*. 34(1):18–24.

Engebretson SP, Hey-Hadavi J, Ehrhardt FJ, et al. 2004. *J Periodontol*. 75(9):1203–08.

Grossi SG. 2001. *Ann Periodontol*. 6(1):138–45.

Grossi SG, Skrepcinski FB, DeCaro T, et al. 1997. *J Periodontol*. 68(8):713–19.

Guthmiller JM, Hassebroek-Johnson JR, Weenig DR, et al. 2001. *J Periodontol*. 72(11):1485–90.

Iacopino AM. 2001. *Ann Periodontol*. 6(1):125–37.

Iwamoto Y, Nishimura F, Nagakawa M, et al. 2001. *J Periodontol*. 72(6):774–78.

Jansson H, Lindholm E, Lindh C, et al. 2006. *J Clin Periodontol*. 33(6):408–14.

Katz J, Bhattacharyya I, Farkhondeh-Kish F, et al. 2005. *J Clin Periodontol*. 32(1):40–44.

Kuroe A, Fukushima M, Nakai Y, Seino Y. 2006. *Horm Metab*. 38(8):530–35.

Lalla E, Cheng B, Lal S, et al. 2006. *Diabetes Care*. 29(2):295–99.

Lalla E, Cheng B, Lal S, et al. 2007. *J Periodontal Res*. 42(4):345–49.

Lalla E, Kaplan S, Yang J, et al. 2007. *J Periodontal Res*. 42(3):274–82.

Lalla E, Lamster IB, Feit M, et al. 2000. *J Clin Invest*. 105(8):1117–24.

Lamster IB, Lalla E, Borgnakke WS, et al. 2008. *J Am Dent Assoc*. 139(suppl):19S–24S.

Madden TE, Herriges B, Boyd LD, et al. 2008. *J Contemp Dent Pract*. 9(5):9–16.

Makiura N, Ojima M, Kou Y, et al. 2008. *Oral Microbiol Immunol*. 23(4):348–51.

Marugame T, Hayasaki H, Lee K, et al. 2003. *Diabet Med*. 20(9):746–51.

Mealey BL, Rose LF. 2008. *Curr Opin Endocrinol Diabetes Obes*. 15(2):135–41.

Meng HX. 2007. *Beijing Da Xue Xue Bao*. 39(1):18–20.

Nassar H, Kantarci A, van Dyke TE. 2007. *Periodontol 2000*. 43:233–44.

Navarro-Sanchez AB, Faria-Almeida R, Bascones-Martinez A. 2007. *J Clin Periodontol*. 34(10):835–43.

Negishi J, Kawanami M, Terada Y, et al. 2004. *J Int Acad Periodontol*. 6(4):120–24.

Nibali L, D'Aiuto F, Griffiths G, et al. 2007. *J Clin Periodontol*. 34(11):931–37.

Nishimura F, Iwamoto Y, Mineshiba J, et al. 2003. *J Periodontol*. 74(1):97–102.

Novak MJ, Potter RM, Blodgett J, et al. 2008. *J Periodontol*. 79(4):629–36.

O'Connell PA, Taba M, Nomizo A, et al. 2008. *J Periodontol*. 79(5):774–83.

Pontes Andersen CC, Flyvbjerg A, Buschard K, et al. 2007. *J Periodontol*. 78(3):559–65.

Rodrigues DC, Taba MJ, Novaes AB, et al. 2003. *J Periodontol*. 74(9):1361–67.

Ryan ME, Carnu O, Kamer A. 2003. *J Am Dent Assoc*. 134(spec):34S–40S.

Salvi GE, Beck JD, Offenbacher S. 1998. *Ann Periodontol*. 3(1):40–50.

Salvi GE, Collins JG, Yalda B, et al. 1997. *J Clin Periodontol*. 24(1):8–16.

Saito T, Murakami M, Shimazaki Y, et al. 2006. *J Periodontol*. 77(3):392–97.

Schara R, Medvescek M, Skaleric U. 2006. *J Int Acad Periodontol*. 8(2):61–66.

Schmidt AM, Weidman E, Lalla E, et al. 1996. *J Periodontal Res*. 31(7):508–15.

Schulze A, Schonauer M, Busse M. 2007. *J Periodontol*. 78(12):2380–84.

Ship JA. 2003. *J Am Dent Assoc*. 134(spec):4S–10S.

Takahashi K, Nishimura F, Kurihara M, et al. 2001. *J Int Acad Periodontol*. 3(4):104–11.

Takedo M, Ojima M, Yoshioka H, et al. 2006. *J Periodontol*. 77(1):15–20.

Taylor GW. 2003. *J Am Dent Assoc*. 134(spec):41S–48S.

Tsai C, Hayes C, Taylor GW. 2002. *Community Dent Oral Epidemiol*. 30(3):182–92.

Watanabe K, Petro BJ, Schlimon AE, et al. 2008. *J Perodontol*. 79(7):1208–16.

Chapter 3 Osteonecrosis of the Jaw

Jean-Pierre Dibart, MD

Osteonecrosis of the jaw is a rare disease. It is generally induced by bisphosphonates treatment for patients with cancer or osteoporosis and is mainly caused by

- excess bone turnover suppression,
- impaired vascularization, and
- bone infections.

The majority of cases of osteonecrosis of the jaw are related to the treatment of cancers, including intravenous administration of bisphosphonates. Some rare cases are also related to the treatment of osteoporosis. Osteonecrosis of the jaw occurs mainly after a local trauma and surgery, but sometimes may occur spontaneously without any bisphosphonate medication. In case of osteonecrosis, jaw bone becomes hypovascular and hypodynamic because of the action of the antiresorptive bisphosphonate treatment, and is no longer able to repair correctly after a mechanical stress or an infection.

CLINICAL SYMPTOMS

Osteonecrosis of the jaw is generally represented by following clinical symptoms:

- Exposed necrotic bone, generally in the mandible, but sometimes in the maxilla or palate
- Necrotic lesions that are slow to heal
- Swelling, both with pain or without pain
- Bone infection such as osteomyelitis.

Osteonecrosis of the jaw generally occurs after a long therapy and is associated with a 38.7-month mean duration of bisphosphonate treatment. Radiographic imaging or magnetic resonance imaging confirms the sites of jaw osteonecrosis. The pathogenesis consists of an altered bone remodeling with suppression of the normal cycle of bone resorption and formation due to the bisphosphonate treatment (Raje et al. 2008).

RISK FACTORS

Some jaw osteonecrosis risk factors are as follows:

- Cancer
- Duration of bisphosphonates therapy
- Dental disease or infection
- Corticosteroid use
- Advanced age
- Dental procedure or extraction
- Administration of bisphosphonates intravenously
- Radiotherapy
- Chemotherapy
- Smoking
- Poor oral hygiene
- Alcohol abuse
- Diabetes mellitus

OSTEOPOROSIS TREATMENT

In patients receiving bisphosphonates for postmenopausal osteoporosis treatment, the prevalence of jaw osteonecrosis is low, affecting especially the mandible and then the maxilla. Patients are generally female because of the prevalence of osteoporosis after menopause. They are aged over 60 years old and have generally undergone dental surgery or had an oral trauma (Pazianas et al. 2007). Jaw osteonecrosis after osteoporosis treatment represents 5% of all the cases. The estimated incidence of jaw osteonecrosis in patients receiving bisphosphonate treatment for osteoporosis is less than 1 per 100,000 person-years (Khan et al. 2009).

ONCOLOGY TREATMENT

Oncology treatment causes 94% of the osteonecrosis cases. Patients with multiple myeloma or metastatic carcinoma receiving high doses of intravenous bisphosphonates are at high risk for osteonecrosis of the jaw. The mandible is more

Practical Osseous Surgery in Periodontics and Implant Dentistry, First Edition. Edited by Serge Dibart, Jean-Pierre Dibart.
© 2011 John Wiley & Sons, Inc. Published 2011 by John Wiley & Sons, Inc.

commonly affected secondary to a surgical procedure. The pathogenesis is the oversuppression of bone turnover by bisphosphonate treatment (Woo, Hellstein, and Kalmar 2006). Osteonecrosis of the jaw is dependent on the dose and the duration of therapy. The incidence varies from 1% to 12% of the treated patients at 36 months of bisphosphonate treatment exposure (Khan et al. 2009). The incidence among multiple myeloma patients is estimated to be 3.2%. Some other osteonecrosis risk factors are significant: longer duration of pamidronate therapy (intravenous bisphosphonate), dental extraction, cyclophosphamide therapy (chemotherapy), prednisone therapy (corticosteroid), erythropoietin therapy, low hemoglobin level, renal dialysis, and advanced age (Jadu et al. 2007).

BISPHOSPHONATES

There are two categories of bisphosphonates:

1. Nitrogen-containing bisphosphonates or amino bisphosphonates. These are more effective as resorption inhibitors and for fracture prevention. These bisphosphonates are more often used in therapy and include alendronate, risedronate, ibandronate, pamidronate, and zoledronate. They interfere with enzymes such as farnesyl pyrophsphate synthase. Intravenous forms of pamidronate and zoledronate are statistically more often associated with osteonecrosis of the jaw (Aapro et al. 2008).

2. Non-nitrogen-containing bisphosphonates. These bisphosphonates include etidronate, tiludronate, and clodronate; they are less effective and rarely used in therapy. They are incorporated into adenosine triphosphate-containing compounds to inhibit cell function (Aapro et al. 2008).

OSTEONECROSIS TREATMENT

Prevention

Before beginning a bisphosphonate treatment for osteoporosis and especially for cancer, patients should undergo a dental examination, and all oral infections must be treated. After bisphosphonates treatment has started, patients should be informed about the risk of osteonecrosis. They should follow a regular program of dental care, all oral infections must be prevented and treated. If possible invasive procedures should be avoided during therapy (Shenker and Jawad 2007). All sites of potential infection should be treated before beginning bisphosphonates treatment (Woo, Hellstein, and Kalmar 2006). Implant treatment may be a risk for osteonecrosis because of osteotomy and bone regeneration. Instead of implants, periodontal, endodontic, or nonimplant procedures should be discussed. Endodontics instead of extraction and bridges instead of implants should also be discussed if possible. In case of surgery, conservative techniques should

be used, chlorexidine rinses should be taken before and after surgery, and antibiotics may be used in case of an extensive procedure or presence of other osteonecrosis risk factors (Expert Panel 2006).

There is a reduction in the incidence of osteonecrosis from 3.2% to 1.3% of the patients with the use of these prevention programs. Preventive measures with regular dental examination can significantly reduce the incidence of jaw necrosis in cancer patients receiving bisphosphonates treatment (Ripamonti et al. 2009). Prevention should focus on maintaining good oral hygiene during bisphosphonate treatment (Khan et al. 2006).

Treatment

After jaw osteonecrosis diagnosis, the bisphosphonates treatment should be immediately stopped, although there are long-lasting effects of bisphosphonates, which are able to remain in bone cells for several months, or years.

After jaw osteonecrosis is diagnosed, the following treatment is necessary:

- Conservative debridement of osteonecrotic bone
- Good pain control
- Efficacious treatment of infections
- Antimicrobial rinses and antibiotics,
- Withdrawal of bisphosphonates (Woo, Hellstein, and Kalmar 2006).

The treatment should focus generally on conservative surgical procedures (Khan et al. 2006).

REFERENCES

Aapro M, Abrahamsson PA, Body JJ, et al. 2008. *Ann Oncol.* 19(3):420–32.

Expert Panel Recommendations. 2006. *J Am Dent Assoc.* 137(8):1144–50.

Jadu F, Lee L, Pharoah M, et al. 2007. *Ann Oncol.* 18(12):2015–19.

Khan AA, Sandor GK, Dore E, et al. 2009. *J Rheumatol.* 36(3):478–90.

Pazianas M, Miller P, Blumentals WA, et al. 2007. *Clin Ther.* 29(8):1548–58.

Raje N, Woo S-B, Hande K, et al. 2008. *Clin Cancer Res.* 14(8):2387–95.

Ripamonti CI, Maniezzo M, Campa, T, et al. 2009. *Ann Oncol.* 20(1):137–45.

Shenker NG, Jawad ASM. 2007. *Rheumatology.* 46(7):1049–51.

Woo SB, Hellstein JW, Kalmar, JR. 2006. *Ann Intern Med.* 144(10):753–61.

Chapter 4 Periodontitis and Cardiovascular Disease

Jean-Pierre Dibart, MD

INTRODUCTION

Cardiovascular disease is one of the most common diseases in Western countries. Chronic infections and chronic inflammation are two important risk factors in the development of cardiovascular diseases.

Chronic microbial infection and chronic inflammation caused by the dental plaque in periodontal disease may predispose to atherosclerosis. Microbial dental plaque is the cause of inflammatory oral diseases such as gingivitis and periodontitis. Severe periodontal disease is associated with cardiovascular disease because of low-grade chronic inflammation and periodic systemic bacteremia with migration of bacteria in general circulation responsible for the damage to vascular cells. High prevalence of periodontitis is associated with cardiovascular diseases such as atherosclerosis, myocardial infarction, and stroke. Severe periodontitis is also associated with peripheral arterial disease, and subclinical atherosclerosis defined by the measure of carotid artery intima-media thickness.

Two main mechanisms are responsible for the association between atherosclerosis and periodontitis: the general systemic inflammatory response and the specific effects of periodontal bacteria on vascular host tissues.

Cofactors for periodontitis and cardiovascular disease are the following:

- Hypertension
- Diabetes
- Smoking
- Altered lipid metabolism with high low-density lipoprotein cholesterol, low high-density lipoprotein cholesterol, and high triglycerides
- High body mass index
- Low physical activity
- Genetics
- Stress
- Chronic alcohol abuse

There are many risk factors for the development of atherosclerosis in periodontal disease:

- Chronic inflammatory conditions
- Infections with direct microbial effect or systemic bacteremia and indirect cross-reactivity with microbial antigens
- Oxidative damage of plasmatic lipoproteins or lipid peroxidation
- Vascular endothelium dysfunction
- Platelet activation

Chronic Inflammation

Periodontal inflammation is associated with an elevated systemic inflammatory state and an increased risk of cardiovascular diseases such as atherosclerosis, myocardial infarction, and stroke (Mealey and Rose 2008). Systemic inflammation may contribute in the pathogenesis of atherosclerosis, with accumulation of lipids on the vascular walls.

Periodontitis is responsible for a local progressive inflammation leading to the destruction of the supporting tissues and alveolar bone loss. Periodontitis induces systemic inflammation with increased production of serum cytokines and inflammatory mediators. Most patients present elevated levels of systemic inflammation markers such as C-reactive protein, IL-6, and fibrinogen (Amabile et al. 2008; Amar et al. 2003; Bizzarro et al. 2007; Chen et al. 2008; D'Aiuto 2004; Karnoutsos et al. 2008; Linden et al. 2008; Meurman et al. 2003; Smith et al. 2009).

Infection

Chronic infection is a risk factor in the development of cardiovascular diseases. There are two important pathogenic mechanisms.

Practical Osseous Surgery in Periodontics and Implant Dentistry, First Edition. Edited by Serge Dibart, Jean-Pierre Dibart.

1. Direct microbial infection with direct action of bacteria present in systemic circulation and in vascular walls: The DNA from periodontal pathogens is detected in some atherosclerotic lesions after vascular surgery. The presence of *Actinobacillus actinomycetemcomitans* in atheromatous plaques and periodontal pockets of the same patients may indicate a role for periodontal bacteria in atherosclerosis pathogenesis (Padilla et al. 2006).

2. Cross-reactivity or molecular mimicry between microbial antigens and self-antigens with induction of autoimmunity: Bacterial endotoxins and the action of proinflammatory cytokines such as prostaglandin E2, interleukin-1β (IL-1β), and tumor necrosis factor-α (TNF-α) may play a role in endothelial toxicity. Periodontitis leads to systemic exposure to oral bacteria and production of inflammatory mediators responsible for the development of atherosclerosis and coronary heart disease. Procedures such as dental extraction, periodontal surgery, and tooth scaling may lead to the presence of oral bacteria in systemic circulation.

Periodontal infection, or the response of the host against the infection, may play a role in the pathogenesis of coronary heart disease. Serum antibodies to periodontal pathogens are associated with coronary heart disease. All antibody levels against periodontal pathogens correlate positively with the measure of carotid intima-media thickness. Serum antibody levels to periodontal pathogens are associated with subclinical atherosclerosis and consequently with future incidence of coronary heart disease. Infections caused by *Porphyromonas gingivalis* increases the risk for myocardial infarction. High *P. gingivalis* IgA class antibody levels can predict the risk for myocardial infarction independently from other cardiovascular risk factors (Pussinen et al. 2003, 2004, 2005; Yamazaki et al. 2007).

Dyslipidemia

Periodontal infection is associated with elevated plasma levels of atherogenic lipoproteins. Chronic infection is associated with increased risk of systemic diseases because of metabolic changes. Periodontitis is an independent risk factor of cardiovascular diseases because of the systemic inflammatory reaction and hyperlipidemia. In periodontitis patients, elevated serum levels of lipoprotein associated phospholipase A2, which is a marker of dyslipidemia, is correlated with cardiovascular disease risk (D'Aiuto et al. 2006; Katz et al. 2002; Losche et al 2005; Nibali et al. 2007; Rufail et al. 2005, 2007).

Endothelial Dysfunction

Endothelial dysfunction is one mechanism, which combined with inflammation, is responsible for the development of atherosclerosis. Periodontal disease is associated with endothelial dysfunction because the chronic systemic inflammation may lead to impaired functioning of the vascular endothelium. There is a direct interaction of periodontopathic bacteria with vascular tissues. Endothelial dysfunction present in periodontitis is an important element in the pathogenesis of atherosclerosis. Endothelial dysfunction is tested using flow-mediated dilation of the brachial artery.

Periodontal therapy results in an improvement in endothelial function and a decrease in inflammatory markers. Improvement in endothelial function, as measured by flow-mediated dilation of the brachial artery, is possible through elimination of oral infections by periodontal treatment (Amar et al. 2003; Elter et al. 2006; Seinost et al. 2005; Tonetti et al. 2007).

Platelet Activation

Periodontitis is caused by Gram-negative bacteria. Chronic Gram-negative infections represent a risk factor for thromboembolic events. Bacteria from dental plaque and their products disseminate into circulation and can promote thromboembolic events associated with cardiovascular diseases. Platelets from periodontitis patients are more activated because of regularly occurring bacteremic episodes. This may increase impaired fibrinolysis and be responsible for a prothrombotic state. Plasma levels of markers of a prothrombotic state, such as plasminogen activator inhibitor-1, are elevated in patients with periodontal disease. Platelet-activating factor, an inflammatory phospholipid mediator, is present in elevated levels in inflamed gingival tissues, gingival crevicular fluid, and saliva in periodontitis patients (Antonopoulou et al. 2003; Bizzarro et al. 2007; McManus and Pinckard 2000; Renvert et al. 2006; Sharma et al. 2000).

Patient Management

Oral infections may represent a significant risk factor for systemic diseases. The control of oral diseases is necessary in the prevention of systemic conditions. Health education to encourage better oral hygiene is also an important element in the prevention of cardiovascular diseases. Periodontitis patients may benefit from an intensive therapy in order to reduce coronary artery disease progression.

Dentists and physicians should treat or prevent risk factors for cardiovascular disease. These risk factors include the following:

- Atherosclerosis
- Dyslipidemia
- Hypertension
- Diabetes mellitus
- Cigarette smoking
- High body mass index and high waist-to-hip ratio

- Periodontal disease
- Low physical activity
- Stress

Dentists and physicians should also educate patients about the relationship between cardiovascular disease and periodontitis. They should encourage smoking cessation, low-fat diet, regular exercise, and good oral hygiene. In cases of patients with cardiovascular disease, before oral therapy, dentists should minimize stress and check blood pressure and all of the patients' medical prescriptions.

CHRONIC INFLAMMATORY CONDITIONS

Inflammation Markers and Cytokines

Inflammation markers are as follows:

- C-reactive protein
- Erythrocyte sedimentation rate
- Leukocyte counts
- Fibrinogen
- Serum amyloid A protein.

Inflammatory cytokines are as follows:

- Thromboxane A2
- IL-1β
- IL-6
- Prostaglandin E2
- TNF-α.

Inflammation Markers

C-reactive Protein

Patients with advanced periodontitis present significantly higher serum levels of high-sensitivity C-reactive protein (Amar et al. 2003). Patients with coronary heart disease also show higher levels of serum C-reactive protein (Meurman et al. 2003). Periodontitis is associated with increased levels of C-reactive protein; patients with levels greater than 3 mg/L have 2.49 times higher risk for advanced periodontitis (Linden et al. 2008). Chronic infections such as periodontitis produce inflammatory conditions, and patients with periodontitis show higher levels of serum C-reactive protein than healthy subjects (Bizzarro et al. 2007). Patients with periodontitis have significantly higher levels of serum C-reactive protein, with a median of 2.19 mg/L, compared to healthy people who have a median level of 1.42 mg/L (Briggs et al. 2006). High serum C-reactive protein is significantly associated with a high level of tooth loss, with an odds ratio of 2.17 (Linden et al. 2008). Systemic inflammatory response is more important in periodontitis patients presenting coronary artery lesions, with mean periodontal pocket depth greater than in subjects without coronary lesions. Mean pocket-depth values also correlate significantly with high-sensitivity C-reactive protein and with angiographic score of coronary lesions (Amabile et al. 2008).

Serum C-reactive protein levels are significantly associated with the outcome of periodontal treatment; nonsurgical periodontal therapy significantly decreases serum markers of systemic inflammation, with significant reduction of C-reactive protein levels (D'Aiuto et al. 2004). Intensive periodontal therapy produces significant reduction of inflammatory markers, with significant serum C-reactive protein decrease at 1 and 2 months after treatment (D'Aiuto et al. 2006).

Erythrocyte Sedimentation Rate

Chronic infections such as periodontitis produce inflammatory conditions, with higher serum erythrocyte sedimentation rates (Bizzarro et al. 2007). Patients with coronary heart disease also show higher levels of blood erythrocyte sedimentation rate (Meurman et al. 2003).

Leukocytes

Periodontitis produces inflammatory conditions with higher levels of leukocyte counts (Bizzarro et al. 2006); patients present a low-grade systemic inflammation with significantly increased blood leukocyte counts (Nibali et al. 2007). In periodontitis, the low-grade chronic inflammatory response is characterized by elevated levels of blood neutrophils and monocytes (Smith et al. 2009).

Serum Amyloid A Protein and Fibrinogen

Periodontitis is associated with increased levels of serum inflammation markers such as fibrinogen (Linden et al. 2008). In patients presenting periodontitis and coronary lesions, mean pocket-depth values correlate significantly with serum amyloid A protein and fibrinogen levels (Amabile et al. 2008). Patients with coronary heart disease also show higher levels of serum fibrinogen concentrations (Meurman et al. 2003).

Inflammatory Cytokines

Inflammatory mediators such as TNF-α, IL-1β, and prostaglandin E2 may play an important role in coronary heart disease and atherosclerosis. Monocytes in periodontal tissues react to lipopolysaccharide production of the plaque pathogens by secreting inflammatory mediators:

- TNF-α
- IL-1β

- Prostaglandin E2

- Thromboxane A2

These mediators produce local effects in the periodontal tissues and in the vessels. Inflammatory cytokines promote cholesterol accumulation in monocytes and proliferation of vascular smooth muscle with thickening of vessels, which is responsible for development of atherosclerosis. In periodontitis, inflammatory mediators such as cyclooxygenase 2, TNF-α, and IL-1β are upregulated (Smith et al. 2009). Periodontitis leads to systemic exposure to oral pathogens and production of inflammatory mediators responsible for the pathogenesis of cardiovascular diseases. Cytokines and lipopolysaccharide produced by oral bacteria enter into circulation and promote atherosclerosis. Cytokines produce their effects directly, and lipopolysaccharides induce the production of inflammatory mediators such as TNF-α, IL-1β, and prostaglandin E2 (Karnoutsos et al. 2008). Periodontitis is associated with increased serum TNF-α and IL-6 levels (Chen, Umeda, et al. 2008). Nonsurgical periodontal therapy significantly decreases inflammatory mediators, with significant reductions of IL-6 (D'Aiuto et al. 2004). After intensive periodontal therapy, there is a significant reduction in serum IL-6 concentrations at 1 and 2 months after treatment (D'Aiuto et al. 2006).

Clinical Expression

Coronary Heart Disease

Patients with coronary heart disease generally present more signs of dental infection, and are significantly more likely to be edentulous. The remaining teeth and supporting tissues are more often diseased (Meurman et al. 2003). Patients with coronary heart disease have significantly fewer remaining teeth, and they present significantly more pathological periodontal pockets. Dentures and edentulousness are significantly more frequent (Buhlin et al. 2005). The mean number of pockets and missing teeth is also significantly greater. The proportion of mobile teeth, bleeding sites, and periodontal pockets are also significantly higher (Geerts et al. 2004). Patients with coronary artery disease have significantly deeper pockets and greater attachment loss (Nonnenmacher et al. 2007). Periodontal pocket-depth values correlate significantly with the American College of Cardiology and American Heart Association coronary angiographic scores (Amabile et al. 2008). Thirty-eight percent of the coronary heart disease patients present a significant risk of periodontal disease. In these patients, a higher proportion of sites show significantly more plaque, more bleeding on probing, and more probing depths greater than 4 mm or 6 mm (Briggs et al. 2006).

Patients with gingivitis have a significant 3.37 times higher risk for coronary artery disease (Meurman et al. 2003). There is a linear positive association between incidence of periodontitis and coronary heart disease. The incidence of coronary artery disease is significantly 2.12 times higher when comparing highest versus lowest category of radiographic alveolar bone loss or the sum of probing pocket depths (Dietrich et al. 2008). Periodontitis patients present a significant 1.14 times higher risk of coronary artery disease. In prospective cohort studies, there is a significant 1.24 times higher risk of coronary artery disease in patients with fewer than 10 teeth. In case-control studies, there is a significant 2.22 times greater risk of coronary artery disease in periodontitis. In cross-sectional studies, the prevalence of coronary artery disease is significantly 1.59 times higher in periodontitis (Bahekar et al. 2007). Mean probing depth greater than 2 mm is associated with a 1.6 times increased risk for electrocardiographic abnormalities. Mean attachment loss greater than 2.5 mm is associated with a significant 1.7 times increased risk for electrocardiographic abnormalities. Electrocardiographic abnormalities are left ventricular hypertrophy caused by cardiac muscle dilatation and ST segment depression caused by coronary artery disease. These abnormalities are significantly associated with mean probing depth, mean attachment loss, the number of teeth, and the plaque index (Shimazaki et al. 2004).

Stroke

The association between periodontitis and risk of stroke is high. Nonfatal stroke is associated with attachment levels greater than 6 mm, with an odds ratio of 4 (Sim et al. 2008). Periodontitis is a significant risk factor for nonhemorrhagic strokes and total cerebrovascular accidents. The relative risks for nonhemorrhagic strokes are

- 1.24 for gingivitis,

- 1.41 for edentulousness, and

- 2.11 for periodontitis.

The relative risks for total cerebrovascular accidents (hemorrhagic and nonhemorrhagic) are

- 1.02 for gingivitis,

- 1.23 for edentulousness, and

- 1.66 for periodontitis (Wu et al. 2000).

In patients free from cardiovascular disease, systemic exposure to *P. gingivalis* increases the risk of stroke. Men IgA seropositive for *P. gingivalis* have a multivariate odds ratio of 1.63 for stroke. Women IgG seropositive for *P. gingivalis* present a multivariate odds ratio of 2.3 for stroke (Pussinen et al. 2007).

Atherosclerosis

Ultrasonography is used to measure carotid intima-media thickness generally by high-resolution B-mode ultrasonography at the common carotid artery.

Severe periodontitis is associated with increased cardiovascular risk and subclinical atherosclerosis, defined by elevated values of carotid intima-media thickness. The overall mean carotid intima-media thickness is significantly greater in patients with periodontitis than in healthy subjects (Cairo et al. 2008). High-resolution ultrasonography-Doppler is also used to measure carotid artery plaques in the common carotid artery or internal carotid artery. A 10% significant difference in carotid artery plaque prevalence exists between the lowest and highest tertiles of patients with tooth loss and between the lowest and highest tertiles of patients with clinical attachment loss (Desvarieux et al. 2004). Mean values of common carotid intima-media thickness are significantly higher in women with periodontitis. Subclinical atherosclerosis is also associated with the amount of dental plaque, the gingival inflammation, bleeding on probing, and pocket depth (Soder and Yakob 2007).

INFECTION

Bacterial Detection in Vascular Lesions

The DNA from periodontal pathogens is detected in atherosclerotic plaques from carotid or femoral arteries of patients undergoing vascular surgery. DNA of *Prevotella intermedia* is constantly found, and the DNA of *Prevotella nigrescens* and *P. gingivalis* are found sporadically (Fiehn et al. 2005). *A. actinomycetemcomitans* is isolated in vascular atherosclerotic plaques and in periodontal pockets of the same patients (Padilla et al. 2006). Periodontal bacteria can be detected in 52% of vascular atherosclerotic samples of peripheral arteries after surgery. Patients with severe peripheral arterial disease show a significant higher frequency of *P. gingivalis* presence in atheromatous plaques. Periodontitis increases fivefold the risk of peripheral arterial disease (Chen et al. 2008). *P. intermedia* shows significantly higher mean counts in patients with coronary artery disease (Nonnenmacher et al. 1007). In experimentation, atherosclerotic vascular lesions are more advanced in *P. gingivalis*-inoculated animals. Proximal aortic lesion size is also significantly greater in mice inoculated with *P. gingivalis* (Li et al. 2002).

Lipopolysaccharide

Infection is a risk factor for atherogenesis and thromboembolism. Lipopolysaccharide on the outer membrane of Gram-negative bacteria are responsible for endotoxin properties (Nonnenmacher et al. 2007). Total oral bacterial load is significantly higher in patients with acute coronary syndrome, especially for *P. gingivalis*, *Tannerella forsythensis*, and *Treponema denticola* (Renvert et al. 2006). There is a significant association between periodontal pathogens and coronary artery disease, with an odds ratio of 1.92. There is also a significant association between the number of *A. actinomycetemcomitans* in periodontal pockets and coronary artery disease, with an odds ratio of 2.7 (Spahr et al. 2006).

P. gingivalis induces atherosclerotic lesions by general inflammatory response and specific effects on host tissues. *P. gingivalis* lipopolysaccharide can induce foam cell formation in macrophages in the presence of low-density lipoproteins (Kuramitsu, Kang, and Qi 2003). Microbial pathogens are responsible for the induction of atherosclerosis by the activation of inflammatory markers or mediators and for direct damage to the vessels. Periodontal bacteria can damage the vasculature; *P. gingivalis* can invade epithelial and endothelial cells. Periodontal inflammation can be responsible for an inflammatory response at distant sites. Animals with experimentally induced periodontitis present more important amount of lipid deposition in the aorta, and the severity of periodontitis is positively correlated with the extent of vascular lipid deposition experimentally (Jain et al. 2003).

Elevated Antibody Titer and P. gingivalis

Oral bacteria may promote atherogenesis. There is an association between periodontal infection, with the presence of high antibody serum titer, and coronary artery disease. The antibody response against *P. gingivalis* is the most prevalent (Yamazaki et al. 2007). Patients with coronary artery disease are significantly more often seropositive for *P. gingivalis* IgA and IgG antibody than patients without coronary disease (Pussinen et al. 2005). Coronary artery disease is significantly more frequent among *P. gingivalis* IgG antibody seropositive patients (Pussinen et al. 2003). A high *P. gingivalis* IgA antibody level predicts the risk of myocardial infarction, independently from other cardiovascular risk factors. The risk increases significantly by increasing quartiles of antibody levels. Compared with the first quartile, the odds ratio of myocardial infarction are

- 2.47 in the second quartile,
- 3.3 in the third quartile, and
- 3.99 in the fourth quartile (Pussinen et al. 2004b).

Infections caused by *P. gingivalis* are also associated with stroke. Patients with a history of stroke or coronary disease are more often seropositive for *P. gingivalis* IgA antibody. The *P. gingivalis* seropositive patients also present an odds ratio of 2.6 for secondary stroke (Pussinen et al. 2004a)

A. actinomycetemcomitans

Patients with a high combined antibody response to *A. actinomycetemcomitans* and *P. gingivalis* have a significant odds ratio of 1.5 for prevalent coronary disease (Pussinen et al. 2003). Men with myocardial infarction are significantly more often seropositive for *A. actinomycetemcomitans* IgA. All antibody levels also correlate positively with carotid intima-media thickness and subclinical atherosclerosis (Pussinen et al. 2005).

Infections caused by *A. actinomycetemcomitans* are also associated with stroke. Patients seropositive for *A. actinomycetemcomitans* IgA present a multivariate odds ratio of 1.6 for stroke (Pussinen et al. 2004a).

LIPOPROTEIN PARAMETERS

Periodontitis is associated with increased risk of metabolic modifications. There is an association between severe periodontitis and metabolic risk factors for cardiovascular diseases: periodontitis patients show dyslipidemia that predisposes to atherosclerosis, with significantly lower plasma levels of protective high-density lipoprotein cholesterol, and significantly higher plasma levels of deleterious low-density lipoprotein cholesterol (Nibali et al. 2007). Patients with generalized aggressive periodontitis show significantly

- higher plasma levels of large, medium, and small very low-density lipoprotein;
- higher plasma levels of intermediate density lipoprotein;
- higher plasma levels of small low-density lipoprotein; and
- lower plasma levels of large low-density lipoprotein.

Patients have a significantly greater number of circulating low-density lipoproteins, and their average size is significantly lower (Rufail et al. 2005). Periodontal infection is associated with elevated levels of atherogenic lipoprotein species. Mean periodontal pocket depth correlates positively with very low-density lipoprotein levels. The prevalence of the atherogenic lipoprotein phenotype subclass pattern B, characterized by a predominance of small, dense low-density lipoprotein represents

- 8.3% in healthy people,
- 33.3% in localized aggressive periodontitis patients, and
- 66.6% in generalized aggressive periodontitis patients (Rufail et al. 2007).

Periodontal pockets may be associated with elevated blood lipid levels and atherosclerosis; they are positively associated with higher total cholesterol and higher low-density lipoprotein cholesterol (Katz et al. 2002). Edentulous patients present a more atherogenic serum lipid profile. Edentulous patients have lower protective plasma high-density lipoprotein cholesterol levels. Edentulous women also have significantly higher levels of total cholesterol and triglycerides (Johansson et al. 1994). *P. gingivalis* is responsible for foam cell formation in vascular cell culture. *P. gingivalis*, the outer membrane vesicles, and the lipopolysaccharide induce modifications of low-density lipoproteins. Modified low-density lipoproteins are in turn responsible for cholesterol and lipid accumulation in vascular walls (Kuramitsu et al. 2002). Combined IgG antibody levels to *A. actinomycetemcomitans* and *P. gingivalis* are significantly inversely correlated with plasma high-density lipoprotein cholesterol levels (Pussinen et al. 2003).

Lipoprotein-associated phospholipase A2 is an enzyme that is a risk factor for cardiovascular diseases. Lipoprotein-associated phospholipase A2 and low-density lipoprotein cholesterol levels correlate significantly with clinical parameters of periodontal inflammation. Local periodontal therapy induces a significant reduction of about 10% in plasma levels of lipoprotein-associated phospholipase A2 (Losche et al. 2005). Intensive periodontal therapy produces a significant reduction in plasma total cholesterol level at 2 and 6 months after treatment. After intensive periodontal therapy, there is also a significant decrease in the Framingham cardiovascular risk score at 2 and 6 months (D'Aiuto et al. 2006).

ENDOTHELIAL DYSFUNCTION

Pathogenesis

Endothelial dysfunction is an important element in the pathogenesis of vascular diseases (D'Aiuto et al. 2007). Chronic inflammation of periodontal disease can lead to impaired functioning of vascular endothelium (Elter et al. 2006). Periodontitis is a risk factor for atherosclerosis and thromboembolism. Endothelial function plays an important role in the pathogenesis of atherosclerosis. It is quantified by flow-mediated dilation of the brachial artery, which represents the endothelium-dependent relaxation of the artery due to an increased blood flow.

Activation of endothelial cells by inflammatory cytokines induces the loss of the antithrombotic and vasodilator properties of endothelium. Periodontal pathogens may affect endothelium by two mechanisms: directly because of bacteremia and presence of bacteria in the vascular wall, and indirectly because of induced systemic inflammation (D'Aiuto et al. 2007).

Endothelial function is assessed by measurement of the diameter of the brachial artery during flow, levels of inflammatory mediators, and markers of coagulation and endothelial activation (Tonetti et al. 2007). Flow-mediated dilation of the brachial artery is significantly lower in advanced periodontitis patients because the oral pathogens induce endothelial dysfunction and systemic inflammation. Endothelial dysfunction is associated with coronary artery disease before the development of cardiovascular symptoms (Amar et al. 2003).

Treatment

Improvement in endothelial function is related to the reduction of periodontal lesions. After intensive periodontal therapy, flow-mediated dilation of the brachial artery is significantly greater, and markers of endothelial dysfunction such as plasma-soluble E-selectin are significantly lower (Tonetti et al. 2007). Improvement in endothelial function as measured by flow-mediated dilation is possible after periodontal therapy and elimination of chronic oral infection. Periodontal therapy results in significant improvement in flow-mediated dilation and in significant decrease in plasma inflammatory mediators such as IL-6 (Elter et al. 2006). Treatment of severe periodontitis reverses endothelial dysfunction. Successful periodontal therapy results in significant improvements in flow-mediated dilation of brachial artery and significant decrease in plasma inflammatory marker such as C-reactive protein (Seinost et al. 2005). There is an inverse correlation between plasma C-reactive protein levels and flow-mediated dilation of brachial artery (Amar et al. 2003). Two months after intensive periodontal therapy, there is also a significant decrease in systolic blood pressure (D'Aiuto et al. 2006).

PLATELET ACTIVATION

Platelets from periodontitis patients are more activated. These activated platelets and leukocytes may contribute to increased thrombotic disease. Periodontal pathogens promote platelet aggregation and foam cell formation. The stimulation of host responses can result in vascular damage and thrombotic disease (Renvert et al. 2006). *P. gingivalis* vesicles are able to induce mouse platelet aggregation in vitro. *Streptococcus sanguis* and *P. gingivalis* can also induce platelet aggregation in vitro. Oral plaque bacteria and their products can disseminate into systemic circulation and promote thromboembolism, with the possible consequences of myocardial infarction and stroke (Sharma et al. 2000).

Platelet-activating factor is a phospholipid with proinflammatory action. Platelet-activating factor is increased in the saliva of patients with periodontal disease and correlates with the importance of inflammation. In periodontitis, platelet-activating factor is increased in gingival tissues and in gingival crevicular fluid. This signaling system is responsible for acute inflammation and thromboembolism (McManus and Pinckard 2000). Platelet-activating factor is elevated in inflamed gingival tissues, saliva, and gingival crevicular fluid. The biologically active phospholipid in gingival crevicular fluid is a hydroxyl platelet-activating factor analogue, which plays a role in oral inflammation. Platelet-activating factor and hydroxyl platelet-activating factor analogue may be responsible for increased cardiovascular diseases by inflammation and thromboembolism (Antonopoulou, Tsoupras, et al. 2003). Plasminogen activator inhibitor 1 activity is a marker of a prothrombotic state. Plasminogen activator inhibitor 1 activity plasma levels are significantly elevated in severe periodontitis patients (Bizzarro et al. 2007).

REFERENCES

Amabile N, Susini G, Pettenati-Soubayroux I, et al. 2008. *J Intern Med.* 263(6):644–52.

Amar S, Gokce N, Morgan S, et al. 2003. *Arterioscler Thromb Vasc Biol.* 23(7):1245–49.

Antonopoulou S, Tsoupras A, Baltas G, et al. 2003. *Mediators Inflamm.* 12(4):221–27.

Bahekar AA, Singh S, Saha S, et al. 2007. *Am Heart J.* 154(5):830–37.

Bizzarro S, van der Velden U, ten Heggeler JM, et al. 2006. *J Clin Periodontol.* 34(7):574–80.

Briggs JE, McKeown PP, Crawford VL, et al. 2006. *J Periodontol.* 77(1):95–102.

Buhlin K, Gustafsson A, Ahnve S, et al. 2005. *J Periodontol.* 76(4):544–50.

Cairo F, Castellani S, Gori AM, et al. 2008. *J Clin Periodontol.* 35(6):465–72.

Chen YW, Umeda M, Nagasawa T, et al. 2008. *Eur J Vasc Endovasc Surg.* 35(2):153–58.

D'Aiuto F, Parkar M, Andreou G, et al. 2004. *J Clin Periodontol.* 31(5):402–11.

D'Aiuto F, Parkar M, Nibali L, et al. 2006. *Am Heart J.* 151(5):977–84.

D'Aiuto F, Parkar M, Tonetti MS. 2007. *J Clin Periodontol.* 34(2):124–29.

Desvarieux M, Schwahn C, Volzke H, et al. 2004. *Stroke.* 35(9):2029–35.

Dietrich T, Jimenez M, Krall Kaye EA, et al. 2008. *Circulation.* 117(13):1668–74.

Elter JR, Hinderliter AL, Offenbacher S, et al. 2006. *Am Heart J.* 151(1):47.

Fiehn NE, Larsen T, Christiansen N, et al. 2005. *J Periodontol.* 76(5):731–36.

Geerts SO, Legrand V, Charpentier J, et al. 2004. *J Periodontol.* 75(9):1274–80.

Jain A, Batista EL Jr, Serhan C, et al. 2003. *Infect Immun.* 71(10):6012–18.

Johansson I, Tidehag P, Lundberg V, et al. 1994. *Community Dent Oral Epidemiol.* 22(6):431–36.

Karnoutsos K, Papastergiou P, Stefanidis S, et al. 2008. *Hippokratia.* 12(3):144–49.

Katz J, Flugelmann MY, Goldberg A, et al. 2002. *J Periodontol.* 73(5):494–500.

Kuramitsu HK, Miyakawa H, Qi M, et al. 2002. *Ann Periodontol.* 7(1):90–94.

Kuramitsu HK, Kang IC, Qi M. 2003. *J Periodontol.* 74(1):85–89.

Li L, Messas E, Batista EL Jr, et al. 2002. *Circulation.* 105(7):861–67.

Linden GJ, McClean K, Young I, et al. 2008. *J Clin Periodontol.* 35(9):741–47.

Losche W, Marshal GJ, Apatzidou DA, et al. 2005. *J Clin Periodontol.* 32(6):640–44.

McManus LM, Pinckard RN. 2000. *Crit Rev Oral Biol Med.* 11(2):240–58.

Mealey BL, Rose LF. 2008. *Curr Opin Endocrinol Diabetes Obes.* 15(2):135–41.

Meurman JH, Janket SJ, Ovarnstrom M, et al. 2003. *Oral Surg Oral Med Oral Pathol Oral Radiol Endod.* 96(6):695–700.

Nibali L, D'Aiuto F, Griffiths G, et al. 2007. *J Clin Periodontol.* 34(11):931–37.

Nonnenmacher C, Stelzel M, Suzin C, et al. 2007. *J Periodontol.* 78(9):1724–30.

Padilla C, Lobos O, Hubert E, et al. 2006. *J Periodontal Res.* 41(4):350–53.

Pussinen PJ, Jousilahti P, Alfthan G, et al. 2003. *Arterioscler Thromb Vasc Biol.* 23(7):1250–54.

Pussinen PJ, Alfthan G, Tuomilehto J, et al. 2004. *Eur J Cardiovasc Prev Rehabil.* 11(5):408–11.

Pussinen PJ, Alfthan G, Rissanen H, et al. 2004. *Stroke.* 35(9):2020–23.

Pussinen PJ, Nyysonen K, Alfthan G, et al. 2005. *Arterioscler Thromb Vasc Biol.* 25(4):833–38.

Pussinen PJ, Alfthan G, Jousilahti P, et al. 2007. *Atheroscler.* 193(1):222–28.

Renvert S, Petterson T, Ohlsson O, et al. 2006. *J Periodontol.* 77(7):1110–19.

Rufail ML, Schenkein HA, Barbour SE, et al. 2005. *J Lipid Res.* 46(12):2752–60.

Rufail ML, Schenkein HA, Koertge TE, et al. 2007. *J Periodontal Res.* 42(6):495–502.

Seinost G, Wimmer G, Skerget M, et al. 2005. *Am Heart J.* 149(6):1050–54.

Sharma A, Novak EK, Sojar HT, et al. 2000. *Oral Microbiol Immunol.* 15(6):393–96.

Shimazaki Y, Saito T, Kiyohara Y, et al. June 2004. *J Periodontol.* 75(6):791–97.

Sim SJ, Kim HD, Moon JY, et al. 2008. *J Periodontol.* 79(9):1652–58.

Smith BJ, Lightfoot SA, Lerner MR, et al. 2009. *Cardiovasc Pathol.* 18(1):1–10.

Soder B, Yakob M. 2007. *Int J Dent Hyg.* 5(3):133–38.

Spahr A, Klein E, Khuseyinova N, et al. 2006. *Arch Intern Med.* 166(5):554–59.

Tonetti MS, D'Aiuto F, Nibali L, et al. 2007. *N Engl J Med.* 356(9):911–20.

Wu T, Trevisan M, Genco RJ, et al. 2000. *Arch Intern Med.* 160(18):2749–55.

Yamazaki K, Honda T, Domon H, et al. 2007. *Clin Exp Immunol.* 149(3):445–52.

Chapter 5 Periodontitis, Arthritis, and Osteoporosis

Jean-Pierre Dibart, MD

INTRODUCTION

Pathogenesis

Clinical Parameters

Arthritis is a common disease in the general population, and women are more often affected. Rheumatoid arthritis is a chronic polyarthritis including synovial inflammation, pain, swelling, tenderness, synovium hypertrophy, and excess joint synovial fluid. Joint destruction is due to the degradation of tissues, ligaments, tendons, and capsules. The serum of rheumatoid arthritis patients generally contains rheumatoid factors, which are autoantibodies. The presence of high rheumatoid factor titers is the sign of an aggressive rheumatic disease and the presence of extra-articular manifestations. Serum anticitrullinated peptide autoantibodies (ACPA) are more specific of rheumatoid arthritis, but less sensitive than rheumatoid factors. Serum acute-phase reactants such as erythrocyte sedimentation rate, C-reactive protein, and fibrinogen are generally elevated because of systemic inflammation. Magnetic resonance imaging and radiographs generally show the articular cartilage degradation, bone erosions, and juxta-articular bone loss. Disease severity is characterized by:

- the number of swollen joints,
- high erythrocyte sedimentation rate,
- high titer rheumatoid factors,
- bone erosions, and
- phenotype HLA DRB1*0401 and HLA DRB1*0404.

Medical therapy generally includes prescription of analgesics, nonsteroidal anti-inflammatory drugs, corticosteroids, disease-modifying antitheumatic drugs (DMARDS).

Chronic Inflammation

Autoimmune diseases are mediated by the humoral immune response with the action of B lymphocytes, by immune cell–mediated response with T lymphocytes and monocytes, and phagocytosis with macrophages and leukocytes.

Immune response to pathogens is composed of lymphocytes T and B, macrophages, natural killer cells, neutrophils, eosinophils, and basophils. There are many phases in the immune response:

- migration of leukocytes to antigens
- recognition of pathogens by macrophages
- recognition of antigens by lymphocytes T and B
- amplification of response by effector cells
- destruction of antigens by phagocytosis or cytotoxicity.

An infectious microorganism can be the cause of a chronic inflammatory arthritis. Many mechanisms may explain this phenomenon, such as persistent or chronic infection and pathologic immune cross-reactions between microbial antigens and some joint molecules. An altered immune response can be produced against a persistent microbial antigen such as *Chlamydia*, a modified autoantigen such as filaggrin, and an immunoglobulin or a heat shock protein. Joints are infiltrated by a majority of T lymphocytes CD4$^+$ and B lymphocytes with antibody-producing plasma cells. Synovial fibroblasts produce destructive enzymes such as collagenases and cathepsins. CD4$^+$ lymphocytes induce the production of interferon gamma, and macrophages produce cytokines such as interleukin-1 (IL-1) and tumor necrosis factor-α (TNF-α). Cytokines are responsible for regulation and activation of the immune system and inflammatory response. There are many categories of cytokines: IL-2, interferon, IL-10, IL-1α, IL-1β, IL-18, IL-17, chemokines, and IL-8. There is an increased migration of leukocytes in synovial tissues with production of reactive oxygen species and cytokines. IL-1 and TNF-α induce the production of collagenases and the activation of osteoclasts, which are the bone-resorbing cells.

Major Histocompatibility Complex

The major histocompatibility complex is composed of HLA class I and class II genes; they play a certain role in many autoimmune diseases. Class II major histocompatibility allele HLA-DR4 is a genetic risk factor for rheumatoid arthritis, and

---

Practical Osseous Surgery in Periodontics and Implant Dentistry, First Edition. Edited by Serge Dibart, Jean-Pierre Dibart.
© 2011 John Wiley & Sons, Inc. Published 2011 by John Wiley & Sons, Inc.

related alleles HLA-DRB1*0401 and HLA-DRB1*0404 are associated with a greater disease risk. HLA molecules play a role in T lymphocyte activation. They bind antigenic peptides and present them to T lymphocytes to induce an immune response. Class I genes are composed of different alleles: HLA-A, HLA-B, and HLA-C. Class II genes are composed of different regions: HLA-DR, HLA-DQ, and HLA-DP. Resistance to pathogens is based on differences of HLA genotype; certain HLA alleles are associated with autoimmune diseases (Kasper et al. 2008).

Class I alleles HLA-B27 are associated with spondyloarthropathies, HLA-Cw6 with psoriasis, and class II alleles HLA-DRB1 locus and HLA-DPB1 locus are associated with juvenile idiopathic arthritis. HLA-DRB1*0401 and HLA-DRB1*0404 genes are associated with rheumatoid arthritis. These genes encode a distinctive sequence of DRB molecule called the shared epitope, which is a disease severity risk factor.

HLA DR4 antigens are associated with both periodontitis and rheumatoid arthritis (Fauci et al. 2008).

Periodontitis and Arthritis

Rheumatic diseases and periodontitis are common inflammatory diseases. Autoimmune diseases include immunological and inflammatory modifications of connective tissues. Many cytokines are produced in synovium: TNF-α, IL-1, IL-6, IL-8. Prostaglandins and matrix metalloproteinases are responsible for connective tissue destruction.

There are many rheumatic diseases:

- Rheumatoid arthritis
- Ankylosing spondylitis and spondylarthropathies of different origins
- Sjögren syndrome
- Juvenile idiopathic arthritis

Rheumatoid arthritis is a chronic inflammatory disease of synovial tissues with some extra-articular symptoms. Rheumatoid arthritis, juvenile idiopathic arthritis, and sometimes Sjögren syndrome may be associated with periodontitis. Rheumatoid arthritis is a systemic autoimmune disease with joint destruction by chronic inflammation and synovial hyperplasia. Patients with severe rheumatoid arthritis have an increased risk for periodontitis, and patients with periodontitis present a higher prevalence of arthritis.

There are some similar features in the inflammatory response between periodontitis and rheumatoid arthritis, in periodontitis ligaments and bone around teeth are destructed; in arthritis there is joint bone, ligament, and cartilage tissue destruction. Patients may present with a dysregulation of the inflammatory response. The medical complications due to chronic arthritis can also affect oral health; these patients need attention from dentists for regular care and periodontitis prevention. Patients with rheumatic diseases sometimes present alterations in saliva flow rate and saliva composition. Patients with rheumatoid arthritis present higher serum inflammatory markers when arthritis is associated with periodontal disease. Localized oral infection induces periodontal tissue inflammation and bone loss because of the action of osteoclast cells responsible for bone resorption. In arthritis and periodontitis, the bone loss is due to an excess of bone resorption. In periodontitis, bone loss is mediated by leukocytes, with aspects of tissue destruction similar to those seen in arthritis. Excessive neutrophil activation induces periodontal tissue damage and articular destruction, secondary to the excess of neutrophil degranulation and the release of reactive oxygen species such as superoxide radical. Periodontitis may also be responsible for the dissemination of pathogens in general circulation. The presence of bacterial products, cells, and enzymes in circulation is responsible for an immune response, producing increased levels of antibodies and cytokines present either in serum or in gingival fluid.

There are some similarities between the two diseases, and the treatment of one of them may influence the evolution of the other (Mercado, Marshall, and Bartold 2003). The treatment of periodontal disease may have a beneficial effect on the clinical and biological markers of arthritis disease activity. Periodontal treatment can improve the systemic rheumatic disease markers for rheumatoid arthritis patients presenting with severe periodontitis. Inflammatory markers are increased in gingival crevicular fluid, and their levels are lower after anti-inflammatory treatment (Abou Raya et al. 2007; Abou Raya, Naim, and Abuelkheir 2007; Al Katma et al. 2007; Bartold, Marshall, and Haynes 2005; Ebersole et al. 1997; Havemose-Poulsen et al. 2006; Kasser et al. 1997; Mercado et al. 2000; Miia et al. 2005; Miranda et al. 2003; Moen 2005 et al.; Ribeiro, Leao, and Novaes 2005; Welbury et al. 2003; Zhang et al. 2005).

PERIODONTITIS AND ARTHRITIS

Periodontitis and Rheumatoid Arthritis

Clinical Manifestations

There are some similarities between periodontitis and rheumatoid arthritis. Patients with rheumatoid arthritis present oral manifestations such as missing teeth and a high percentage of deeper pockets (Mercado et al. 2001). They are more likely to be edentulous and to have periodontal disease (de Pablo, Dietrich, and McAlindon 2008). These patients have a higher percentage of sites with probing depth greater than 4 mm, a higher percentage of attachment loss greater than 2 mm, and radiographic alveolar bone loss greater than 2 mm. These parameters are correlated with serum IgM and IgA rheumatoid factor levels (Havemose-Poulsen et al. 2006). Rheumatoid arthritis prevalence is significantly increased in periodontitis, and rheumatoid arthritis patients also present advanced forms of periodontal disease (Mercado et al. 2000). C-reactive protein levels, erythrocyte sedimentation rate levels, fibrinogen, and TNF-α are elevated in rheumatoid arthritis patients also presenting with periodontitis (Abou Raya, Naim, and Abuelkheir 2007). In patients with rheumatoid arthritis and periodontitis, erythrocyte sedimentation rate, high-sensitivity C-reactive protein, fibrinogen, and TNF-α are higher (Abou Raya et al. 2007). Periodontal disease is more frequent among rheumatoid arthritis patients. The presence of moderate to severe alveolar bone loss is associated with some arthritis manifestations:

- Longer morning joint stiffness
- Accelerated erythrocyte sedimentation rate
- Elevated C-reactive protein (Zhang et al. 2005)

Patients with rheumatoid arthritis present more severe periodontitis because of the excess production of inflammatory cytokines and matrix metalloproteinases, inducing both periodontal bone and articular joint destruction (Bartold, Marshall, and Haynes 2005). Some clinical manifestations of rheumatic diseases, such as the ability to control oral hygiene, xerostomia (or dry mouth), temporomandibular joint disease, and some medical treatments such as corticosteroids or immunomodulators, may influence oral and dental care (Treister and Glick 1999). Rheumatoid arthritis and advanced age are two significant predictors of periodontitis. Rheumatoid arthritis patients have a significant 8.05 times increased odds ratio of having periodontal disease, and they present significantly increased periodontal attachment loss (Pischon et al. 2008). Rheumatoid arthritis patients have more gingival bleeding, and they present more tooth loss and alveolar bone loss. Severity of periodontitis correlates with arthritis disease duration, the number of tender and swollen joints, serum C-reactive protein level, and erythrocyte sedimentation rate. Alveolar bone loss also correlates with the percentage of radiographic articular erosions (Abou Raya, Abou Raya, and El Kheir 2004). Rheumatoid arthritis is associated with connective tissue destruction and cartilage and bone erosions. Active rheumatoid arthritis is associated with the following:

- Greater prevalence of periodontitis
- Higher rate of gingival bleeding
- Greater probing depth and attachment loss
- Higher number of missing teeth (Kasser et al. 1997).

Pathophysiology

There is an association between rheumatoid arthritis and periodontitis. Rheumatoid arthritis and periodontal disease may have a common pathobiology because they are both chronic inflammatory diseases (Abou Raya et al. 2007).

Genetic Factors

Genetic factors may influence disease severity in rheumatoid arthritis, especially HLA-DR antigens and the shared epitope. Wrist destruction is correlated with periodontal bone degradation. Presence of dry mouth syndrome is associated with greater wrist and periodontal bone destruction. Positivity of the HLA-DR–shared epitope also induces greater wrist and periodontal bone destruction (Marotte et al. 2006).

Microvascular Circulation

Microvascular circulation may be involved in some autoimmune diseases such as systemic sclerosis or rheumatoid arthritis. Capillary circulation is assessed by capillaroscopy. Periodontal capillaroscopy in rheumatoid arthritis patients shows reduced capillary caliber and greater number of elongated capillaries. Capillaries and microcirculation are altered in rheumatoid arthritis, which may in turn worsen the evolution of periodontitis (Scardina and Messina 2007).

Chronic Inflammation

Bone destruction is induced by dysregulation of the immune response secondary to autoimmune diseases or microbial gingival infection. Elevation of IL-1, IL-6, and TNF-α induce the production of matrix metalloproteinases responsible for articular destruction, periodontal destruction, and alveolar bone loss. Activation of receptor activator of nuclear factor kappa B ligand and production of matrix metalloproteinases are responsible for tissue destruction (Golub et al. 2006). Cytokines are responsible for bone resorption induced by inflammation; cytokines and kinins activate prostaglandins synthesis. Stimulation of cytokines and kinins with increased receptor activator of nuclear factor kappa B ligand expression is responsible for the inflammation and bone resorption seen in rheumatoid arthritis and periodontal disease (Bernhold Brechter 2007). Bone metabolism markers such as alkaline phosphatase levels in gingival crevicular fluid are correlated with probing depth and gingival index. Osteocalcin concentration, which is a bone formation marker, is correlated with gingival index (Nakashima, Roehrich, and Cimasoni 1994). Receptor activator of nuclear factor kappa B and its ligand activate osteoclastic resorption; on the contrary, osteoprotegerin has an inhibitory effect on osteoclast activity. Higher levels of receptor activator of nuclear factor kappa B ligand and lower levels of osteoprotegerin are present in periodontitis tissues, with the consequence of increased alveolar bone loss (Crotti et al. 2003). Periodontitis is due to oral tissue destruction, and arthritis is due to articular tissue destruction caused by synovitis. Arthritis is often associated with periodontitis because of excess systemic inflammation and possible interaction between the two diseases (Chieko et al.

2003). Serum antiphospholipid antibodies are sometimes found in arthritis patients; they are responsible for vascular thrombosis in autoimmune diseases, especially lupus disease. One of them is anticardiolipin autoantibody, which is increased in case of chronic or generalized periodontitis. Anticardiolipin is associated with increased periodontal pocket depth and attachment loss (Schenkein et al. 2003).

Matrix Metalloproteinases

Matrix metalloproteinases or MMPs are collagenases responsible for extracellular matrix degradation. There are inhibitors called tissue inhibitor of metalloproteinases or TIMP. In progressive periodontitis, the matrix metalloproteinase-13 level is elevated, and the tissue inhibitor of metalloproteinase-1 level is decreased (Hernandez et al. 2007). Matrix metalloproteinases induce connective tissue degradation. Matrix metalloproteinase-3 action is mediated by IL-1 and TNF-α. Matrix metalloproteinase-3 is responsible for the degradation of proteoglycans and type IV collagen in periodontitis and arthritis, with the consequence of increased periodontal tissue and bone destruction (Borghaei, Sullivan, and Mochan 1999). Rheumatoid arthritis and periodontitis are diseases modulated by cytokines, interleukins, chemokines, and interferons. They activate fibroblasts to produce matrix metalloproteinases. IL-1 stimulates fibroblasts to produce matrix metalloproteinase-1 or collagenase and matrix metalloproteinase-3 or stromelysin. They are responsible for the degradation of connective tissues in both arthritis and periodontitis (Thornton et al. 2000).

Microbial Pathogenesis of Rheumatoid Arthritis

Arthritis may be triggered by the immune response to some bacterial cell wall fragments or some bacterial DNA. There are more bacterial species that are found at high concentrations in synovial fluid samples of rheumatoid arthritis patients (Moen et al. 2005). Several pathogens may play a role in triggering an immune response in rheumatoid arthritis, such as Epstein-Barr virus, parvovirus B19, periodontopathic bacteria, and especially *Porphyromonas* and *Prevotella*. Higher levels of IgG antibodies against *B. forsythus* and *P. intermedia* are present in joint synovial fluid samples of rheumatoid arthritis patients. Serum pyridinoline cross-linked carboxyterminal telopeptide of type 1 collagen (CTX1) is a bone resorption marker; CTX1 levels are elevated in periodontitis and are associated with the presence of microbial pathogens such as *Prevotella intermedia*, *Prevotella nigrescens*, *Prevotella denticola*, *Porphyromonas gingivalis*, and *Bacteroides forsythus* (Palys et al. 1998). An immune response may occur with capture of the microbial DNA, microbial protein, or toxin and the production of inflammatory mediators. The presence of increased levels of antibodies against oral pathogens in serum and synovial fluid of rheumatoid arthritis patients may indicate a link between rheumatoid arthritis and periodontitis (Moen et al. 2003). Serum IgG

antibody titers to the DNA from *Actinobacillus actinomycetemcomitans* are higher in rheumatoid arthritis patients and may be a factor in the pathogenesis of the disease (Yoshida et al. 2001). Antibody titers to *P. gingivalis* above 800 are more common in rheumatoid arthritis patients. Antibodies to *P. gingivalis* show a significant correlation with serum C-reactive protein levels and with autoantibodies to cyclic citrullinated peptides. Antibodies to cyclic citrullinated peptides (ACPA) are specific to rheumatoid arthritis, which may indicate a role of antibodies to *P. gingivalis* in arthritis disease risk and progression (Miklus et al. 2009). Mean number of oral bacteria found in joint synovial fluid is more elevated in arthritis patients; also *P. gingivalis*, *T. forsythensis*, and *P. intermedia* are identified in arthritis synovial fluid samples. Higher concentrations of DNA are found in synovial fluid, which may suggest a link between the presence of oral pathogens and arthritis (Moen et al. 2006). Oral bacterial DNA is found at higher concentrations in joint synovial fluid of arthritis patients and may induce excess joint inflammation. *Actinobacillus*, *Tannerella*, Eubacterium, *Streptococcus*, *Prevotella*, and *Actinomyces* are found at high concentrations in synovial fluid (Moen et al. 2005). The mechanism of autoimmunity against oral pathogens may be explained by the fact that *P. gingivalis* possess an enzyme called peptidyl arginine deiminase, which is responsible for the deimination of fibrin and the activation of anti-citrullinated peptide autoantibodies, which are very specific to rheumatoid arthritis. Deimination of fibrin induces an autoimmune response against joint tissues with production of ACPA and the articular joint destruction specific to rheumatoid arthritis (Rosenstein et al. 2004).

Treatment

Treatment of periodontal disease may have beneficial effects on inflammation marker levels of rheumatoid arthritis patients. Full-mouth scaling and root planing can induce a great reduction in serum erythrocyte sedimentation rate levels (Ribeiro, Leao, and Novaes 2005). Scaling, root planning, and plaque control can improve disease severity in rheumatoid arthritis. After mouth scaling, root planing, and oral hygiene, a majority of these patients show an improvement of clinical and biological parameters of arthritis disease severity. They show an improvement of the disease activity score called DAS28 and also a reduction of erythrocyte sedimentation rate levels (Al Katma et al. 2007). Mouth scaling and root planing followed by periodontal surgery induce a decrease in serum C-reactive protein and TNF-α levels (Chieko et al. 2003). Periodontal treatment is associated with a decrease in systemic inflammation and serum inflammatory markers. After periodontal nonsurgical therapy, serum C-reactive protein and IL-6 levels are decreased (D'Aiuto et al. 2004).

Arthritis therapy may also improve periodontal inflammation. After treatment of rheumatoid arthritis, inflammatory markers such as IL-1beta levels show a decrease in gingival crevicular fluid (Miranda et al. 2007). Gold salts are old medications for rheumatoid arthritis. In experimental periodontitis, gold salts–treated subjects present significantly smaller areas of infiltrated supracrestal connective tissues, less attachment loss, and less alveolar bone loss (Novak, Polson, Freeman 1984). Omega-3 fatty acids are sometimes prescribed for dietary supplementation in cardiovascular diseases and inflammatory conditions such as periodontitis or rheumatoid arthritis. There are three omega-3 fatty acids: eicosapentaenoic acid and docosahexaenoic acid, which are found in fish oil, and alphalinolenic acid, which is found in vegetables. These fatty acids are precursors of prostaglandins and lipoxins, and they have some anti-inflammatory action and antithrombotic effects. Omega-3 fatty acids can modulate inflammatory process, and they may have some beneficial effects on gingival inflammation and bone destruction. Resolvins are anti-inflammatory agents derived from omega-3 fatty acids. Resolvin E1 is derived from eicosapentaenoic acid and blocks reactive oxygen species such as superoxide radical produced by leukocytes. Local oral treatment with Resolvin E1 at the sites of surgery prevents periodontal destruction and bone loss (Hasturk et al. 2006).

Periodontitis and Sjögren Syndrome

Sjögren syndrome is an autoimmune disease affecting salivary glands, characterized by xerostomia (or dry mouth). There are two Sjögren syndrome categories: primary Sjögren syndrome and secondary Sjögren syndrome. Primary Sjögren syndrome patients often present xerostomia and may consequently present many oral symptoms (Pers et al. 2005). Some autoimmune diseases are also associated with secondary Sjögren syndrome with oral clinical manifestations such as dry mouth, low saliva flow rate, and increased dental caries. Periodontitis is more frequent in arthritis patients. They present saliva modifications with increased albumin, protein, IgG, and IgM concentrations (Miia et al. 2005). Some Sjögren syndrome patients also present dry mouth, low saliva secretion, and a higher percentage of missing teeth (Jorkjend et al. 2003).

Periodontitis and Juvenile Idiopathic Arthritis

Arthritis that affects children and adolescents is called juvenile idiopathic arthritis. Juvenile idiopathic arthritis patients should receive good oral hygiene education because poor oral hygiene induces many dental problems, especially with such an immunocompromised situation. Juvenile idiopathic arthritis patients present generally poor oral hygiene, more caries, and more missing teeth (Welbury et al. 2003). Juvenile idiopathic arthritis is accompanied by poor oral health status (Walton et al. 2000). Juvenile idiopathic arthritis patients present higher plaque index and more sites with attachment loss (Reichert et al. 2006). They also share some human leukocyte antigens in common with periodontitis patients.

HLA-DRB3 occurs more frequently in females with juvenile idiopathic arthritis and chronic periodontitis, HLA-A01 and HLA-A01-DRB3 are present in cases of increased attachment loss (Reichert et al. 2007). Juvenile idiopathic arthritis patients present a higher percentage of attachment loss greater than 2 mm and more sites with probing depth of 4 mm (Miranda et al. 2003). They also present significantly high levels of IL-1β and IL-18, especially in cases of attachment loss. These factors may explain the early attachment loss seen in juvenile idiopathic arthritis patients presenting periodontitis (Miranda et al. 2005).

PERIODONTITIS AND OSTEOPOROSIS

General skeletal osteoporosis, oral bone loss, and periodontal disease are related diseases. Osteoporosis is characterized by a low bone mass of the skeleton and an increased incidence of fractures. Alveolar bone loss is associated with periodontal disease because of localized periodontal inflammation responsible for bone resorption and systemic inflammation. Osteoporosis is a phenomenon that is increased by inflammation of periodontal tissues. In consequence, maxillar bone mineral density is low and alveolar bone loss is accelerated. Periodontal inflammation induces the production of inflammatory cytokines interacting on IL-1, receptor activator of nuclear factor kappa B ligand, and TNF-α, which in turn accelerate bone resorption. Bone mass is dependent on bone formation by osteoblast cells and bone resorption by osteoclast cells. Bone turnover can be measured by biological markers of bone formation and bone resorption.

For mandibular osteoporosis, mandibular bone density can be evaluated by the measure of the mandibular cortical shape and width on panoramic x-rays. For general osteoporosis, vertebral and hip bone mineral density is generally evaluated by dual x-ray absorptiometry, or DEXA, with determination of T-score and Z-score necessary for osteoporosis diagnosis, and the FRAX score can also be helpful (Krejci and Bissada 2002; Lerner 2006a; Lerner 2006b; Reddy 2002; Taguchi et al. 2003; von Wovern 2001; Wactawski et al. 1996).

PERIODONTITIS AND POSTMENOPAUSAL OSTEOPOROSIS

Periodontitis and postmenopausal osteoporosis are common diseases, and their incidence increases with age. There is a correlation between a low skeletal bone mineral density and periodontal disease. Severity of osteoporosis is associated with the loss of alveolar crestal height and tooth loss in postmenopausal women (Wactawski et al. 1996). Osteoporosis induces low oral bone mineral density and facilitates periodontal disease progression. Treatment of osteoporosis may in consequence improve oral bone mineral density and reduce alveolar bone loss (Reddy 2002). Postmenopausal osteoporosis is responsible for increased clinical attachment loss and increased periodontitis incidence (Krejci and Bissada 2002). In periodontitis, the chronic inflammation induces an excessive bone resorption with increased alveolar bone loss. In postmenopausal osteoporosis, the physiological lack of estrogen is responsible for general accelerated bone resorption by osteoclast cells and also with increased alveolar bone loss (Lerner 2006). Lack of estrogen is responsible for a decreased bone mass because of the upregulation of inflammatory process and accelerated bone resorption. Prevalence of osteoporosis increases with age and may in consequence promote the progression of periodontal disease (Lerner 2006).

The determination of jaw osteoporosis necessitates the measurement of the jaw bone mineral density or the bone mineral content using radiological equipment dedicated to the diagnosis of oral osteoporosis. Periodontal bone loss or presence of dental implants may also modify the bone mineral density (von Wovern 2001). Dental panoramic radiographs may help diagnose postmenopausal osteoporosis, and mandibular cortical measurement of shape and width may assess bone mineral density. Mandibular cortical erosion is associated with general osteoporosis. It is associated with lower vertebral bone mineral density on absorptiometry DEXA, and with increased serum markers of bone turnover. Mandibular inferior cortical width on panoramic x-rays is correlated with the measure of vertebral bone mineral density on absorptiometry (Taguchi et al. 2003).

Vitamin D

Vitamin D posseses some immunomodulatory effects and may reduce gingival inflammation because of the possible anti-inflammatory effects of vitamin D. Patients presenting the highest serum circulating levels of vitamin D, called 25-hydroxy D3, are less likely to bleed on probing (Dietrich et al. 2005). Vitamin D can also affect periodontal status because of the effects of vitamin D on improvement of bone mineral density. Circulating levels of vitamin D or 25-hydroxy D are inversely associated with attachment loss. Vitamin D can improve bone mineral density and also immunity, which may explain in periodontitis patients the positive correlations between the low levels of circulating vitamin D and the presence of periodontal disease (Dietrich et al. 2004).

Bisphosphonates Therapy

Bisphosphonates are medications often used for the treatment of osteoporosis. Bisphosphonates modify the bone resorption by inhibition of osteoclast cell action. They induce an increase in alveolar bone density and an improvement of teeth mobility scores and pocket depth. They may be beneficial in the therapy of periodontitis because of the inhibition of bone resorption and improvement in periodontal disease.

Unfortunately they can also promote jaw osteonecrosis in some patients, especially those presenting cancer disease (Takaishi et al. 2001).

REFERENCES

Abou Raya S, Abou Raya A, El Kheir HA. 2004. Presentation at Congress of EULAR 2004, Berlin, Germany, June 9–12, 2005.

Abou Raya S, Abou Raya A, Naim H, et al. 2008. *Clin Rheumatol.* 27(4):421–27.

Abou Raya S, Naim A, Abuelkheir H. 2007. *Ann NY Acad Sci.* 1107(1):56–67.

Aiuto FD, Parkar M, Andreou G, et al. 2004. *J Dent Res.* 83(2):156–60.

Al Katma MK, Bissada NF, Bordeaux J, et al. 2007. *J Clin Rheumato.* 13(3):134–37.

Bartold PM, Marshall RI, Haynes DR. 2005. *J Periodontol.* 76(11):2066–74.

Bernhold Brechter A. 2007. "Kinins: important regulators in inflammation induced bone resorption." PhD diss., Umea University, Sweden.

Borghaei RC, Sullivan C, Mochan E. 1999. *J Biol Chem.* 274(4):2126–31.

Chieko K, Takayuki K, Fusanori N, et al. 2003. *Jpn J Cons Dent.* 46(1):110–17.

Crotti T, Smith MD, Hirsch R, et al. 2003. *J Periodontal Res.* 38(4):380–87.

de Pablo P, Dietrich T, McAlindon TE. 2008. *J Rheumatol.* 35(1):70–76.

Dietrich T, Joshipura KJ, Dawson-Hughes B, et al. 2004. *Am J Clin Nutr.* 80(1):108–13.

Dietrich T, Nunn M, Dawson-Hughes B, et al. 2005. *Am J Clin Nutr.* 82(3):575–80.

Ebersole JL, Machen RL, Steffen MJ, et al. 1997. *Clin Exp Immunol.* 107(2):347–52.

Fauci AS, Braunwald E, Kasper DL, et al. 2008. *Harrison's Principles of Internal Medicine.* 17th edition. New York: McGraw Hill.

Golub LM, Payne JB, Reinhardt RA, et al. 2006. *J Dent Res.* 85(2):102–105.

Hasturk H, Kantarci A, Ohira T, et al. 2006. *FASEB J.* 20:401–03.

Havemose-Poulsen A, Westergaard J, Stoltze K, et al. 2006. *J Periodontol.* 77(2):280–88.

Hernandez M, Martinez B, Tejerina JM, et al. 2007. *J Clin Periodontol.* 34(9):729–35.

Jorkjend L, Johansson A, Johansson AK, et al. 2003. *J Oral Rehabil.* 30(4):369–78.

Kasser UR, Gleissner C, Dehne F, et al. 1997. *Arthritis Rheum.* 40:2248–51.

Krejci CB, Bissada NF. 2002. *J Am Dent Assoc.* 133(3):323–29.

Lerner UH. 2006a. *J Dent Res.* 85(7):584–95.

Lerner UH. 2006b. *J Dent Res.* 85(7):596–607.

Marotte H, Farge P, Gaudin P, et al. 2006. *Ann Rheum Dis.* 65:905–09.

Mercado FB, Marshall RI, Bartold PM. 2003. *J Clin Periodontol.* 30(9):761–72.

Mercado FB, Marshall RI, Klestov AC, et al. 2000. *J Clin Periodontol.* 27(4):267–72.

Mercado FB, Marshall RI, Klestov AC, et al. 2001. *J Periodontol.* 72:779–87.

Miia L, Helenius J, Meurman JK, et al. 2005. *Acta Ondol Scand.* 63(5):284–93.

Mikuls TR, Payne JB, Reinhardt RA, et al. 2009. *Int Immunopharmacol.* 9(1):38–42.

Miranda LA, Fischer RG, Sztajnbok FR, et al. 2003. *J Clin Periodonto.* 30(11):969–74.

Miranda LA, Fischer RG, Sztajnbok FR, et al. 2005. *J Periodontol.* 76:75–92.

Miranda LA, Islabao AG, Fischer RG, et al. 2007. *J Periodontol.* 78(8):1612–19.

Moen K, Brun JG, Eribe ERK, et al. 2005. *Microb Ecol Health Dis.* 1:2–8.

Moen K, Brun JG, Madland TM, et al. 2003. *Clin Diagn Lab Immunol.* 10(6):1043–50.

Moen K, Brun JG, Valen M, et al. 2006. *Clin Exp Rheumatol.* 24(6):656–63.

Nakashima K, Roehrich N, Cimasoni G. 1994. *J Clin Periodontol.* 21(5):327–33.

Novak MJ, Polson AM, Freeman E. 1984. *J Periodontol.* 55(2): 69–77.

Palys MD, Haffajee AD, Socransky SS, et al. 1998. *J Clin Periodontol.* 25(11):865–71.

Pers JO, D'Arbonneau F, Devauchelle Pensec V, et al. 2005. *Arthritis Rheumatism.* 52(8):2411–14.

Reddy MS. 2002. *Compend Contin Educ Dent.* 23(10suppl):21–28.

Reichert S, Machulla HKG, Fuchs C, et al. 2006. *J Clin Periodontol.* 33(5):317–23.

Reichert S, Stein J, Fuchs C, et al. 2007. *J Clin Periodontol.* 34(6):492–98.

Ribeiro J, Leao A, Novaes AB. 2005. *J Clin Periodontol.* 32(4): 412–16.

Rosenstein ED, Greewald RA, Kushner LG, et al. 2004. *Inflammation.* 28(6):311–18.

Scardina GA, Messina P. 2007. *Clin Hemorheol Microcirc.* 37(3):229–35.

Schenkein HA, Berry CR, Burmeister JA, et al. 2003. *J Dent Res.* 82(11):919–22.

Taguchi A, Sanada M, Krall E, et al. 2003. *J Bone Miner Res.* 18:1689–94.

Takaishi Y, Miki T, Nishizawa Y, et al. 2001. *J Int Med Res.* 29(4):355–65.

Thornton RD, Lane P, Borghaei RC, et al. 2000. *Biochem J.* 350:307–12.

Treister N, Glick BA. 1999. *J Am Dent Assoc.* 130(5):689–98.

Von Wovern N. 2001. *Clin Oral Investig.* 5(2):71–82.

Wactawski Wende J, Grossi SG, Trevisan M, et al. 1996. *J Periodontol.* 67(10 suppl):1076–84.

Walton AG, Welbury RR, Thomason JM, et al. 2000. *Rheumatology.* 39:550–55.

Welbury RR, Thomason JM, Fitzgerald JL, et al. 2003. *Rheumatology.* 42:1445–51.

Yoshida A, Nakano Y, Yamashita Y, et al. 2001. *J Dent Res.* 80:346–50.

Zhang DZ, Zhong DY, Deng J, et al. 2005. *The Affiliated Hospital, Medical College of Qingdao University, China.* 23(6):498–501.

Section 2
Osseous Surgery in Periodontal Therapy

Chapter 6 Resective Osseous Surgery

Oreste Zanni, DDS

HISTORY

As periodontists we currently have many treatment options available.

At present we have the advantage of newer techniques not available in the past, such as dental implants, bone regeneration and augmentation, sinus lifts, etc. Implant treatment is one option that has been quite predictable and fairly successful. These advances allow us to expand our treatment options. However, sometimes these modalities cannot be used for any number of reasons. Therefore, it is important to have other options available when needed. After all, our main objective has been, whenever feasible, to maintain the patient's natural dentition in a healthy state. This chapter is intended to elaborate on one particular treatment option available to us to obtain this goal of maintaining a healthy periodontium.

Osseous surgery has had a controversial history as a modality of periodontal treatment. Recently, however, it has experienced a renaissance at Boston University Henry M. Goldman School of Dental Medicine. The concept of using a flap to visualize the alveolar bone was not controversial but whether or not to "touch" the bone has been. In 1884, Robicsek described a procedure to allow access to the bone (Stern, Everett, and Robicsek 1965). In the 1920s, Zentler, Zemsky, and Neuman reported that access to the bone was necessary to remove necrotic or infected bone (Zentler 1918; Zemsky 1926). Kronfield (1935) reported that bone was neither necrotic nor infected. Orban (1939) introduced the gingivectomy procedure in 1939. However, recurrence of pockets was frequently observed. Schluger's (1949) classic article defined the principles of osseous surgery. He outlined the basic principles of osseous resection in periodontal surgery. The goal was to create a form to the bone that resembles an ideal architectural form. The purpose, therefore, was to reestablish physiologic contours to the bone and establish shallow gingival pockets. Lindhe and Nyman published 5-year results in 1,620 teeth in 75 patients who had advanced periodontal disease and were treated with surgical pocket elimination (Lindhe and Nyman 1975). The authors concluded that pocket elimination surgery, along with good oral hygiene, resulted in periodontal health. Becker et al.

This chapter is in memory of my wife, Paula M. Zanni.

(1988) published results comparing root planning and scaling, osseous resective surgery, and modified Widman flap. They concluded that 1 year later modified Widman and osseous resective surgery resulted in effective pocket reduction.

Scaling was not as effective in reducing pocket depth. There have also been numerous studies demonstrating that surgical and nonsurgical therapy were both viable treatments. However, studies do show that the deeper the pockets, the poorer the plaque removal (Waerhaug 1978). Waerhaug found that most reliable means of allowing for adequate plaque control was to eliminate the pathological pockets. However, in moderate to deep pockets, if maximum pocket reduction is accepted as the main objective in periodontal therapy, then surgery and not curettage would be the treatment of choice (Knowles et al. 1979, 1980). Another study (Olsen Simmons 1985) compared flap curettage with no osseous therapy and flap surgery with osseous therapy (Olsen, Simmons 1985). Split-mouth random surgery was done. Pocket depth with flap surgery only returned to preoperative levels. The deeper the pocket is preoperatively, the more effective osseous surgery is at reducing and maintaining pocket depth. They demonstrated that if minimal pocket depth is the clinical objective, then osseous resective surgery is the procedure of choice. It would seem reasonable that osseous resective surgery may be the most predictable "pocket" reduction procedure.

DEFINITIONS

Osseous surgery is accomplished with a combination of ostectomy and osteoplasty, as classified by Friedman (1955). Osseous surgery, therefore, is intended for the elimination of osseous defects and elimination of periodontal pockets in order to make the area more amenable to self-maintenance as well as maintenance by the patient. Patients cannot perform adequate oral physiotherapy on teeth surfaces that are adjacent to osseous defects. The walls of the bony defect support the overlying gingiva and hinder attempts to clean the apical portion of the teeth. *Osteoplasty* is defined as reshaping alveolar bone to achieve a more physiological form

Practical Osseous Surgery in Periodontics and Implant Dentistry, First Edition. Edited by Serge Dibart, Jean-Pierre Dibart.
© 2011 John Wiley & Sons, Inc. Published 2011 by John Wiley & Sons, Inc.

without removal of supporting bone. *Ostectomy* is the excision of bone (American Academy of Periodontology 1992). Both are subtraction procedures. Minor osteoplasty does not remove supporting bone. However, ostectomy does remove supporting bone. Some have criticized the technique of osseous surgery because of the possibility of excessive osseous loss. Selipsky reported an average of 0.6 mm of supporting bone loss (Selipsky 1976). Also, mobility increased markedly after osseous surgery but did gradually return to below presurgical levels at 1 year. He also noted that the reshaping of thickened margins does not reduce any portion of the attachment apparatus. The use of these procedures, therefore, requires sound clinical judgment. All osseous surgery is aimed at allowing the patient to adequately remove plaque, which is essential in preventing periodontal disease. In fact, it is the author's opinion that surgical treatment should not be discarded in favor of chemotherapeutics when time has shown surgical techniques to be successful for the long term.

Ochsenbein and Bohannan (1964) classified craters. Class 1 comprised craters of 2–3 mm osseous concavity with relatively thick buccal and lingual walls. These were treated with palatal ramping. Class 2 comprised 4–5 mm osseous concavity with a wide orifice and thinner walls. These were treated with buccal and palatal ramping. Class 3 were concavities 6–7 mm and were treated with both palatal and buccal ramping. Class 4 were lesions of variable depth with thin buccal and palatal walls. Therefore, ostectomy is used to treat shallow (1–2 mm) to medium (3–4 mm) intrabony and hemiseptal osseous defects (Goldman and Cohen 1958; Ochsenbein 1969, 1986; Ariaudo and Tirrell 1957). Osteoplasty is generally done to treat buccal and lingual bony ledges, buccal and lingual minimal intrabony lesions, and incipient furcation involvement (Ariaudo and Tirrell 1957; Friedman 1955; Ochsenbein 1958, 1977; Pritchard 1961). The result with osteoplasty, along with an apically positioned flap, allows better tissue adaptation when suturing. The end result of ostectomy is the elimination of the intrabony pocket. An apically positioned buccal flap and a thinned palatal flap are necessary in conjunction with the above (Ochsenbein 1958). Osseous periodontal surgery is a combination of ostectomy and osteoplasty to reestablish osseous contours that resemble normal or physiologic bone. In other words, the interproximal bone is coronal to the buccal and lingual radicular bone (Ochsenbein 1986).

CONSIDERATIONS AFFECTING SURGICAL TECHNIQUE

In periodontitis there is resorption of bone with an apical migration of connective tissue and junctional epithelium (Page and Schroeder 1976). This forms a "defect" in the bone adjacent to the root. The surrounding bone that is in a more coronal position forms the walls of the defect (an intrabony defect). If, on the contrary, the alveolar housing is thin, the osseous lesion would be all encompassing. In this case, the gingival margin would be unsupported (Oschenbein 1958; Goldman and Cohen 1958), and dependent upon the thickness of the soft tissue, a suprabony pocket with increased pocket depth would occur or, more often than not, the gingival margin would recede. Normally the connective tissue and epithelial attachments average 2 mm in width and are coronal to or adjacent to osseous margins apically in the base of intrabony defects and coronally over the walls of the defect (Oschenbein 1958; Goldman and Cohen 1958; Gargiulo, Wentz, and Orban 1961). Osseous surgery is done to remove the walls of bone that make up the defect and place the gingival architecture in a more apical position. The removal of supporting bone (ostectomy) and nonsupporting bone (osteoplasty) with the use of an apically positioned flap is osseous resective surgery. The flap's final position should be at the crest of bone. Therefore, precise placement of the flap at this level necessitates a split-thickness flap on the buccal, and a thinned palatal flap allows precise placement by periosteal suturing. The probing depths and amounts of attached gingiva will determine the initial incision for flap design. If there is an adequate dimension of attached gingiva, the distance of the primary incision from the gingival margin is proportional to the difference in probing depths of the adjacent teeth. The apical positioning of the flap allows the gingival margin to coincide with the osseous crest. See Figure 6.1.

TECHNIQUES TO ELIMINATE OSSEOUS DEFECTS

Osseous resective surgery, as stated previously, is done to reshape abnormal bone architecture resulting from periodontitis to recreate a more physiologic alveolar anatomy. A knowledge of the morphology of healthy periodontium is a prerequisite for osseous therapy. An awareness of local anatomy of the surgical area and good clinical sense is essential to determine the amount and location of osseous removal. In most areas of the mouth, the gingiva and alveolus follow the same architectural pattern. Marginal radicular bone is usually thin at the tooth junction whereas interproximal septa are coronal in relation to marginal bone on the buccal and lingual surfaces, creating a scalloped appearance. So if there were a two-walled interproximal crater that was centrally located bucco-lingually, the base of the crater would be selected as the location for the crest of the septa. In this case, ostectomy would be needed on both the buccal and lingual. If only one of the osseous walls of the crater was removed, bone support would be much less affected. Ostectomy would be on only one side, and the crest of bone interproximally would be positioned either to the buccal or lingual side of the contact area. However, lingual angulation of teeth and the location of the osseous defect may dictate bone removal in

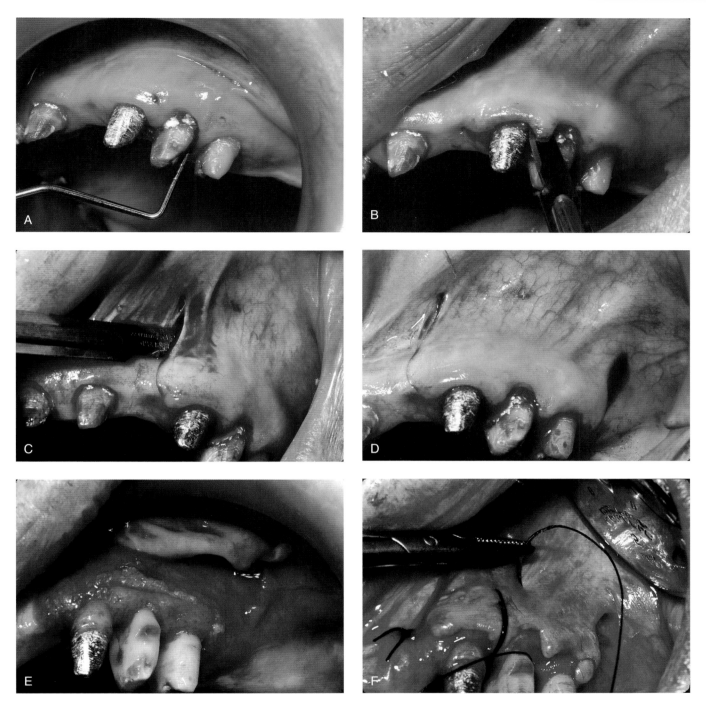

Figure 6.1 Partial-thickness flap. (A) probing the site for pocket depths. (B) Sharp intrasulcular incision to demonstrate dissection needed to "split" the periosteum. (C) Vertical releasing incision initiated. (D) Releasing incisions completed mesially and distally. (E) Split-thickness flap elevated. (F) Periosteal suturing initiated. (G) Palatal suturing. (H) Buccal suturing. (I) Occlusal view demonstrating buccal and palatal flaps placed apically to crest of bone to gain increase in amount of attached gingiva.

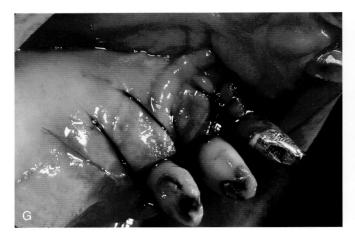

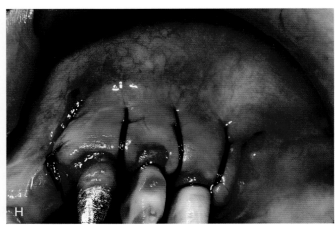

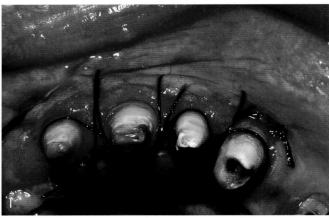

Figure 6.1 *Continued*

a way that creates an asymmetrical slope. For example, mandibular molars are usually inclined lingually and the lingual furcation and cemental-enamel junctions (CEJ) are more apical than the buccal. Often, interproximal defects on mandibular molars are located more to the lingual. Therefore if there were a crater interproximally closer toward the lingual, more of the lingual portion of the crater could be removed resulting in a sloping from the buccal to the lingual ("ramping"). In the maxilla, a palatal approach is often indicated for similar situations. Ochsenbein and Bohannan proposed a palatal approach to osseous craters on maxillary molars (Ochsenbein and Bohannan 1964). We often see interproximal craters and no deep pockets on the buccal and palatal sides. If the removal of the crater is attempted, then reverse gingival architecture could occur on the buccal. Also, if the buccal bone is removed to avoid this reverse architecture, exposure of furcations becomes a possible problem. This ramping avoids the thin bone usually found on buccal roots of maxillary molars as well as avoiding the possibility of exposing the buccal furca.

Other factors to consider include the shape of the interproximal bone. In the incisor region, interdental septa tend to be

prominent and convex, whereas in the molar regions they tend to be flatter. O'Connor and Biggs studied the bucco-lingual interproximal bone contours of 118 skulls (O'Connor and Biggs 1964). They noted that convex bony interproximal areas were noted far less in molar regions (flatter) and increased as they progressed anteriorly. There are many other factors that determine the morphology of the periodontium. These include alignment of teeth, tooth-size versus jaw size, tilting of teeth, exostoses, enamel projections, and so on. It is extremely important to be familiar with the many factors that influence and determine the topography of the alveolar bone. This is why emphasis should be placed on the clinician doing a thorough sextant analysis prior to initiating any osseous surgery.

LONG-TERM HEALING AFTER OSSEOUS SURGERY

Selipsky (1976) reported average bone loss after osseous surgery to be 0.6 mm. There was an increase in mobility that returned to presurgical levels by the end of the first year. He claimed that reshaping the ledges and thickened margins did not reduce any portion of the attachment apparatus.

Wilderman concluded 0.8 mm average crestal bone loss (Wilderman et al. 1970). Moghaddas determined interdental bone loss at 0.23 mm, interradicular bone loss at 0.55 mm, and furcal bone loss at 0.88 mm (Moghaddas and Stahl 1980). Both authors claimed that the thickness of bone was an important factor to determine postoperative bone loss. Olsen (Olsen, Ammons, and van Belle 1985) compared apically positioned flaps with osseous surgery versus apically positioned flaps without osseous surgery. Osseous surgery showed 67% more reduction at 5 years. The deeper the pockets (>4 mm) the more effective osseous surgery is in reducing and maintaining pocket depth at 5 years. He concluded that osseous recontouring is more effective in reduc-

ing and maintaining pocket depths while it reduces a minimal amount of bone. Crestal bone loss from resorption during healing after flap elevation with or without osseous surgery is summarized in Figure 6.2.

Recently we have begun to use piezosurgery for osseous recontouring (Figure 6.3). There are limited studies at present. One animal study by Vercellotti and colleagues demonstrates that there may be a slight increase in osseous with the piezosurgery (Vercellotti et al. 2005). Piezosurgery may provide a more favorable osseous response than traditional carbide and diamond burs. Again, the use of piezosurgery during osseous resection is still in the early stages of study.

Crestal bone loss from resorption during healing after flap elevation with or without osseous surgery		
Authors	Full thickness flap	Full thickness flap with osseous surgery
Aeschlimann et al.	0.16 mm	0.28 mm
Moghaddas & Stahl		0.23-0.88 mm
Smith et al.	0.2 mm	0.2-0.3 mm
Donnenfeld et al.		0.6-1.00 mm
Wood et al.	0.62 mm	
Friedman & Levine	None	0.25-0.3 mm

Carnevale, G. Kaldahl, WB. Osseous resective surgery. Periodontology 2000. 22: 59-87, 2000 Feb

Figure 6.2 Osseous surgery comparisons table.

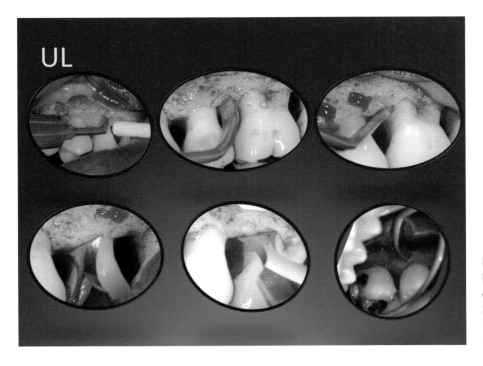

Figure 6.3 Piezoelectric instruments being used for osseous surgery instead of high-speed carbide or diamond burs. Lower left and lower middle images use conventional hand instruments for comparison.

CLINICAL STEPS FOR OSSEOUS SURGERY

The objective of osseous surgery, as previously stated, is to eliminate the osseous defect and provide soft tissue contours that are amenable to adequate cleansing by the patient. The crest of the interdental bone is normally located coronal to the marginal bone over the roots of the teeth. Terms used to describe this type of bony architecture include *physiologic*, *positive*, *flat*, and *ideal*. If after the completion of osseous surgery you are successful, the term *definitive therapy* could be used. If not, the terms *compromised therapy* or *nondefinitive therapy* would be used. Bone loss in the interdental area creates an environment that is opposite to the above. This is termed *reverse architecture* or *negative architecture*. In performing osseous surgery, we want to have the base of the defect become the crest of the interdental area. The morphology of the defects that we previously discussed determines whether or not we can recreate "normal architecture." Sound and prudent judgment is required by the clinician so as to prevent removal of too much supporting bone that would cause too much weakening of tooth support. The amount of bone that can be removed is dependent on the numerous factors listed in the preceding section.

SEQUENCE

It is important for the clinician to have knowledge of the underlying bone prior to flap elevation for proper flap design. During the sextant analysis phase, the clinician must gain as much indirect information as possible. Then, if an osseous lesion is amenable to treatment, the following steps, in general, would serve as an adequate guide.

Vertical Grooving

Vertical grooving is done to reduce the thickness of radicular bone. Alveolar bone on the buccal and lingual aspects of the interproximal bone is removed in order to create these vertical grooves (also called *sluiceways*). In relation to the interdental osseous, the teeth then become more prominent. This first step can create the general thickness and subsequent form of the alveolar housing. Vertical groove formation along with the next step also facilitates flap adaptation. The quantity of bone removed requires considerable clinical judgment. The clinician does not want to compromise the teeth by removing or thinning too much bone. The surgery should not diminish aesthetics or increase mobility. In other words osseous surgery has limitations. This creation of vertical grooves (sluiceways) is usually performed with high-speed rotary instruments. Carbide burs and coarse diamonds can be used to reduce the bulk of bone. Copious irrigation of the surgical site is essential when using these rotary cutting instruments. See Figure 6.4.

Radicular Blending

The next phase, radicular blending, is a continuation of vertical grooving. This is done to blend the alveolar surface into the vertical grooves to achieve "physiologic" shape and allow better flap adaptation (Figure 6.5). Obviously, if the radicular bone is very thin or fenestrated, this step is not necessary. Again, this requires clinical judgment. These first two steps, vertical grooving and radicular blending, are osteoplastic in nature, and thus no supporting bone is removed. In cases of shallow interdental craters, thick radicular ledges, and class 1 and early class 2 furcas, these two steps usually suffice.

Interdental Crater Removal

The next sequential step, if necessary, would be elimination of interdental craters (Figure 6.6). This is done to reposition the interdental bone in a more coronal position than that of the radicular bone. Again, as before, the clinician's awareness is critical since this step involves ostectomy. If a two-walled interproximal crater is more toward the lingual, then to eliminate it more of the lingual bone wall would be removed rather than the buccal to create an apical slope of the crest of the interproximal bone from buccal to lingual (also called *ramping*). This step is also done with high-speed rotary burs.

Blending the Marginal Bone

This final step also involves minimal ostectomy. This step, however, is usually done with hand instruments. These include but are not limited to chisels (e.g., Oschenbein, Wedelstaedt, Rhodes, back and side action), files, rongeurs, etc. Bone removal is minimal but necessary to prevent repocketing. These small bony discrepancies at the margins of the teeth (also called *widows peaks*) must be removed. Failure to do this step would allow the gingival tissue at these points to remain at a higher level than the base of bone, and this would allow repocketing to occur. As with the preceding three steps, clinical prudence is required so as not to nick or gouge the roots of teeth. To do so could result in sensitivity and create a nidus for bacterial accumulation. See Figures 6.7 and 6.8.

LIMITATIONS

As I have stated repeatedly, performing osseous surgery requires sound clinical judgment. A clinician would not want to do osseous surgery if radicular bone is thin. Vertical grooving and, in particular, radicular blending would have to be modified. Also, one would not want to compromise the prognosis of teeth by thinning too much and creating open furcations. The surgery should not be the cause of increasing mobility or cause any other detriment to the long-term prognosis of the dentition. Therefore, osseous surgery has its limitations. For example, if ideal osseous surgery were done on maxillary molars with palatal furcation involvement, this could open and worsen the furcal problem. Some compro-

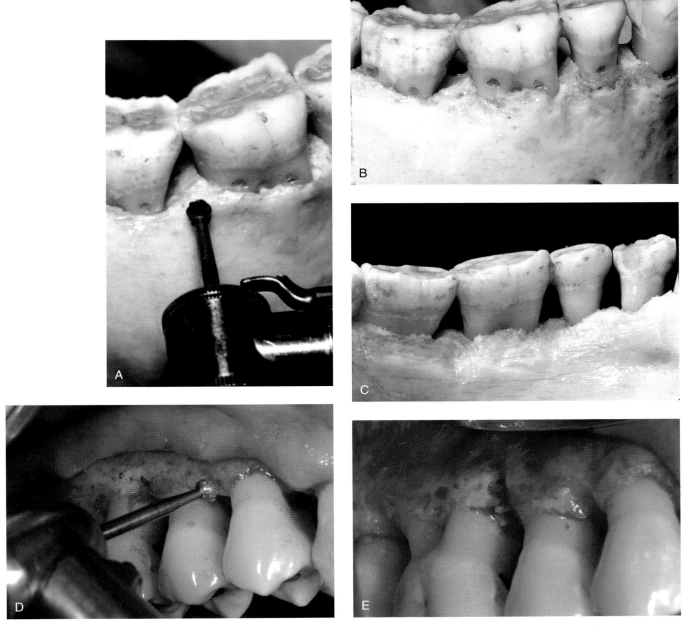

Figure 6.4 Vertical grooving. (A) Dry skull specimen used to demonstrate high-speed rotary carbide to initiate sluiceways on buccal side. (B) Dry skull specimen showing buccal grooving completed. (C) Dry skull specimen showing lingual grooving. (D) High-speed rotary diamond to initiate sluiceway clinically. (E) Clinical example of created sluiceways.

mise would be necessary, or perhaps a root amputation or implant placement would be a better choice. See Figure 6.9.

Radicular furcations on molars in the maxilla or mandible can be treated as if they were two individual teeth (e.g., two bicuspids). Osteoplasty in this situation would create a double scalloped appearance. This is commonly referred to as a *double parabola*. See Figure 6.10.

Thus, sometimes the severity of the defect limits the amount of osseous correction. Partial and incomplete defect elimination that results in shallower but still present pockets (i.e., compromised therapy) may sometimes be the treatment of choice. One is able to realize, therefore, that the surgeon may be a critical factor where prognosis is concerned. The patient's plaque control is the other critical factor in long-term success. Rosling and Nyman showed that following osseous

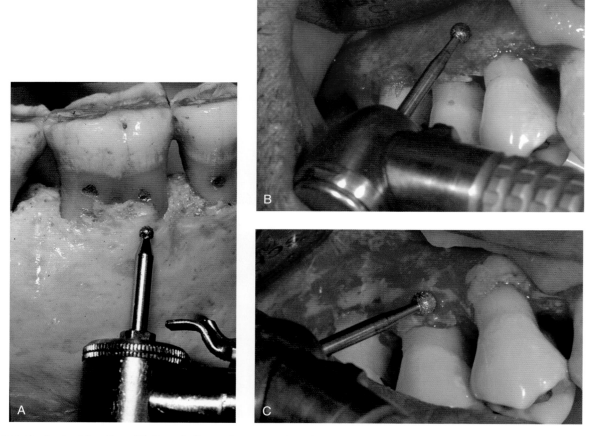

Figure 6.5 Radicular blending. (A) Dry skull specimen used to demonstrate use of high-speed rotary diamond to radicular blending. (B) Clinical initiation of blending using high-speed diamond. (C) Completion of radicular blending clinically.

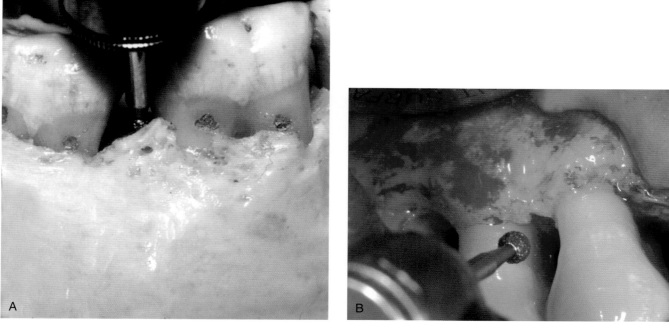

Figure 6.6 Interdental crater removal. (A) Dry skull showing interdental crater elimination with high-speed rotary. (B) Clinical use of high-speed diamonds for interdental craters.

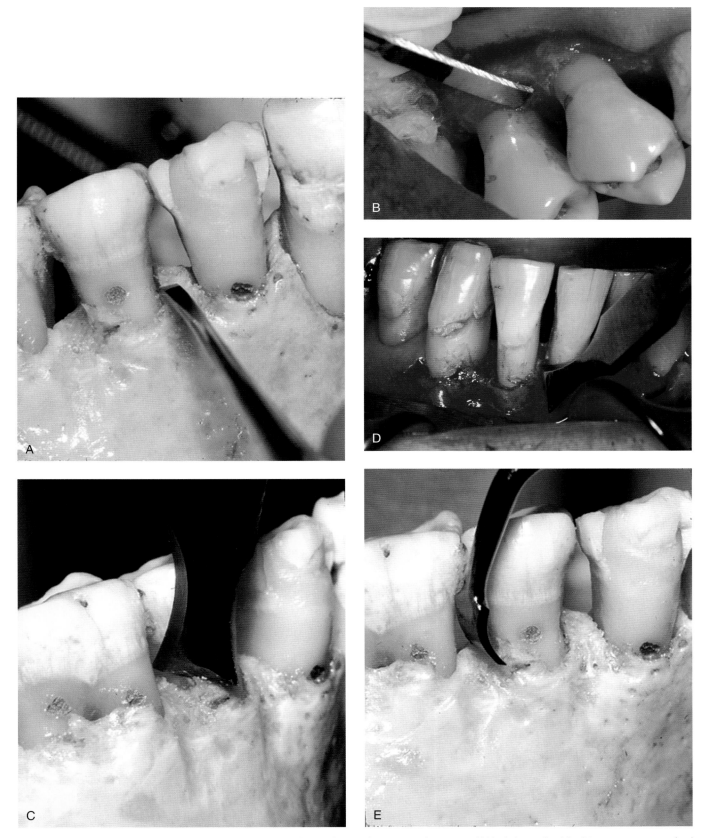

Figure 6.7 Blending the marginal bone. (A) Dry skull specimen demonstrating use of Wedelstaedt chisel to remove marginal bone (widow's peaks). Prudence is needed so as to not damage root surface. (B) Wedelstaedt chisel in clinical use. (C) Dry skull specimen demonstrating use of the Ochsenbein chisel. (D) Ochsenbein chisel in clinical use. Diligence needed not to force cutting edge of the chisel into root of tooth. (E) Dry skull specimen demonstrating use of Rhodes back-action chisel.

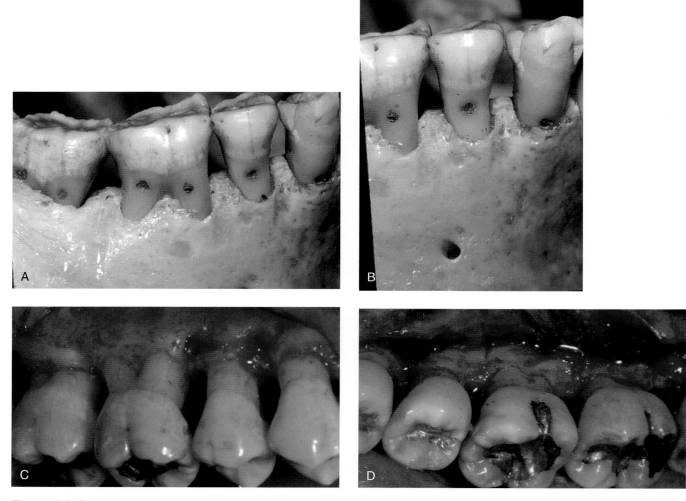

Figure 6.8 Completion of osseous surgery. (A) Dry skull specimen demonstrating completion of osseous surgery. Note the restoration of physiologic architecture molar area. (B) Dry skull specimen demonstrating completion of osseous surgery. Note the restoration of physiologic architecture premolar area. (C) Clinical example of completed osseous on buccal aspect posterior showing restoration of positive architecture. (D) Palatal view at completion in clinical situation.

surgery, patients with good home care and maintenance therapy remained stable (Rosling et al. 1976l Nyman, Lindhe, and Rosling 1977). Those with inadequate home care had a continuation of progressive periodontitis.

POSTSURGICAL MANAGEMENT

Once the osseous therapy is completed, the surgical site should be examined again for meticulous cleansing and be irrigated prior to flap replacement. The flaps are positioned at the crest of bone via precise suturing, including periosteal suturing. Sometimes, in order to gain an increase in attached gingiva, the flaps may be apically repositioned. This can easily be accomplished if a partial-thickness flap (split flap) was initi-

ated prior to flap elevation. Following suturing, the surgical site is covered with a periodontal pack. Pack removal, as well as suture removal, is usually done 7–10 days later. At this time, the area is irrigated again and checked for adequate healing. The patient is instructed to resume normal oral hygiene physiotherapy at the time clinical healing is adequate, usually also at 7–10 days.

SUMMARY

Osseous surgery is performed in order to eliminate osseous defects and eliminate pocket depth by recreating a more physiologic architecture conducive to self-maintenance as well as maintenance by the patient. Various factors that influ-

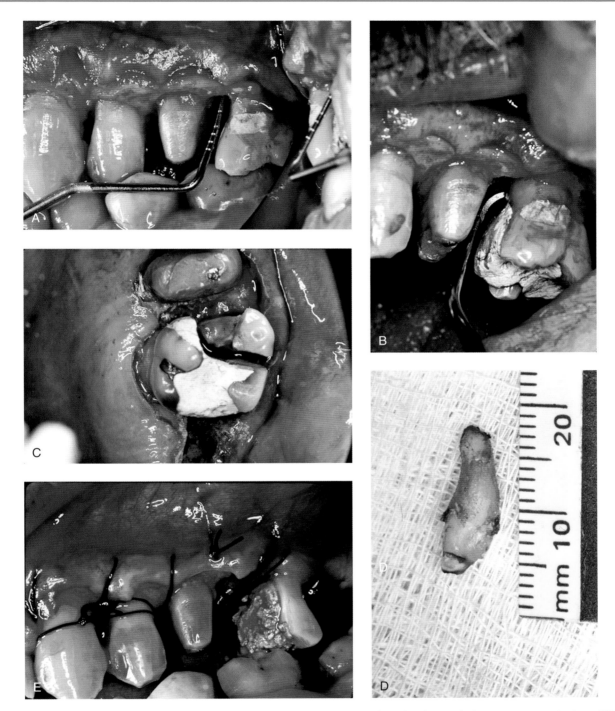

Figure 6.9 Root amputation. (A) Periodontal probings to determine pocket depths and demonstrate cratering. (B)Shows cratering and furcation involvement. Communication of mesial and buccal furcations (through-and-through). (C)Sectioning of the mesio-buccal root. No remnants of furca should remain. (D) Sectioned root removal. (E) Flaps apically repositioned in order to create more attachment and eliminate pockets. (F) Palatal flap sutured at crest. (G) Suturing of distal wedge.

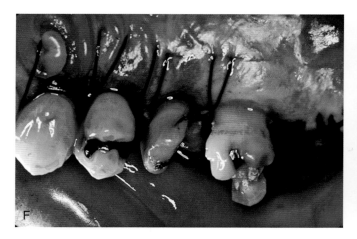

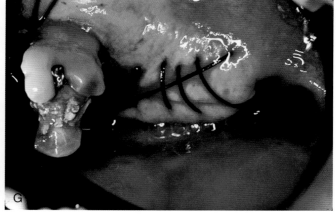

Figure 6.9 *Continued*

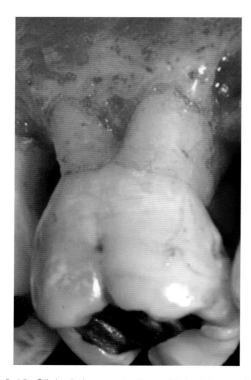

Figure 6.10 Clinical demonstration of "double parabola" on maxillary first molar.

ence the clinician to choose a particular path of treatment have been outlined in this chapter. One must always keep in mind that being successful in osseous surgery requires full knowledge and control over all etiologic factors prior to surgery. Sextant analysis is recommended. Flap designs and types should be determined prior to surgery initiation. Guidelines are not set in stone, which emphasizes that the clinician is a critical factor. Yet, osseous resective surgery has been the most predictable pocket reduction technique when

used judiciously. Flap surgery with osseous recontouring allows the patient to maintain adequate home care by reshaping soft and hard tissues to attain a normal (physiologic) topography. This is deemed necessary to allow adequate home care by the patient. Those of us who use osseous surgery do not feel that a long junctional epithelium is a resistant due to its weaker epithelial attachment to the tooth. A more reliable and stable result would be to create a shallow sulcus. Other studies have shown that moderate pockets can be maintained with meticulous home care and frequent recalls (pros and cons of pocket elimination) (Weeks 1980). "Zero" pocket depths (i.e., pocket elimination), however, allow complete removal of all irritants and accept the fact that even in the best of patients home care may be lacking or insufficient at times. As we have listed earlier, there are numerous studies indicating the efficacy of this type of surgery. However, I would like to cite one final reference from my former mentor, Dr. Gerald M. Kramer, "The Case for Ostectomy" (Kramer 1995), a time-tested therapeutic modality in selected periodontal sites. In this article he stated that although ostectomy has been proven in numerous studies to be an effective means of pocket reduction, some clinicians still question its merits. In this study, 870 radiographs of sites treated by ostectomy were examined. The radiographs spanned a time period of 5–30 years and again demonstrated that ostectomy is an effective and predictable technique for intercepting the progressive loss of attachment in selected sites with periodontitis. After digesting this chapter, it is hoped that you will find some merit to this therapeutic modality.

REFERENCES

Aeschlimann C, Robinson P, Kaminski E. 1979. A short-term evaluation of periodontal surgery. *J Periodontal Res.* 14:182–84.

American Academy of Periodontology. *Glossary of periodontal terms*, 3rd edition. 1992. Chicago. American Academy of Periodontology. 34–35.

Ariaudo AA, Tirrell HA. 1957. Repositioning the increasing the zone of attached gingival. *J Periodontol*. 28:106–10.

Becker W, Becker B, Ochsenbein C, et al. 1988. A longitudinal study comparing scaling, osseous surgery and modified Widman procedures: Results after one year. *J Periodontol*. 59:351–65.

Carnevale G, Kaldahl WB. 2000. Osseous resective surgery. *Periodontol*. 22:59–87.

Carranza FA, Carranza Jr FA. 1956. The management of the alveolar bone in the treatment of the periodontal pocket. *J Periodontol*. 27:29–35.

Donnenfeld OW, Hoag PM, Weissman DP. 1970. A clinical study on the effects of osteoplasty. *J Periodontol*. 41:131–41.

Friedman N. 1955. Periodontal Osseous Surgery: Osteoplasty and ostectomy. *J Periodontol*. 26:257–69.

Friedman N, Levine H. 1964. Experimental periodontal surgery in human beings. A clinical histologic (preliminary) study. *J Dent Res.* 43(spec issue):791–92 (abstr 13).

Gargiulo AW, Wentz FM, Orban B. 1961. Dimensions and relations of the dentogingival junction in humans. *J Periodontol*. 32:261–67.

Goldman HM, Cohen DW. 1958. The infrabony pocket: Classification and treatment. *J Periodontol*. 29:272–91.

Knowles J, Burgett F, Morrison E, et al. 1980. Comparison of results following three modalities of periodontal therapy related to tooth type and initial pocket depth. *J Clin Periodontol*. 7:32–47.

Knowles J, Burgett F, Nissle R, et al. 1979. Results of periodontal treatment related to pocket depth and attachment level. *J Periodontol*. 50:225–33.

Kramer GM. 1995. The case for ostectomy: A time tested therapeutic modality in selected periodontitis sites. *Int J Periodont Restorat Dent.* 3:228–37.

Kronfeld R. 1935. Condition of alveolar bone underlying periodontal pockets. *J Periodontol*. 6:22.

Lindhe J, Nyman S. 1975. The effects of plaque control and surgical pocket elimination on the establishment and maintenance of periodontal health: A longitudinal study of periodontal therapy in cases of advanced disease. *J Clin Periodontol*. 1:67–79.

Moghaddas H, Stahl S. 1980. Alveolar bone remodeling following osseous surgery. A clinical study. *J Periodontol*. 51:376–81.

Nyman S, Lindhe J, Rosling B. 1977. Periodontal surgery in plaque-infected dentitions. *J Clin Periodontol*. 4:240–49.

O'Connor TW, Biggs NL. 1964. Interproximal bone contours. *J Periodontol*. 35:326–30.

Ochsenbein C. 1958. Osseous resection in periodontal surgery. *J Periodontol*. 29:15–26.

Ochsenbein C, Ross S. 1969. A reevaluation of osseous surgery. *Dent Clin North Am*. 13:87–102.

Ochsenbein C. 1977. Current status of osseous surgery. *J Periodontol*. 48:577–86.

Ochsenbein C. 1986. A primer for osseous surgery. *International Int J Periodon Restorat Dent*. 6:8–47.

Olsen C, Ammons W, van Belle G. 1985. A longitudinal study comparing apically positioned flaps, with and without osseous surgery. *Int J Periodont Restorat Dent*. 5:11–39.

Orban B. 1939. Gingivectomy or flap operation? *J Am Dent Assoc*. 26:1276–83.

Ochsenbein C, Bohannan HM. 1964. The palatal approach to osseous surgery. II. Clinical application. *J Periodontol*. 35:54–58.

Page RC, Schroeder HE. 1976. Pathogenesis of inflammatory periodontal disease. A summary of current work. *Lab Invest*. 36:235–49.

Pritchard J. 1961. Gingivoplasty, gingivectomy, and osseous surgery. *Int J Periodont Restor Dent*. 32:275–82.

Rosling B, Nyman S, Lindhe J, et al. 1976. The healing potential of periodontal tissues following different techniques of periodontal surgery in plaque-free dentitions. *J Clin Periodontol*. 3:233–50.

Schluger S. 1949. Osseous resection—A basic principle in periodontal surgery. *Oral Surg Oral Med Oral Pathol*. 2:316–25.

Selipsky H. 1976. Osseous surgery: How much need we compromise? *Dent Clin North Am*. 20:79–106.

Stern IB, Everett F, Robicsek K. 1965. Robicsek—A pioneer in the surgical treatment of periodontal disease. *J Periodontol*. 36:265.

Tibbetts Jr LS, Ochsenbein C, Loughlin DM. 1976. Rationale for the lingual approach to mandibular osseous surgery. *Dent Clin North Am*. 20:61–78.

Vercellotti T, Nevins ML, Nevins M, et al. 2006. Osseous response following resective therapy with piezosurgery. *Int J Periodont Restorat Dent*. 25:543–49.

Waerhaug J. 1978. Healing of the dentoepithelial junction following subgingival plaque control: As observed in human biopsy material. *J Periodontol*. 49:1–8, 119–34.

Weeks PR. 1980. Pros and cons of pocket elimination procedures. *J West Soc Perio Abst*. 28:4–16.

Wilderman M, Pennel B, King K, et al. 1970. Histogenesis of repair following osseous surgery. *J Periodontol*. 41:551–65.

Wood DI, Hoag PM, Donnenfeld OW, et al. 1972. Alveolar crest reduction following full and partial thickness flaps. *J Periodontol*. 43:141–44.

Zemsky JL. 1926. Surgical treatment of periodontal disease. *Dent Cosmos*. 68:465.

Zentler, A. 1918. Suppurative gingivitis with alveolar involvement: A new surgical procedure. *JAMA*. 71:1918.

Chapter 7 Regenerative Osseous Surgery: The Use of Growth Factor–Enhanced Bone Grafts

Ulrike Schulze-Späte, DMD, PhD, Rayyan Kayal, DMD, DSc

Growth factors are proteins secreted by cells that act on the appropriate target cell or mediator cells to carry out a specific action. Their function involves a vast cellular communications network that influences such critical processes as cell division, matrix synthesis, and tissue differentiation. The results of experimental studies have established that growth factors play an important role in bone and cartilage formation, osseous healing, and regeneration. With the advent of recombinant proteins, there has been considerable interest in the use of growth factors as therapeutic agents in the treatment of skeletal injuries and in augmentation techniques. As growth factors become available as therapeutic agents, it is essential for surgeons to understand their biological characteristics and clinical potential.

BIOLOGY BEHIND GROWTH FACTOR ACTION

Growth Factors and their specific Profile of Action

Growth factors can cause a cellular response in three different ways: autocrine, paracrine and endocrine.

1. *Autocrine:* A growth factor acts on the same cell that produced it or on cells of the same phenotype (e.g., a growth factor produced by an osteoblast influences the activity of another osteoblast).

2. *Paracrine:* A growth factor acts on an adjacent or neighboring cell that is different from its cell of origin (e.g., a growth factor produced by an osteoblast stimulates differentiation of an undifferentiated nonrelated cell).

3. *Endocrine:* A growth factor influences a cell that is different from its cell of origin and located at a remote anatomical site (e.g., a growth factor produced by neural tissue in the central nervous system stimulates osteoblast activity).

Thus growth factors might have effects on multiple cell types and induce an array of cellular functions in a variety of tissues (Lieberman, Daluiski, and Einhorn 2002; Barnes et al. 1999).

Mechanisms Behind Cellular Responses Induced by Growth Factors

Growth factors act through binding to specific receptors on the target cell. This binding is referred to as ligand-receptor interaction. Once a growth factor binds to a target cell receptor, this receptor is activated by a change in its conformation. Receptors usually have an extracellular domain that bind to the ligand and an intracellular domain that activates the signal transduction system. Generally, activation of the transduction system results in modulation of transcription factors, which are intracellular proteins that are part of the overall signaling pathway. The activated transcription factor travels to the cell nucleus where it binds to nuclear DNA and induces transcription of specific mRNA. This results in expression of a new gene or set of genes. It is the expression of these new genes that ultimately changes the characteristics of a particular cell (Lieberman, Daluiski, and Einhorn 2002).

GROWTH FACTORS INVOLVED IN BONE METABOLISM

Signaling molecules, which are important during bone healing, can be categorized into three groups:

1. proinflammatory cytokines such as interleukin-1 (IL-1), interleukin-6 (IL-6), and tumor necrosis factor-α (TNF-α);

2. transforming growth factor (TGF-β) superfamily, especially bone morphogenetic proteins (BMPs), platelet-derived growth factor (PDGF), fibroblast growth factor (FGF), and insulin-like growth factor (IGF); and

3. angiogenic factors such as vascular endothelial growth factor (VEGF), angiopoietins, and matrix metalloproteinases (MMPs) that degrade bone and cartilage and, therefore, enable vessel invasion (Dimitriou, Tsiridis, and Giannoudis 2005).

Cytokines IL-1, IL-6, and TNF-α are involved early in the repair cascade. These cytokines are secreted by macrophages and mesenchymal cells present in the periosteum and respond to injury with a peak in expression during the

Practical Osseous Surgery in Periodontics and Implant Dentistry, First Edition. Edited by Serge Dibart, Jean-Pierre Dibart.
© 2011 John Wiley & Sons, Inc. Published 2011 by John Wiley & Sons, Inc.

first 24 hours. However, they are also active in the remodeling phase of healing. In addition, these cytokines exert chemotactic activity on inflammatory cells, enhance cellular matrix synthesis, and stimulate angiogenesis (Dimitriou, Tsiridis, and 2005; Kon et al. 2001).

TGF-β is produced by osteoblasts. It stimulates expression of bone matrix proteins and suppresses the degrading activity of matrix metalloproteinases and other enzymes. TGF-β also induces proliferation or differentiation of osteoblastic cells while inhibiting the formation of osteoclast precursors and, in greater concentrations, may exert an inhibitory effect on mature osteoclasts. A subgroup of the TGF-β superfamily, called BMPs, are involved in cell growth, migration, and differentiation and play a regulatory role in tissue homeostasis and repair in adult organisms (Overall, Wrana and Sodek 1991; Wrana et al. 1988; Kingsley 1994).

PDGF is a potent mitogen for mesenchymal cells. Platelets, monocytes, macrophages, endothelial cells, and osteoblasts produce this growth factor. In the early stages of bone healing, PDGF is a powerful chemotactic agent for inflammatory cells and a stimulus for osteoblasts and macrophages. Another growth factor involved in bone healing is FGF, which is produced by monocytes, macrophages, mesenchymal cells, chondrocytes, and osteoblasts. FGF is important in chondrogenesis and bone resorption. The target cells are mesenchymal and epithelial cells as well as chondrocytes and osteoblasts (Dimitriou, Tsiridis, and Giannoudis 2005; Hollinger et al. 2008).

The role of IGF in bone formation has been disputed. Sources of IGF are bone matrix, endothelial cells, osteoblasts, and chondrocytes. There are two isoforms, IGF-1 and IGF-2. IGF-1 is the more potent and involved in bone matrix formation (Lieberman, Daluiski, and Einhorn 2002; Barnes et al. 1999; Fowlkes et al. 2006).

In the late phases of healing and bone remodeling, cartilage and bone are degraded by MMPs. This allows angiogenic factors to regulate vessels in growth by either the VEGF-dependent pathway or the angiopoietin-dependent pathway. VEGF is found in four isoforms (A, B, C, and D). Several cells, including macrophages, smooth muscle cells, and osteoblasts, produce the protein (Gerstenfeld et al. 2003). See Table 7.1 for growth factor function in the bone and cell.

This chapter focuses on the group of growth factors that are associated with bone formation and maturation. These include TGF-β, BMPs, PDGF, FGF, and IGF.

Transforming Growth Factor

The TGF-β superfamily of growth factors contains over 30 members, and it is vital for development and homeostasis. The ligands and their downstream pathway components regulate diverse cellular functions, such as growth, adhesion, migration, apoptosis, and differentiation (Wu and Hill 2009).

The TGF-β superfamily ligands are secreted as precursors composed of prodomain and a C-terminal mature polypeptide. The prodomains are required for the formation of dimers via disulfide bonds. The ligands are activated when the prodomains are cleaved by proteases. Ligand dimers bind and activate heteromeric complexes of type I and type II receptors. Activated receptors then phosphorylate the intra-

Table 7.1. Effect of growth factors on bone formation and remodeling.

Growth Factor	Cell Source	Function in Bone
TGF-β	Platelets, osteoblasts, bone marrow stromal cells, chondrocytes, endothelial cells, fibroblasts, macrophages	1. Undifferentiated mesenchymal cell proliferation. 2. Osteoblast precursor recruiting. 3. Osteoblast and chondrocyte differentiation. 4. Bone matrix production. 5. Recruitment of osteoclast precursors.
BMP	Osteoproginator cells, osteoblasts, chondrocytes, endothelial cells	1. Differentiation of mesenchymal cells into chondrocytes and osteoblasts. 2. Migration and differentiation of osteoprogenitors into osteoblasts. 3. Influences skeletal pattern formation. 4. Induction of matrix synthesis.
PDGF	Platelets, osteoblasts, endothelial cells, monocytes, macrophages	1. Osteoprogenator migration 2. Proliferation and differentiation.
IGF	Osteoblasts, chondrocytes, hepatocytes, endothelial cells	1. Osteoprogenator proliferation and differentiation. 2. Osteoblast proliferation. 3. Bone matrix synthesis. 4. Bone resorption.
FGF	Macrophages, monocytes, bone marrow stromal cells, chondrocytes, osteoblasts, endothelial cells	1. Chondrocyte maturation. 2. Osteoblast proliferation and differentiation 3. Inhibition of apoptosis of immature osteoblasts. 4. Induction of apoptosis of mature osteocytes. 5. Bone resorption.

cellular mediators (Smads), which form complexes with each other and other proteins to modulate transcription of target genes in the nucleus (Wu and Hill 2009).

TGF-β superfamily members require two different serine/threonine kinase receptors to signal, a type I and a type II. There are seven type I receptors (ALKs 1–7) and five type II receptors in the human genome. The ligand brings the receptors together in a heterotetrameric complex in which the type II receptors phosphorylate and activate the type I receptors. In the case of the TGF-β receptors, the ligand–receptor interaction is highly cooperative. The ligand–receptor complexes assemble through the recruitment of the low-affinity type I receptor by the ligand-bound high-affinity type II receptor, facilitated by direct type I–type II interactions at the composite ligand–type II interface (Wu and Hill 2009; Groppe et al. 2008).

The most studied signaling pathway downstream of TGF-β superfamily receptors is the Smad pathway. The Smads are a group of intracellular signaling molecules comprising the receptor-regulated Smads (R-Smads) Smad1, 2, 3, 5, and 8; the co-Smad, Smad-4; and the inhibitory Smads, Smad-6 and -7. Upon ligand stimulation, the R-Smads are phosphorylated by the type I receptors and form both homomeric and heteromeric complexes with Smad-4 that accumulate in the nucleus and directly regulate the transcription of target genes. Although the Smads are the best understood signal transducers downstream of TGF-β superfamily receptors, other signaling pathways can also be activated directly in response to TGF-β, such as ERK MAP kinase (MAPK) signaling pathway, JNK and p38 MAPK signaling, and the kinase PAK2 (Kinglsey 1994; Wu and Hill 2009).

TGF-β has three isoforms, TGF-β1, -β2, and -β3. All three isoforms are detected in bone, but the TGF-β1 isoform is the most abundant at the protein level. In neonatal human bone, all isoforms can be found at sites of endochondral and intramembranous ossification, but the patterns of expression differ. At sites of endochondral bone formation, TGF-β1 and TGF-β3 are detected in proliferative and hypertrophic zone chondrocytes, and TGF-β2 is detected in all zones of the cartilage. During intramembranous bone formation, TGF-β1 and -β2 are present at sites of mineralization, whereas TGF-β3 is more widely distributed. Osteoclasts also express TGF-β, mostly TGF-β1, in high amounts. It is also important to note that expression of all three TGF-β isoforms is upregulated during fracture healing, suggesting that their roles are not restricted to embryonic bone development, but extend to adult bone remodeling (Ai-Aql et al. 2008; Janssens et al. 2005).

TGF-β1 increases bone formation mainly by recruiting osteoblast progenitors and stimulating their proliferation, thus increasing the number of committed osteoblasts, as well as by promoting the early stages of differentiation. On the other hand, it blocks later phases of differentiation and mineralization. These later stages are regulated by other growth factors such as the BMPs. TGF-β1 also blocks apoptosis of osteoblasts and promotes maintenance of survival during differentiation into osteocytes. Interestingly, recruitment of osteoclast precursors to the bone environment, differentiation to the mature osteoclast, bone resorption, and osteoclast apoptosis are also modulated by TGF-β1 either directly or indirectly through osteogenic cells (Janssens et al. 2005).

Bone Morophogenic Proteins

In 1965 Marshall R. Urist recognized the concept that there is a substance in bone that can induce new bone formation when he observed that bone had formed after the implantation of demineralized bone matrix in a muscle pouch in rat model. He termed this phenomenon the *bone induction principle* and later identified the protein responsible for this effect, which took on the name *bone morphogenetic protein.* In 1988, Wozney et al. identified the genetic sequence of BMP, which led to the identification of its various isoforms. With this genetic information, it is now possible to produce various BMPs using recombinant gene technology. (Urist 1965; Wozney et al. 1988)

BMPs are members of the TGF-β superfamily, and there are at least 30 individual molecules that have been identified so far. Of these, BMP-2 to BMP-8 show high osteogenic potential. BMP-2, -4, and -7 are known to play a critical role in bone healing by means of their ability to stimulate differentiation of mesenchymal cells to an osteochondroblastic lineage. In vitro studies show that mesenchymal stem cells exhibit a great number of BMP receptors. Mesenchymal stem cells also synthesize the BMP antagonists noggin, gremlin, follistatin, and sclerostin, which are capable of blocking osteogenesis as mesenchymal stem cells differentiate into osteoblasts. Osteoblasts secrete BMPs as well as their antagonists by a delicate regulatory mechanism during bone formation and remodeling. When BMPs are secreted from cells, they have one of several fates: they may immediately exert their actions locally; they may be bound up by extracellular antagonists present at the site of BMP secretion; or, they may interact with extracellular matrix proteins that serve to sequester or enhance BMP activity by anchoring it to make it more available to target cells (Barnes et al. 1999; Abe 2006; Rosen 2006).

BMPs use the same serine/threonine kinase receptor complex to initiate cell signaling. BMP receptors are classified as type I or type II based on sequence homology. Three type I BMP receptors have been identified, Alk3, Alk6, and Alk2, and the BMP type I receptor mainly determines the specificity of the intracellular signals. Type II receptors that exhibit BMP binding are BMP RII and Act RII and IIb. Unlike TGF-β receptors, the BMP receptor complex does not assemble cooperatively, which means that both type I and type II BMP receptors can bind BMPs in the absence of the other receptor. Also in contrast to other TGF-β family members, there is no direct connection between the extracellular domains of the individual receptors. BMP ligand binding to type I receptor triggers the intracellular association of type I and type II receptors, allowing the constitutively phosphorylated type II receptor to phosphorylate the type I receptor. Once activated, type I receptors can recognize and phosphorylate pathway-specific R-Smads that will then associate with Smad 4. The R-Smad/Smad4 complex then translocates to the nucleus where it recruits DNA-binding transcription factors, coactivators, and corepressors to a single genomic locus, providing a way in which many nuclear components can interact with Smads, producing both positive and negative regulation of gene expression (Wu and Hill 2009; Rosen 2006).

BMPs play a critical role in cell growth and bone formation. Mice deficient in BMP-2, -4, and -7 die either early during embryonic development or soon after birth. Mice deficient in BMP-2 have developmental abnormalities of the skull, hind limb, and kidney. Mice deficient in BMP-5 have short-ear deformities, and BMP-7 deficiency has been associated with hindlimb polydactyly and renal agenesis (Lieberman, Daluiski, and Einhorn 2002; Barnes et al. 1999).

Although different BMPs are closely related structurally and functionally, they exhibit different temporal patterns of expression during bone healing. In studies of murine fracture healing, BMP-2 mRNA expression showed maximal levels within 24 hours of injury, suggesting that this BMP plays a role in initiating the repair cascade. Consistent with this finding are recent studies showing that BMP-2 is necessary for postnatal bone repair and is genetically associated with the maintenance of normal bone mass. Other in vitro studies examining marrow stromal stem cell differentiation have shown that BMP-2 controls the expression of several other BMPs, and when its activity is blocked, marrow stromal stem cells fail to differentiate into osteoblasts (Lieberman, Daluiski, and Einhorn 2002; Barnes et al. 1999; Ai-Aql et al. 2008).

Platelet-Derived Growth Factor

The PDGF family of growth factors includes PDGF-A, -B, -C, and -D, encoded by four genes located on different chromosomes. PDGF-A and PDGF-B can form both homodimers and heterodimers, whereas PDGF-C and PDGF-D exist as homodimers. When circulating in the blood, PDGF has a half-life of approximately 30 minutes, which indicates that local delivery of the growth factor is critical to achieving success (Hollinger et al. 2008; Alvarez, Kantarjian, and Cortes 2006).

Following bone injury and hemorrhage, the coagulation cascade is activated, and a blood clot is formed at the site of injury. Platelets aggregate and release their cytokines,

including PDGF, into the developing blood clot. The PDGFs act early in the wound-healing process by initially attracting and activating neutrophils and macrophages, which are key cell mediators of early tissue repair. These cells then serve as an ongoing source of PDGFs and other growth factors that are responsible for the formation of granulation tissue, which is the next step in endochondral bone repair. Chemotaxis and mitogenesis of a variety of cells of mesenchymal origin, including fibroblasts, osteoblasts, chondrocytes, and smooth muscle cells, are also accomplished by the local release of PDGF (Hollinger et al. 2008; Gerstenfeld et al. 2003).

The PDGF molecules signal through two cell surface tyrosine kinase receptors, termed PDGFR and PDGFR, which are capable of forming homodimers as well as heterodimers. The different isoforms of PDGF have different binding specificities to the two receptors. PDGFR/dimers bind PDGF-AA, -AB, -BB, and -CC; PDGFR/dimers bind PDGF-AB, -BB, -CC, and -DD; and PDGFR/dimers bind PDGF-BB and -DD. This allows different cell types to respond more or less strongly to the different PDGF isoforms depending on the level of expression of the two receptors. PDGF-BB can bind to all known PDGF receptor isotypes. That is why it is considered a universal PDGF (Alvarez, Kantarjian, and Cortes 2006).

Osteogenic progenitor cells respond to PDGF ligand binding by activation of Src tyrosine kinases as well as activation of the AKT protein kinase and Grb2-mediated extracellular regulated kinase signaling. As a consequence, PDGF is able to increase the pool of osteogenic cells at the injury site, acting as both a chemotactic agent and a mitogen (Hollinger et al. 2008).

PDGF also effects bone regeneration indirectly by increasing the expression of angiogenic factors such as VEGF, hepatocyte growth factor (HGF), and the proinflammatory cytokine IL-6. Local application of PDGF-BB will destabilize blood vessels, probably by attracting pericytes or vascular smooth muscle cells via a PDGF chemotactic gradient. This allows blood vessels to "sprout," and a filamentous web of neovasculature penetrates into the granulation tissue. PDGF-BB, VEGF, and FGF were shown to be dependant on one another when it comes to corneal and ischemic limb revascularization. The mechanism involves the upregulation of PDGF receptors-α and -β by basic FGF, leading to improved survival of endothelial cells, increased proliferation of smooth muscle cells, and subsequent stabilization of newly formed capillaries. Moreover, PDGF-BB can increase VEGF expression in mural cells, which in turn target endothelial cells and induce a potent angiogenic response (Hollinger et al. 2008; Alvarez, Kantarjian, and Cortes 2006).

In bone, PDGFs can modulate the responsiveness of osteogenic cells to BMPs by increasing the expression of the BMP inhibitory protein gremlin and enhancing IGF signaling. The responsiveness of osteogenic cells to PDGFs can also be regulated by the inflammatory cytokine interleukin-1, which inhibits PDGFR expression in human osteoblastic cells (Hollinger et al. 2008).

Fibroblast Growth Factor

The FGFs are a family of nine structurally related polypeptides that are characterized by their affinity for the glycosaminoglycan heparin and are known to play a critical role in angiogenesis and mesenchymal cell mitogenesis. The most abundant FGFs in normal adult tissue are acidic fibroblast growth factor (FGF-1 or α-FGF) and basic fibroblast growth factor (FGF-2 or β-FGF). Both FGF-1 and FGF-2 promote growth and differentiation of a variety of cells, including epithelial cells, myocytes, osteoblasts, and chondrocytes. FGF-1 plays a role in chondrocyte proliferation, and FGF-2, which is important for the maturation of chondrocytes and bone resorption, is generally more potent than FGF-1 (Lieberman, Daluiski, and Einhorn 2002; Barnes et al. 1999).

The FGF family of peptides transduces signals through a group of four receptors that contain distinct membrane-spanning tyrosine kinases. Each of these receptors shows variable affinity to different members of the FGF family of growth factors, and they are expressed in wide variety of tissue types, including bone. The activation of the receptor occurs through dimerization in response to ligand binding. The major downstream signaling pathways include signals generated through the RAS/RAF (retrovirus-associated DNA sequence/factors), MEK (MAP kinase kinase), and mitogen-activated protein kinase (MAPK) pathway. Mutations in the FGF receptors have been associated with abnormalities in endochondral ossification and intramembranous ossification (Lieberman, Daluiski, and Einhorn 2002; Barnes et al. 1999).

Both FGF-1 and FGF-2 activity have been identified during the early stages of bone healing. The most likely source could be macrophages and other inflammatory cells, which were shown to express FGFs in granulation tissue. Subsequently, FGFs are expressed by mesenchymal cells, chondrocytes, and osteoblasts and have been demonstrated to enhance TGF-β expression in osteoblasts. Since these factors are associated with angiogenesis and chondrocyte and osteoblast activation, there has been interest in their ability to enhance skeletal repair (Barnes et al. 1999).

Insulin-Like Growth Factor

Approximately 50 years ago, Salmon and Daughaday discovered the presence of a soluble factor induced by growth hormone that had insulin-like properties; subsequently, this factor was identified as IGF. Two IGFs have been identified: IGF-1 and IGF-2. Although IGF-2 is the most abundant growth factor in bone, IGF-1 has been found to be more potent and has been localized in healing fractures in rats and humans. Therefore, studies evaluating the role of IGFs in fracture healing have concentrated on IGF-1 (Lieberman, Daluiski, and Einhorn 2002; Andrew et al. 1993; Salmon and Daughaday, 1957).

IGF is regulated through a system composed of the ligands (IGF-1 and IGF-2), the IGF receptors 1 and 2 (IGF-1R and IGF-2R), IGF-binding proteins (IGFBPs) 1 through 6, and the acid-labile subunit (ALS). IGF-1 can be found in the circulation bound in a complex with IGFBPs and ALS. Some of these complexes, such as IGFBP-3, increase the half-life of circulating IGF-1 and target the ligand to its receptor, whereas other binding proteins, such as IGFBP-1, inhibit IGF-1 bioactivity due to their greater affinity for IGF-1 than the IGF-1R. The redundancy exerted by the IGFBPs in the IGF regulatory system provides an additional level of regulation and can be used to deliver IGF-I in an endocrine fashion (Rosen 1999; Kawai and Rosen 2008; Pass et al. 2009).

IGF-1 exerts its action by binding to the IGF-1 receptor, which induces receptor autophosphorylation in the intracellular kinase domain. Upon receptor activation, a number of protein substrates, including insulin receptor substrate-1 (IRS-1) and Src homology and collagen protein (SHC), are activated and transduce multiple signaling pathways, including the PI3K/PDK-1/Akt pathway and the Ras/Raf-1/MAPK pathway. Activation of the PI3K/PDK-1/Akt pathway has been shown to be important in skeletal acquisition in vitro and in vivo and the Ras/Raf-1/MAPK pathway is critical for cell proliferation (Kawai and Rosen 2008).

The role of circulating IGF-1 in bone cell metabolism and bone turnover has been the subject of tremendous research interest. Alterations in circulating IGF-1 could play a role in modulating bone remodeling and thereby affect bone mass and fracture risk. In fracture healing, IGF-1 was found to stimulate both chondrocyte clonal expansion and hypertrophy, and consequently, bone growth in an autocrine/paracrine manner (Andrew et al. 1993; Kawai and Rosen 2008; Pass et al. 2009).

CLINICAL APPLICATION

Growth Factor Carriers

Growth factor therapy involves delivering the growth factor to the desired site so that it will induce a specific biological effect. The success of the delivery system may depend on the anatomic location, the vitality of the tissue envelope, and the mechanical stability of the site. The kinetics of the growth factor's release may vary depending on the chemistry of the factor or the delivery system and the influence of the host environment. For instance, direct injection of the growth factor in soluble form into a regeneration site is generally not effective due to rapid diffusion of the protein away from the injection site. Therefore, delivery to the bone regeneration site is obtained through a carrier matrix, which may also support osteogenic cell growth (Devescovi et al. 2008).

Certain conditions must be considered when selecting an appropriate carrier or delivery system: (1) the ability of the system to deliver the growth factor at the appropriate time and in the proper dose, (2) the presence of a substratum that will enhance cell recruitment and attachment and will potentiate chemotaxis, (3) the presence of a void space to allow for cell migration and to promote angiogenesis, and (4) the ability of the delivery system to biodegrade without generating an immune or inflammatory response and without producing toxic waste products that would inhibit the repair process (Lieberman, Daluiski, and Einhorn 2002).

A number of carrier and delivery systems have been used to deliver recombinant proteins in experimental and clinical models, including type-1 collagen, synthetic polymers, and hyaluronic acid gels. A variety of so-called bone graft substitutes are also potential carriers for recombinant proteins, including demineralized bone matrix, calcium phosphate–containing preparations (such as hydroxyapatite and coralline hydroxyapatite), and Bioglass (Lieberman, Daluiski, and Einhorn 2002; Devescovi et al. 2008).

Use of Growth Factor BMP-2 in Oral Maxillofacial Procedures

Over the years, research focused on refining the use of growth factors in clinical applications. Out of a variety of factors, Cheng et al. described the isoforms BMP-2, -6, and -9 as having a very high osteogenic potential (Cheng et al. 2003). Especially, recombinant human BMP-2 (rhBMP-2) has been studied extensively in preclinical and clinical settings; rhBMP-2 has been commercially available since July 2002 in the United States (INFUSE Bone Graft/LT-CAGE Lumbar Tapered Fusion Device, Medtronic Inc., Memphis, TN). Initially, it was approved by the U.S. Food and Drug Administration for its use in interbody spinal fusion inside a threaded titanium fusion device. The approved indication was later expanded and now includes two additional clinical indications: fresh tibial fractures and certain oral maxillofacial procedures (maxillary sinus floor augmentation and ridge augmentation associated with extraction sockets). The approvals were based on prospective, randomized clinical trials involv-ing an absorbable collagen sponge (ACS) carrier and rhBMP-2 at a concentration of 1.5 mg/mL. Boyne et al. investigated its use in maxillary sinus floor augmentation. They found a similar level of new bone formation with rhBMP-2/ACS as compared to autograft at 4 months, 10.2 mmm versus 11.3 mm, respectively (Boyne et al. 2005; Nevins et al. 1996). Several preclinical trials evaluating rhBMP-2 in oral bone grafting procedures had preceded this study. Schwartz et al. used rhBMP-2/ACS to induce bone formation in the maxillary sinus of goats (Nevins et al. 1996). Furthermore, in studies of dogs and non-human primates with large mandibular defects, rhBMP-2 induced new bone formation without the addition of bone grafts (Cochran et al. 1997; Hanisch et al. 1997; Zellin and Linde 1997). In line with this finding, Fiorellini et al. did a randomized, placebo-controlled multicenter clinical study to investigate bone formation in extraction sites after placement of collagen sponges (ACS) soaked in rhBMP-2 (Fiorellini et al. 2005). They found that rhBMP-2/ACS produced more bone in extraction sites than was formed in untreated control patients with comparable defects ($p < 0.05$).

The rhBMP-2 hydrated ACS sponge is soft and pliable; it can be easily compressed during surgical implantation or from overlying soft tissue. This would ultimately result in inadequate bone formation. Therefore, space maintenance and a relatively compression-free environment are key for successful inducing of bone growth after rhBMP-2/ACS application. Augmentation of the maxillary sinus floor and extraction sites allow placement of rhBMP-2/ACS in areas where it is protected from compressive forces. However, this could also be achieved by using the aid of a device such as titanium mesh or additional bone graft material.

We will describe the use of rhBMP-2/ACS in more detail in the following case reports. Both patients had been edentulous in the respective areas for a long period of time and presented with an amount of bone that would make implant placement impossible without additional grafting. Surgical informed consent was obtained from both patients after providing detailed information, including possible risks and complications.

Case 1: Maxillary Sinus Floor Augmentation Using rhBMP-2/ACS

A 45-year-old patient presented for rehabilitation of his dentition in the posterior maxilla. The patient's medical history was noncontributory. He did not have any known drug or food allergies, did not smoke, and drank alcohol only occasionally. Computer tomography (CT) revealed severe bone loss in both posterior areas of the maxilla (see Figure 7.2, below). It was decided to augment the upper right side with rhBMP-2/ACS and the upper left side with an allograft (DynaBlast, Keystone Dental, Burlington, MA). Briefly, a midcrestal incision was made with mesial and distal releasing incisions extending well into the buccal fold. The mucoperiosteal flap was reflected in a full-thickness manner, and care was taken to completely release the tissue for a tension-free access to the lateral wall of the maxillary sinus. A lateral window, which is situated between the alveolar crest and zygomatic buttress, was chosen to enter the maxillary sinus (Boyne et al. 1980; Smiler et al. 1997)

The Schneiderian membrane was elevated away from its bony surface, and the newly created space was filled with the respective grafting material (Figure 7.1).

Case 1: *Continued*

The upper left side was grafted with rhBMP-2/ACS and the product was prepared according to manufacturer's recommendation (Infuse, Medtronic). The sponge (ACS) was soaked for 15 minutes in the solution containing rhBMP-2. Afterward, several layers of ACS were placed into the space created by lifting up the Schneiderian membrane. In the rhBMP-2/ACS application, no collagen membrane is needed to protect the lateral access window. The mucoperiosteal flap was positioned back to cover the surgical site and secured with nonresorbable suture material (Gore-Tex suture 4.0, Gore Medical, Flagstaff, AZ) using single interrupted sutures. The patient was prescribed antibiotics (500 mg amoxicillin three times daily for 7 days) and chlorhexidine digluconate mouth rinse twice a day for 21 days postoperatively.

Six weeks after sinus augmentation, CT scans were taken to evaluate both grafted sites (see Figure 7.2). Dental implants can be placed approximately 4–6 months after maxillary sinus floor augmentation (Boyne at al. 2005).

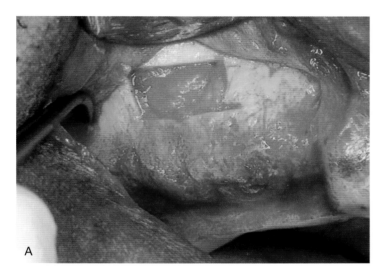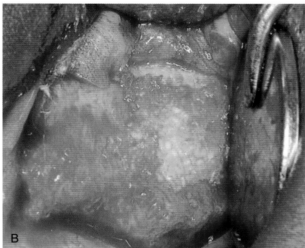

Figure 7.1 Maxillary sinus was accessed over a lateral window. (A) Right maxillary sinus floor was augmented with rhBMP-2/ACS. (B) Left maxillary sinus floor was augmented with an allograft.

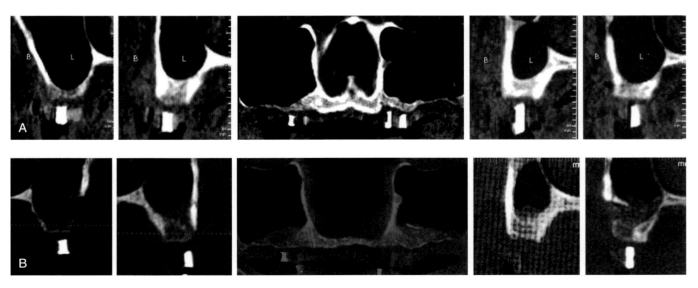

Figure 7.2 CT scan evaluation of the posterior maxilla. (A) CT scan was taken before augmentation and depicts insufficient bone height in the posterior maxilla. (B) CT scan was taken 6 weeks after augmentation. Graft material increases bone height in the posterior maxilla.

Case 2-Alveolar Ridge Augmentation Using rhBMP-2/ACS

A 31-year-old patient was referred for restoring the edentulous maxillary and mandibulary incisor area. The patient's medical history was noncontributory. He did not have any known drug or food allergies, did not smoke, and drank alcohol only occasionally. It was decided to replace those missing teeth with implant-supported restorations. The area was temporized with a bridge that used the adjacent canines as abutments. Intraoral examination and CT scan evaluation revealed severe vertical bone loss at the future implant sites (see Figures 7.3, 7.4).

Therefore, it was proposed to augment both areas using rhBMP-2/ACS covered by titanium mesh. The mesh will act as a space protector and protect the pliable sponge. As part of the preoperative treatment planning, alginate impressions were taken to create casts that allowed preoperative bending of the titanium mesh (see Figure 7.5).

At the time of surgery, midcrestal incisions were made with vertical releasing incisions at the distal line angles of the canines. Full mucoperiosteal flaps were elevated and the bone was decorticated to access the bone marrow space (see Figures 7.6A, 7.7A and B). Sponges were soaked for 15 minutes in rhBMP-2 solution and lightly packed on the ridges (see Figure 7.7C). The preformed titanium meshes were placed over the sponges and secured with self-tapping screws (see Figures 7.6B–D, 7.7D–H). The periosteum of the mucoperiosteal flaps was released, and the flaps were positioned back to cover the surgical sites. The mucoperiosteal flaps were secured with nonresorbable suture material (Gore-Tex suture 4.0) (see Figures 7.6F, 7.7I). The patient was prescribed antibiotics (500 mg amoxicillin 3 times daily for 7 days), and chlorhexidine digluconate mouth rinse twice a day for 21 days postoperatively. Sites will be ready for implant placement 6 months after augmentation.

At 7 months postsurgery, the mesh was removed revealing a nice bony ridge underneath made of vital bone (Figure 7.8A–E). The area is now ready to receive an implant.

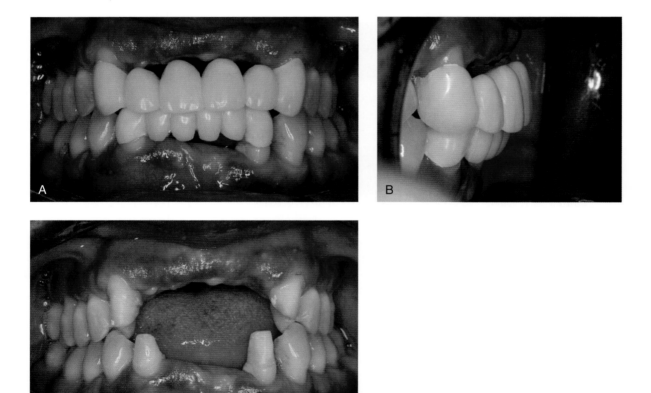

Figure 7.3 Intraoral view of maxillary and mandibulary incisor area. (A, B) A temporary bridge was fabricated using the adjacent canines as abutments. (C) Intraoral examination revealed severe bone loss in the edentulous areas.

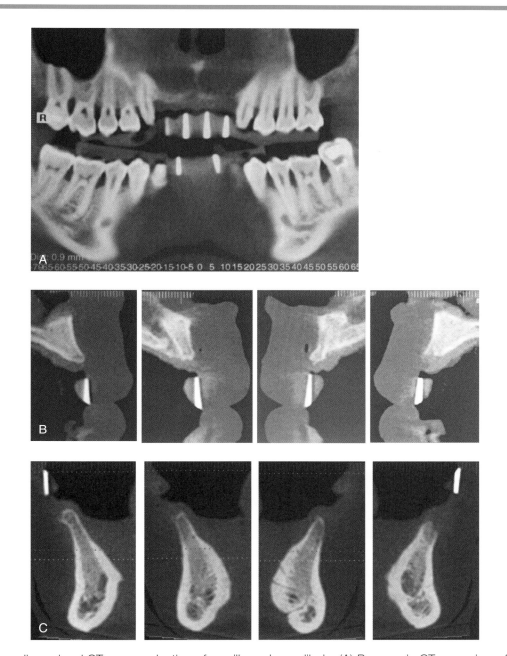

Figure 7.4 Three-dimensional CT scan evaluation of maxilla and mandibula. (A) Panoramic CT scan view of the edentulous areas reveals their bony dimensions. (B) CT scan sections of maxillary incisors depict insufficient bone in the areas of future implant placement. (C) CT scan sections of mandibulary incisors reveal insufficient bone in the areas of future implant placement.

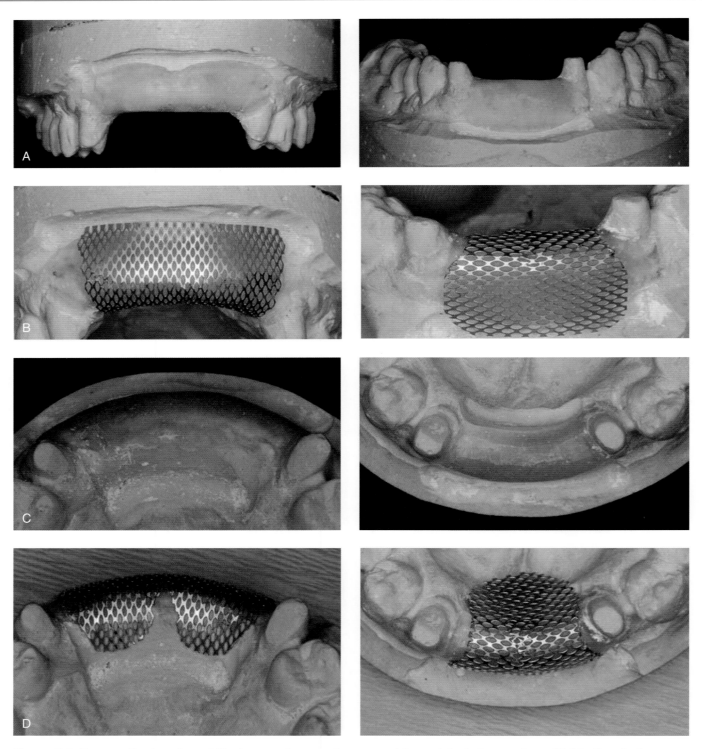

Figure 7.5 Preoperative bending of titanium mesh on casts prepared from alginate impressions. (A) Maxillary incisor area. (B) Mandibulary incisor area.

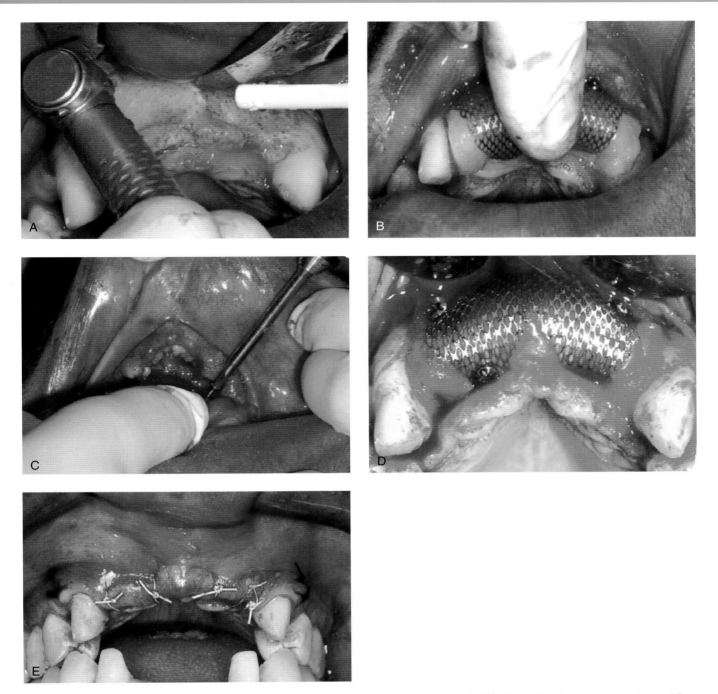

Figure 7.6 Alveolar ridge augmentation (maxillary incisor area) using rhBMP-2/ACS. (A) After reflecting a mucoperiosteal flap, the bone was decorticated with a round carbide bur. (B) The rhBMP-2–soaked sponge was placed in several layers on the ridge and protected with the pre-bent titanium mesh. (C) Self-tapping screws were placed to secure the titanium mesh to the bone. (D) The titanium mesh protects the rhBMP-2–hydrated sponge. (E) The mucoperiosteal flap was secured with a nonresorbable suture.

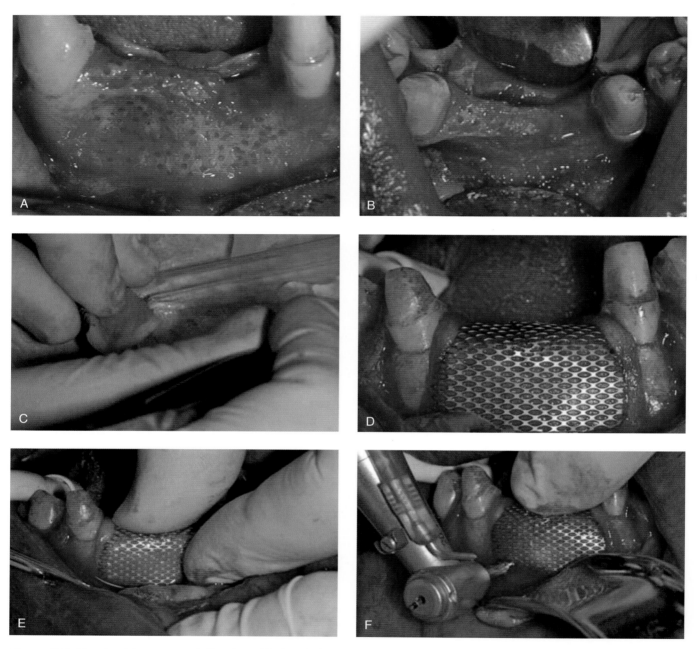

Figure 7.7 Alveolar ridge augmentation (mandibulary incisor area) using rhBMP-2/ACS. (A) After reflecting a mucoperiosteal flap, the bone was decorticated. (B) The alveolar ridge is severely resorbed. (C) The sponge was hydrated with rhBMP-2 for 15 minutes and placed over the ridge in several layers. (D, E) The rhBMP-2–soaked sponge was protected with the pre-bent titanium mesh. (F, G) Self-tapping screws were placed to secure the titanium mesh to the bone. (H) The titanium mesh protects the rhBMP-2–hydrated sponge. (I) The mucoperiosteal flap was secured with a nonresorbable suture.

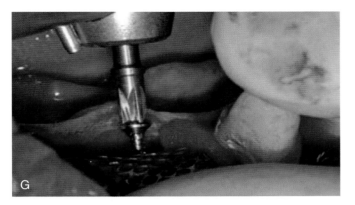

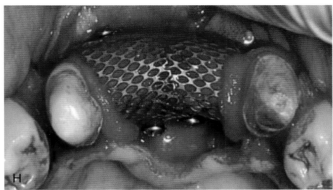

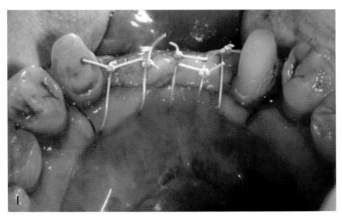

Figure 7.7 *Continued*

Growth factors can facilitate bone grafting by increasing cellular interactions on a molecular level. Today's research aims to expand its use in clinical applications to utilize its benefits and at the same time reduce the amount of grafting material needed in conventional bone-augmentation procedures. In the cases described here, we used rhBMP-2/ACS to create sufficient implant beds in areas that had presented with bony dimensions insufficient for future implant-supported restorations. Nevertheless, the field of growth factor–facilitated bone grafting is still young, and further studies need to be done to refine applications and to completely understand molecular mechanisms associated with it.

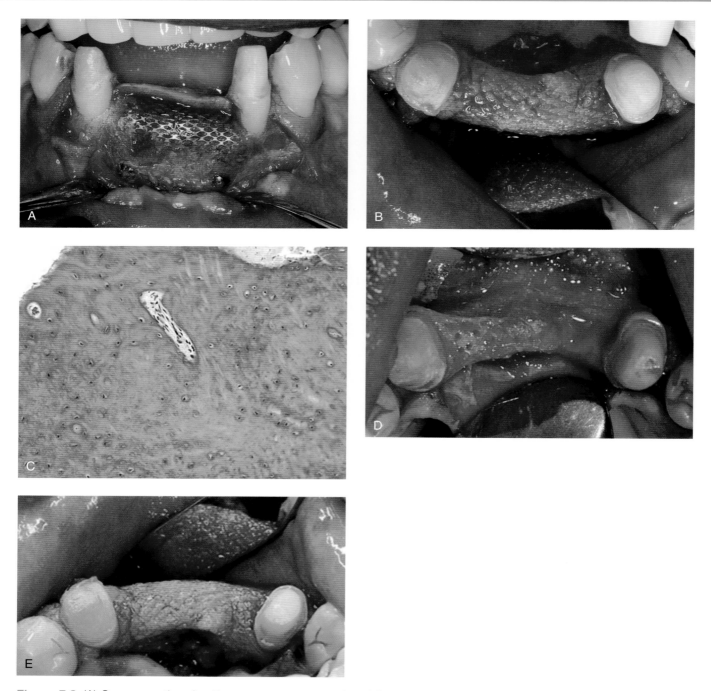

Figure 7.8 (A) Seven months after the surgery, a mucoperiostal flap is elevated to expose and remove the titanium mesh. (B) The ridge (after the mesh removal) has been augmented horizontally and vertically. (C) Biopsy tissue taken at that time shows vital bone. (D) The ridge prior to regenerative surgery. (E) The ridge after regenerative surgery. Notice the three-dimensional changes.

REFERENCES

Abe E. 2006. Function of BMPs and BMP antagonists in adult bone. *Ann N Y Acad Sci.* 1068:41–53.

Ai-Aql ZS, et al. 2008. Molecular mechanisms controlling bone formation during fracture healing and distraction osteogenesis. *J Dent Res.* 87(2):107–18.

Alvarez RH, et al. 2006. Biology of platelet-derived growth factor and its involvement in disease. *Mayo Clin Proc.* 81(9):1241–57.

Andrew JG, et al. 1993. Insulin like growth factor gene expression in human fracture callus. *Calcif Tissue Int.* 53(2):97–102.

Barnes GL, et al. 1999. Growth factor regulation of fracture repair. *J Bone Miner Res.* 14(11):1805–15.

Boyne PJ, et al. 2005. De novo bone induction by recombinant human bone morphogenetic protein-2 (rhBMP-2) in maxillary sinus floor augmentation. *J Oral Maxillofac Surg.* 63(12):1693–707.

Cheng H, et al. 2003. Osteogenic activity of the fourteen types of human bone morphogenetic proteins (BMPs). *J Bone Joint Surg Am.* 85-A(8):1544–52.

Boyne PJ, James RA. 1980. Grafting of the maxillary sinus floor with autogenous marrow and bone. *J Oral Surg.* 38(8):613–16.

Cochran DL, et al. 1997. Radiographic analysis of regenerated bone around endosseous implants in the canine using recombinant human bone morphogenetic protein-2. *Int J Oral Maxillofac Implants.* 12(6):739–48.

Devescovi V, et al. 2008. Growth factors in bone repair. *Chir Organi Mov.* 92(3):161–68.

Dimitriou R, et al. 2005. Current concepts of molecular aspects of bone healing. *Injury.* 36(12):1392–404.

Fiorellini JP, et al. 2005. Randomized study evaluating recombinant human bone morphogenetic protein-2 for extraction socket augmentation. *J Periodontol.* 76(4):605–13.

Fowlkes JL, et al. 2006. Effects of systemic and local administration of recombinant human IGF-I (rhIGF-I) on de novo bone formation in an aged mouse model. *J Bone Miner Res.* 21(9):1359–66.

Gerstenfeld L, et al. 2003. Fracture healing as a post-natal developmental process: Molecular, spatial, and temporal aspects of its regulation. *J Cell Biochem.* 88(5):873–84.

Groppe J, et al. 2008. Cooperative assembly of TGF-beta superfamily signaling complexes is mediated by two disparate mechanisms and distinct modes of receptor binding. *Mol Cell.* 29(2):157–68.

Hanisch O, et al. 1997. Bone formation and reosseointegration in peri-implantitis defects following surgical implantation of rhBMP-2. *Int J Oral Maxillofac Implants.* 12(5):604–10.

Hollinger JO, et al. 2008. Recombinant human platelet-derived growth factor: biology and clinical applications. *J Bone Joint Surg Am.* 90(Suppl1):48–54.

Janssens K, et al. 2005. Transforming growth factor-beta1 to the bone. *Endocr Rev.* 26(6):743–74.

Kawai M, Rosen, CJ. 2008. Insulin-like growth factor-I and bone: Lessons from mice and men. *Pediatr Nephrol.* 24(7):1277–85

Kingsley DM. 1994. The TGF-beta superfamily: New members, new receptors, and new genetic tests of function in different organisms. *Genes Dev.* 8(2):133–46.

Kon T, et al. 2001. Expression of osteoprotegerin, receptor activator of NF-kappaB ligand (osteoprotegerin ligand) and related proinflammatory cytokines during fracture healing. *J Bone Miner Res.* 16(6):1004–14.

Lieberman JR, et al. 2002. The role of growth factors in the repair of bone. Biology and clinical applications. *J Bone Joint Surg Am.* 84-A(6):1032–44.

Nevins M, et al. 1996. Bone formation in the goat maxillary sinus induced by absorbable collagen sponge implants impregnated with recombinant human bone morphogenetic protein-2. *Int J Periodontics Restorative Dent.* 16(1):8–19.

Overall CM, et al. 1991. Transcriptional and post-transcriptional regulation of 72-kDa gelatinase/type IV collagenase by transforming growth factor-beta 1 in human fibroblasts. Comparisons with collagenase and tissue inhibitor of matrix metalloproteinase gene expression. *J Biol Chem.* 266(21):14064–71.

Pass C, et al. 2009. Inflammatory cytokines and the GH/IGF-I axis: novel actions on bone growth. *Cell Biochem Funct.* 27(3):119–27.

Rosen CJ. 1999. Serum insulin-like growth factors and insulin-like growth factor-binding proteins: Clinical implications. *Clin Chem.* 45(8 Pt 2):1384–90.

Rosen V. 2006. BMP and BMP inhibitors in bone. *Ann N Y Acad Sci.* 1068:19–25.

Salmon WD Jr, Daughaday WH. 1957. A hormonally controlled serum factor which stimulates sulfate incorporation by cartilage in vitro. *J Lab Clin Med.* 49(6):825–36.

Smiler DG. 1997. The sinus lift graft: Basic technique and variations. *Pract Periodontics Aesthet Dent.* 9(8):885–93; quiz 895.

Urist MR. 1965. Bone: Formation by autoinduction. *Science.* 150(698):893–99.

Wozney JM, et al. 1988. Novel regulators of bone formation: Molecular clones and activities. *Science.* 242(4885):1528–34.

Wrana JL, et al. 1988. Differential effects of transforming growth factor-beta on the synthesis of extracellular matrix proteins by normal fetal rat calvarial bone cell populations. *J Cell Biol.* 106(3):915–24.

Wu MY, Hill CS. 2009. Tgf-beta superfamily signaling in embryonic development and homeostasis. *Dev Cell.* 16(3):329–43.

Zellin G, Linde A. 1997. Importance of delivery systems for growth-stimulatory factors in combination with osteopromotive membranes. An experimental study using rhBMP-2 in rat mandibular defects. *J Biomed Mater Res.* 35(2):181–90.

Section 3
Osseous Surgery in Implant Therapy

Chapter 8 Introduction, History, and Emergence of Prosthetically Driven Implant Placement

Steven M. Morgano, DMD

Modern implant dentistry began in North America with the 1982 Toronto Conference on Osseointegration in Clinical Dentistry (Zarb and Schmitt 1991). The implant method used by Zarb and Schmidt was developed by Branemark et al. (1969) in Sweden. Prior to this conference, dental implants had not been well accepted by U.S. prosthodontists because of the relatively high failure rate reported for previous implant designs and techniques (Schnitman and Shulman 1980).

TREATMENT OF THE EDENTULOUS MANDIBLE

In the Toronto study, edentulous patients who could not adapt to well-made complete dentures were treated with mandibular implant-supported, metal-acrylic resin, screw-retained fixed complete dentures. Because these complete dentures were fixed restorations that were made with materials and techniques commonly employed for removable complete dentures, the slang term "hybrid prosthesis" was commonly used to describe these dentures (Academy of Prosthodontics 1987).

These mandibular dentures were designed with long transmucosal abutments that were attached to the implant platforms, raising the inferior border of the prosthesis well above the ridge crest in an attempt to facilitate cleaning (Figure 8.1). However, this design often created a flat shelf on the inferior border of the prosthesis with wide-open spaces that were difficult to clean (Figure 8.2). Five implants were commonly used to retain and support the prosthesis, and these implants were commonly placed by the surgeon freehand (McCartney 1993), without regard to the design of the final prosthesis. The ability to make a complete denture that was rigidly fixed was a revolutionary development in dentistry, and few dentists concerned themselves with precision during implant placement. Because the prosthesis was retained with screws, screw-access channels were placed over the center of each implant. The location of these screw-access channels was dictated by the location and angulation of the implants beneath them, and the openings of the access channels

could compromise aesthetics and occlusion (Hebel and Gajjar 1997) (Figure 8.3).

With time, the design of this prosthesis evolved, as treatment planning became prosthetically driven. Implants were placed to ensure favorable location of all access-channel openings and to allow the development of a more cleansable design for the prosthesis. Large open spaces beneath the prosthesis were no longer used (Figure 8.4).

IMPLANT TREATMENT FOR THE EDENTULOUS MAXILLAE

Attempts to use the same protocol to treat the edentulous maxillae were much less successful when compared with the treatment of the edentulous mandible. Problems experienced included lack of adequate lip support, poor aesthetics, phonetic difficulties, and limited access for oral hygiene (Desjardins 1992). The use of implant-supported removable maxillary overdentures was a practical solution to these problems (Figures 8.5).

IMPLANT TREATMENT FOR PARTIALLY EDENTULOUS PATIENTS

The technique originally described by Zarb was further modified to restore partially edentulous patients with implant-supported crowns and fixed partial dental prostheses. With this new development, implant location and angulation became critical, and patients' treatments were planned "from the crown down." The use of cement-retained restorations became more common, and aesthetic outcomes became a major concern. Soft tissue contours in the aesthetic zone were especially important, and techniques were developed to ensure favorable soft tissue contours about implant-supported crowns (Figure 8.6).

Treatment planning for implant-supported restorations must begin with the restorative dentist. Commonly, the restorative dentist or a dental laboratory technician will set an artificial

Practical Osseous Surgery in Periodontics and Implant Dentistry, First Edition. Edited by Serge Dibart, Jean-Pierre Dibart.
© 2011 John Wiley & Sons, Inc. Published 2011 by John Wiley & Sons, Inc.

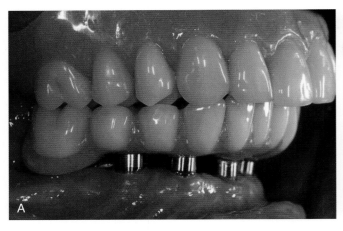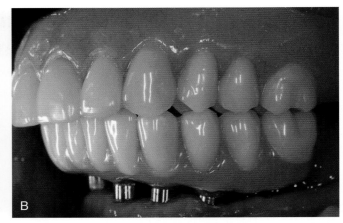

Figure 8.1 Screw-retained fixed complete denture describe by Zarb and Schmidt. (A) Right view; (B) left view. Note the long transmucosal abutments to which the prosthesis is attached.

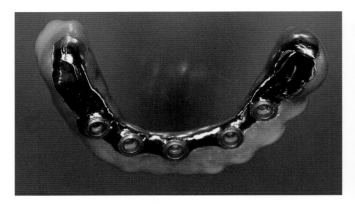

Figure 8.2 Inferior view of prosthesis shown in Figure 8.1. Note shelf-like appearance of this inferior surface that can impede the patient's access to clean this surface.

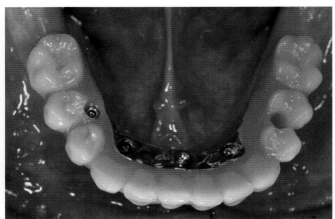

Figure 8.3 Occlusal view of prosthesis shown in Figure 8.1. Screw-access channels will be filled with composite resin after the prosthesis is screwed in place. Access channel openings have minimal effect on aesthetics and occlusal function; nevertheless, the occlusal surfaces of some of the teeth are compromised.

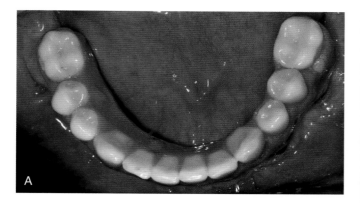

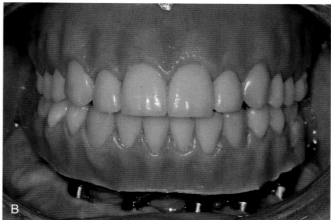

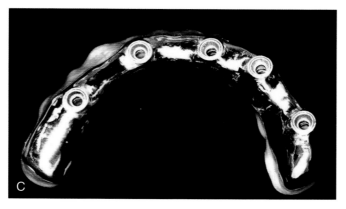

Figure 8.4 Modified prosthetic design. (A) With more precise implant placement, access channel openings do not compromise the occlusal surfaces of the teeth as they do with the prosthesis in Figure 8.3. (B) Large openings above the ridge crest have been eliminated. Note how the denture base acrylic resin tapers toward the implants. A wax trial diagnostic denture was used to determine the desired placement of the artificial teeth. The surgeon removed approximately 5 mm of bone before placing the implants to provide sufficient occluso-gingival space to provide this tapered design. (C) Note lack of shelf on inferior surface of prosthesis, a design that facilitates cleaning.

tooth or teeth on a stone cast in the edentulous area(s) and fabricate an acrylic resin radiological template for a cone-beam computed tomographic (CT) scan with a radiopaque marker for each implant. Each marker indicates the optimal position and angulation of the proposed implant (Figure 8.7). When evaluating the CT scan, angulation problems with implant placement may become obvious, and several options are available. If the angulation problem is minor, a custom abutment or angulated abutment can be used (Figures 8.8). Major angulation problems would require bone augmentation with grafting to improve the configuration of the osseous implant site. If grafting is not practical, an alternative restorative treatment method, other than implant dentistry, should be chosen.

SUMMARY

Although the initial success of mandibular fixed complete dentures supported by osseointegrated implants was very gratifying, attempts at using this technology for other indications were less successful. Totally successful outcomes often were not achievable until innovative implant/prosthetic techniques and components, such as custom abutments, were introduced and treatment planning for implant dentistry became prosthetically driven. See Chapter 18 for a comprehensive review of what every surgeon must know to be able to provide implant surgery that can consistently produce optimal prosthetic results.

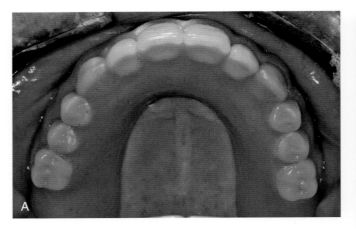

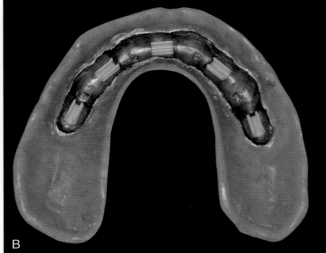

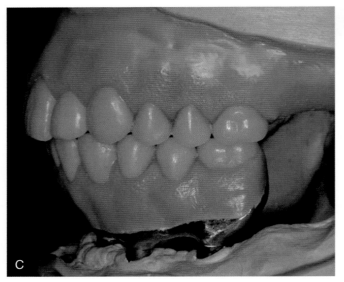

Figure 8.5 (A) Occlusal view of implant-supported, bar-retained maxillary overdenture. Note that prosthesis is U-shaped and does not cover the hard palate. (B) Intaglio of denture with metal reinforcement. (C) Final wax trial arrangement of artificial teeth for maxillary overdenture. Note location of the maxillary anterior teeth and development of a labial flange to provide favorable aesthetics and phonetics.

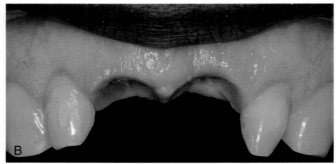

Figure 8.6 (A) Gingival contours about implants supporting maxillary right and left central incisors have been developed. A preprosthetic palatal sliding pedicle graft was performed to ensure adequate bulk of soft tissue in the edentulous area, and provisional restorations were placed to develop the soft-tissue contours. (B) Soft tissue architecture with crowns and abutments removed.

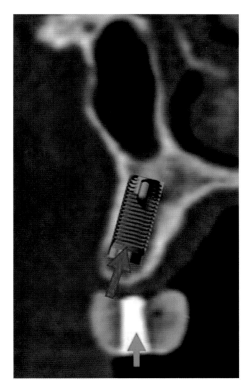

Figure 8.7 Cone-beam CT scan of bone in area of maxillary right second premolar. Radiological marker (green arrow) indicates optimal angulation of planned implant for favorable biomechanics; nevertheless, because of angulation and shape of the alveolar bone, the implant would be angulated differently (red arrow). If angulation of the green arrow is chosen, a bone graft at the apical area of the implant would be required to cover exposed threads. The restorative dentist must plan on compensating for any unfavorable angulation of the implant.

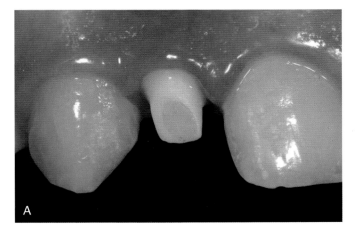
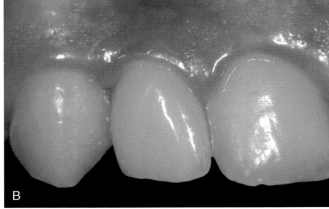

Figure 8.8 (A) Angulation problem with implant for support of maxillary right lateral incisor corrected with the use of custom zirconia abutment. Note that screw-access opening is on facial surface of abutment. (B) Finished cemented crown.

REFERENCES

Academy of Prosthodontics. 1987. Glossary of prosthodontic terms, 5th ed. *J Prosthet Dent.* 58:43.

Branemark PI, Adell R, Breine U, et al. 1969. Intra-osseous anchorage of dental prostheses. 1. Experimental studies. *Scand J Plast Reconstr Surg.* 3:81–100.

Desjardins RP. 1992. Prosthesis design for osseointegrated implants in the edentulous maxilla. *Int J Oral Maxillofac Implants.* 7:311–20.

Hebel KS, Gajjar RC. 1997. Cement-retained versus screw-retained implant restorations: Achieving optimal occlusion and esthetics in implant dentistry. *J Prosthet Dent.* 77:28–35.

McCartney JW. 1993. Line-of-vision surgical guide to implant placement in the anterior mandible. *J Prosthet Dent.* 70:551–52.

Schnitman P, Shulman A. 1980. Dental implants: Benefit and risk. *Proceedings of an NIH-Harvard Consensus Development Conference*, U.S. Department of Health and Human Services. June 12–13, 1978, pp 81–1531.

Zarb GA, Schmitt A. 1991. Osseointegration and the edentulous predicament. The 10-year-old Toronto study. *Br Dent J.* 170:439–44.

Chapter 9 Interpretation of the Preoperative CT Scan: The Relationship of Anatomy and Occlusion to Implant Placement

Albert M. Price, DMD, DSc

The use of endosseous implants to create an aesthetic and biomechanically stable dental prosthesis depends on appropriate sizing and three-dimensional placement of the implants in a relationship that maximizes load distribution. The analysis of the relative intensity, direction, and frequency of forces placed on the plane of occlusion includes consideration of the curves of Wilson and Spee, overbite, overjet, and guidance in excursions from maximum intercuspal position. It is the sum of this loading calculation that gets transmitted through the occlusal plane to the abutments and then in turn to the tooth-ligament or implant-bone attachment (Figure 9.1). The mechanical resistance of these different systems of attachment can be reduced to the following axiom: Compressive forces are well tolerated; lateral forces can be destructive.

Because many reconstructive problems have a mixture of teeth and implant support (Figures 9.2–9.5), a review of the differences between osseointegrated implants and ligament-supported teeth is necessary. Teeth have a collagen-based suspension system embedded within a matrix of extracellular glycoprotein that helps dissipate forces placed on the occlusal table. In addition, the presence of a vascular supply in the ligament space indirectly provides a hydraulic cushion whereas an integrated neural component provides physiologic proprioception and reflex protection against excessive acute force (Figure 9.6).

Normal functional loads on the posterior teeth in the intact dentition are compressive and well tolerated but chronic parafunctional forces can create lateral stress that overloads the periodontal support complex and may result in "physiologic adaption" in the form of mobility and migration of the teeth. Once the posterior teeth "adapt," sometimes referred to as posterior bite collapse, the anterior teeth come under increasing protrusive loads (Figures 9.7 and 9.8). It should be noted that these adaptions protect the individual teeth, not the occlusion. Preservation of occlusal function and aesthetics requires the dental therapist to minimize these "adaptions," otherwise the occlusion becomes disabled and functions at a less than optimal potential. The art and science

of managing occlusal forces acting on an individual arch is a combination of estimating the remaining support (tooth mobility is a good proxy); controlling the location, direction, and distribution of occlusal contacts; and using mechanical load-sharing methods such as splinting or by choosing opposing restorative strength (Figure 9.9). the most vulnerable component in the biology of the natural tooth support system is the vascular net of the periodontal ligament space. The alveolar vascular supply maintains this suspension complex with a pattern of flow directed from inside the bone outward through the ligament space into the gingiva, where it interconnects with the gingival vascular complex (Figure 9.10). If this space is compromised by prolonged or repetitive compressive forces, alveolar bone and root-cemental resorption can occur (Figure 9.11) with a widening of the ligament space; this can result in mobility and migration of teeth (Figures 9.7 and 9.8). Exceeding the elastic limit of these biological materials results in permanent deformation.

Implants do not have a ligament, and they don't have a known proprioceptive response. The implant surface is integrated or is in direct physical contact with the mineralized component of the bone structure (Figure 9.12). The elasticity in this construction depends on both the elastic modulus of the materials involved (Figure 9.13) and the bone, which has a varied three-dimensional architecture (Figure 9.14) and a dynamic state of mineralization. Since in clinical treatment, the details of the bone interface and the stress absorptive capacities of varied bone architectures are not available, the mechanics of the crown-abutment and abutment-implant interface become the focus of our interest for treatment planning. Testing the strength issues involved in these mechanical connections results in the same conclusions found in the analysis of the natural tooth attachment: Compressive forces are well tolerated whereas lateral forces can be destructive (Figure 9.15).

Once implants are integrated, forces that are compressive tend to push the implant components together and are well tolerated whereas lateral forces create mechanical stress by

Practical Osseous Surgery in Periodontics and Implant Dentistry, First Edition. Edited by Serge Dibart, Jean-Pierre Dibart.

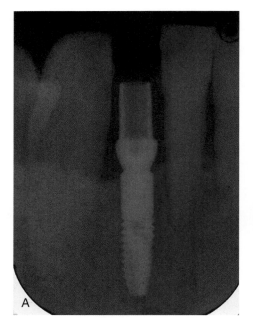

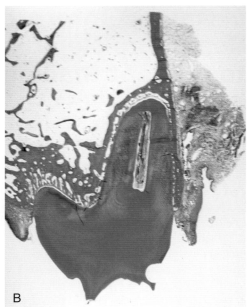

Figure 9.1 (A) Implant-abutement-bone relationship. (B) Natural tooth tissue relationships notch on buccal (monkey).

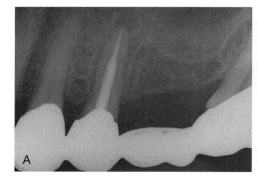

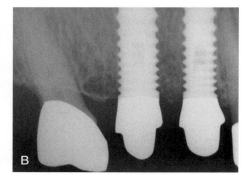

Figure 9.2 (A) Periapical radiograph shows fractured bicuspid beneath four-unit bridge. (B) Periapical postoperative radiograph shows two implants after a sinus lift.

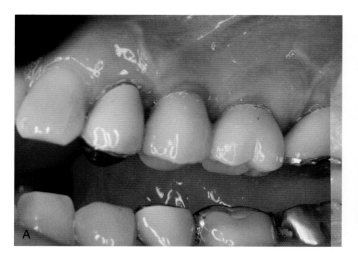

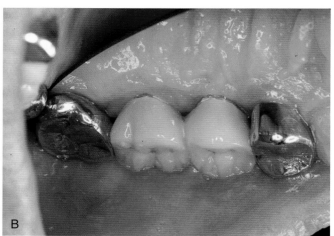

Figure 9.3 Restorative postoperative of case shown in Figure 9.2. (A) Buccal; (B) palatal (restorative courtesy of Dr. Albert Duarte, Cambridge, MA).

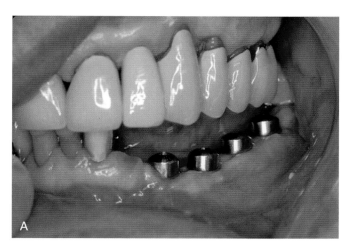

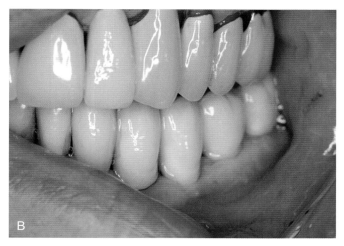

Figure 9.4 (A, B) Four implants placed in narrow ridge to replace #18–23 (restorative courtesy of Dr. Albert Duarte, Cambridge, MA).

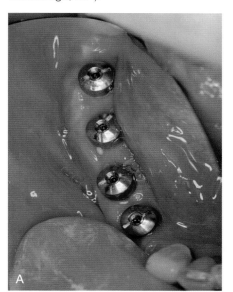

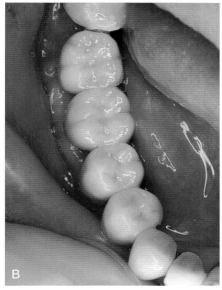

Figure 9.5 (A, B) Occlusual view of Figure 9.4.

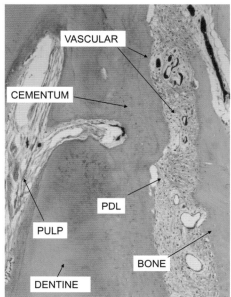

Figure 9.6 Histology near apex of tooth.

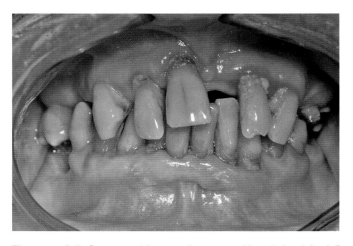

Figure 9.7 Severe bite collapse with "physiologic" adaption.

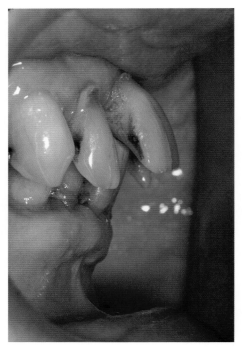

Figure 9.8 Lateral profile same patient as in Figure 9.7. Radiographs in this patient showed 50% or more bone loss, with only teeth #20, 22, 27, and 29 usable.

1 – Periosteal supply
2 – Vessels from bone
3 – Periodontal ligament supply to crest
4 – Papillary loops

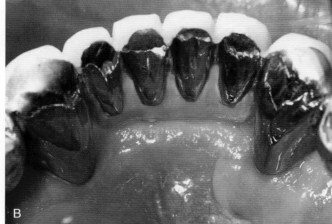

NORMAL VASCULAR SUPPLY

Figure 9.10 Vascular supply to dental/periodontal tissues: distribution of microcirculation and direction of flow.

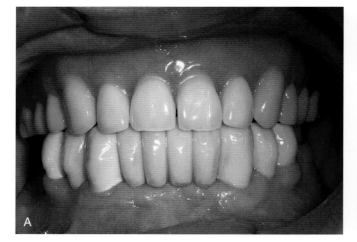

Figure 9.9 (A) Final restorative on patient in Figures 9.7 and 9.8. (B) Lingual, same patient.

bending the connector parts. Where the stress becomes dissipated depends on the nature and arrangement of the parts. In two-piece implant designs such as the classic Branemark external hex platform the abutment screw is the smallest component and most vulnerable to deformation. In an internal attachment design, the weakest link is usually in the collar design (Figures 9.15 and 9.16). With either style, if the connecting interface is strengthened, the result performs more like a one-piece implant, which is the third variation in design. if the occlusal table is overloaded by lateral vectors of force, the stress is focused at the bone crest, which becomes the fulcrum of rotation. In such cases, the implant may experience crestal bone loss (Figure 9.17); the body of the implant itself may break (Figures 9.12 and 9.18); or the implant may experience bone loss and eventual complete loss of integration (Figure 9.19).

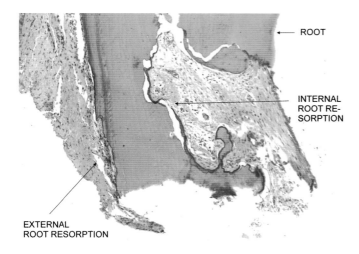

Figure 9.11 Histology-human tooth-INTERNAL and external root resorption-trauma related to occlusal loads. From: Price A. Comparison of the Microvascular Disruption and Regeneration Following Full, Partial, and Modified Partial Thickness Pedicle Flaps in the Alveolar Mucosa of *Macaca mulatta* Monkeys. D.Sc.D. thesis, Boston University, 1974. p. 180.

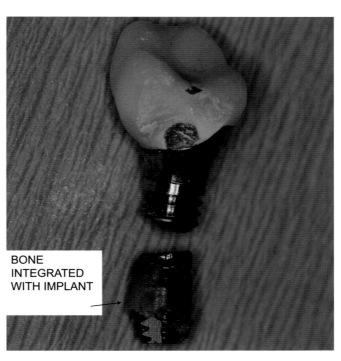

BONE INTEGRATED WITH IMPLANT

Figure 9.12 Note the integration of bone with the fractured implant. Even the increase in leverage after the bone loss at the neck of the implant could not disintegrate the lower portion. It had to be removed by trephine.

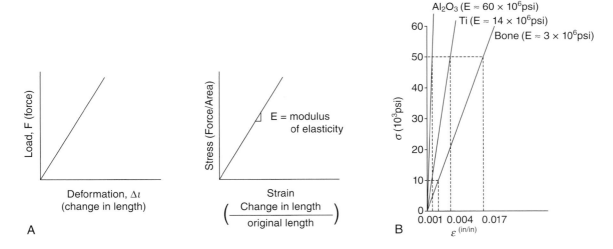

Figure 9.13 (A) Calculation modulus of elasticity. (B) Stress PSI on left. Deformation compared for different material.

THREE-DIMENSIONAL POSITIONING IN THE ALVEOLAR HOUSING

Positioning of the implant within the alveolar housing entails different biological demands when compared to the natural tooth connections. When the buccal-lingual placement of natural teeth is visualized in the alveolous, we find that teeth are often positioned toward the plane of the buccal plate and even beyond it, with minimal bone on the buccal aspect (Figures 9.20 and 9.21). The biology of the periodontal ligament with a rich vascular supply interlinked with the gingival supply supports bone dimensions of less than 1 mm. In mesio-distal positioning of teeth, the interproximal area

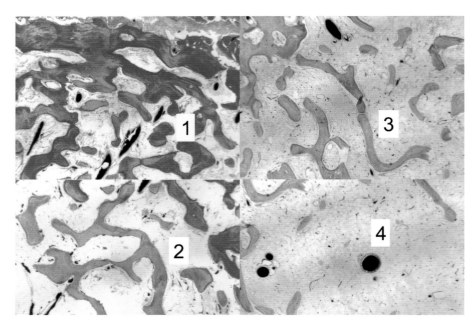

Figure 9.14 Note vascular system is perfused with India ink. "Bone density" when viewed microscopically is revealed to be a product of the relative frequency, distribution, and size of bone trabeculae. In this figure sample 1 would be judged as more dense or "hard," and sample 4 would be sensed as less dense or "soft" when drilling an implant osteotomy.

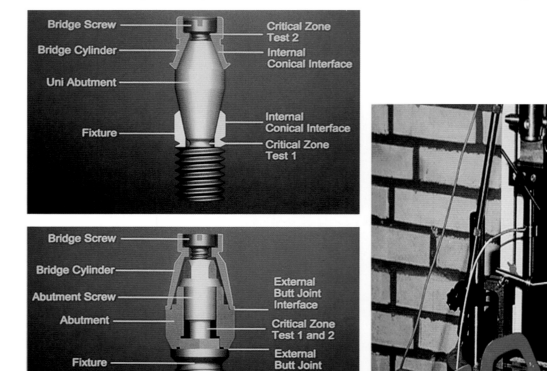

Figure 9.15 Testing deformation on internal vs. external abutment to implant attachments. From: Norton, MR. 1997. An in vitro evaluation of the strength of an internal conical interface compared to a butt joint interface in implant design, *Clinical Oral Implant Research.* 8:290–98.

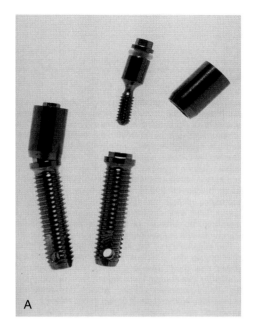
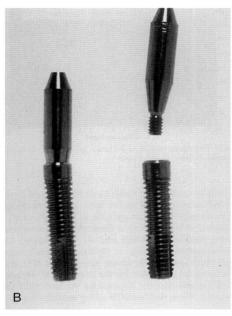

Figure 9.16 (A) Branemark external style. (B) Astra internal style. From Norton, MR. An in vitro evaluation of the strength of an internal conical interface compared to a butt joint interface in implant design. Norton, MR. 1997. An in vitro evaluation of the strength of an internal conical interface compared to a butt joint interface in implant design, *Clinical Oral Implant Research.* 8:290–98.

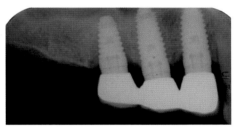

Figure 9.17 Failing implant and bone loss, which may have been an inappropriate fit of framework.

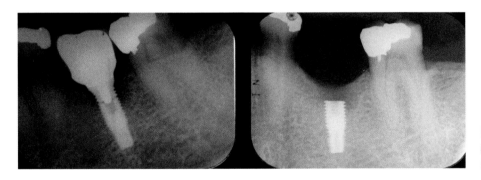

Figure 9.18 Note bone loss to dept of abutment screw and then fracture related to occlusal overload.

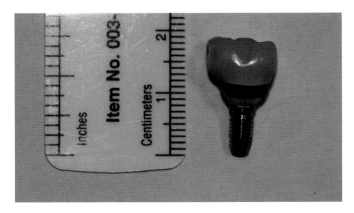

Figure 9.19 Avulse implant/crown restoration. Complete disintegration after 2 years. Note poor crown/root ratio and excessive occlusal table/implant diameter difference.

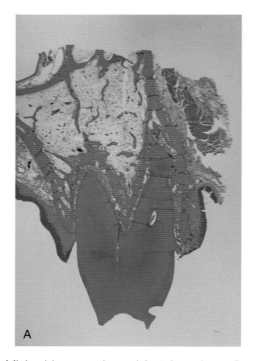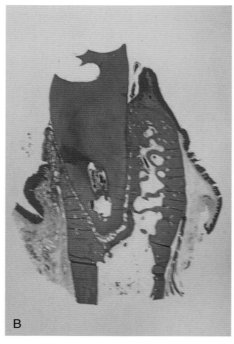

Figure 9.20 (A) Minimal bone on buccal (notch on buccal): maxillary first bicuspid. (B) Minimal bone on buccal (notch on buccal): Mandibular first bicuspid.

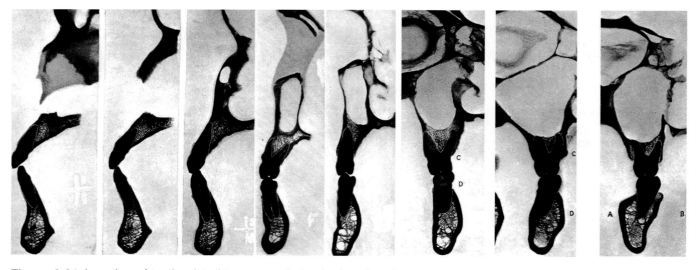

Figure 9.21 Location of teeth related to center of alveolar housing. From: Ash, MM Jr. 1993. *Wheeler's Dental Anatomy, Physiology and Occlusion*, 7th ed. Philadelphia: WB Saunders.

between two teeth has an enriched vascular net from two periodontal ligaments, which also permits closer root proximity and narrow interproximal bone. An edentulous ridge, on the other hand, is quite different and is compromised, with minimal interconnections between the bone marrow and the external gingival supply. Because of these different anatomic relationships, the vascular needs of the bone in a newly integrated implant are derived predominately from endosseous

origins. Branemark's research suggested that 3 mm was the minimum bone needed between implants in the anterior hybrid restoration. This was based on recognition that the residual vascular supply to the interimplant bone conditions after adjacent osteotomies is limited by the presence of highly compact bone with minimal internal circulation. As a general rule, the consensus suggests that an implant should have at least 1 mm of bone on the buccal and lingual and at least

2–3 mm of bone between adjacent implants. The aesthetic needs of a restoration place different demands on spacing. They may require that the implant be placed mesio-distally in the center of the tooth form, and sometimes this results in more than 3 mm between implant bodies. The final proximity can have effects on the interproximal soft tissue and the creation of "black triangles." In addition to these aesthetic needs, a successful osseointegration requires primary stability at the time of surgery, which is best provided by engagement of cortical bone. The hunt for cortex at potential implant sites therefore becomes a primary quest in surgical treatment planning.

The preceding discussion suggests that for both implants and teeth the transfer of forces from the occlusal plane to the support structures is best tolerated if the loads are compressive in nature. To maximize this compressive loading, the placement of the implant or tooth should be oriented perpendicular to the plane of occlusion and close to the center of the occlusal table. To evaluate the available bone and guide this placement, the most useful diagnostic information would provide real-size buccal-lingual and mesial-distal cross sections of the site oriented perpendicular to the plane of occlusion. Various imaging techniques have been applied to this evaluation: periapical, panoramic radiograph, tomograph, and CT scan.

In comparison tests, the periapical radiographs, whether conventional or digital, were found to be affected by inaccuracy of up to 15% (Figure 9.22), whereas panoramic tomographic systems are prone to enlargement and increased distortion of 20–25% (Figure 9.23). Both mediums provide mesio-distal views, but neither of these techniques allows a bucco-lingual cross section. Sequential tomographs using selected focal planes allow an approach to our goal, but increased slice thickness often results in blurry images of poor quality (Figure 9.24). In contrast, computerized axial tomography (CAT scan) approaches 99% accuracy (Figure 9.25), and allows reformated images of both buccal-lingual and mesio-distal dimensions (Figure 9.26). The newer cone beam technology can

provide suitable images, but sometimes lack the consistency and definition of axial technology, especially on curved contour (Figure 9.27). Understanding how the CT scan system generates these images allows them to be used more productively and allows a more accurate interpretation of the results.

THE AXIAL CT

Examining the first generation of axial CT scanners invented by Dr. Godfrey Hounsfield in the 1970s can help to illustrate basic image acquisition (Figure 9.28). In an axial CT, radiation emitters and receivers are arranged in a large ring through which the patient's body is passed while supported by a table (Figure 9.29). The exposure beam is oriented at right angles to the body axis (Thus the term *axial scan*). The beam width is controlled, and the exposure data are recorded in the form of a slice of a uniform thickness (usually in the millimeter or less range). The quantity of transmitted radiation at a particular focal point is measured and used to generate a unit of density called a Hounsfield value for each focal point within the field or slice of the data set (Figures 9.30–9.33). These

July 27, 2006

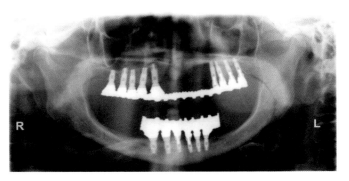

Figure 9.23 Note: All implants are 4.0 mm diameter; distortion can vary in Panorex film.

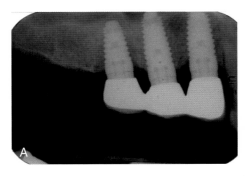
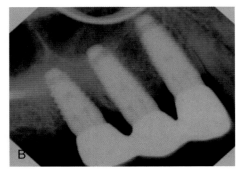

Figure 9.22 A well-aligned conventional periapical is better than a poorly aligned digital image. (A) PA–conventional; distortion = 15% ±. (B) PA–digital; limit two-dimensional.

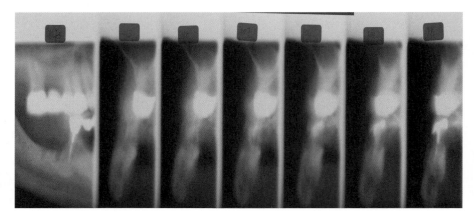

Figure 9.24 Serial tomography. Slice thickness 5 mm with poor resolution of shape and borders.

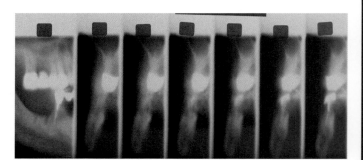

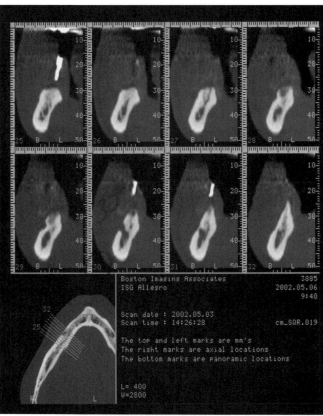

Figure 9.25 Computer automated tomograph (CAT) scan right vs. tomography. (B) Distortion (about 1%) + clear.

numbers in turn can be assigned to a spectrum of gray values (Figure 9.34), which then can be displayed as pixels on a computer screen. (Because the original beam has thickness, the data set actually has three dimensions, and the final data set is stored as small cubes or voxels.) After one slice is acquired, the examination table is moved an incremental distance, and another slice is acquired. The distance between slices is called the slice increment, and this distance is calculated to be in such close proximity that it avoids dead space or voids in information. These slices can be displayed individually in a two-dimensional array or restacked into a three-dimensional visualization (Figure 9.35).

To reinforce this concept of restacked slices of information, an analogy can be made to a common loaf slicer found in most supermarkets (Figure 9.36). If we examine the function of a slicing machine, we see it has a control that regulates slice thickness. Thin or thick slices produced can be restacked

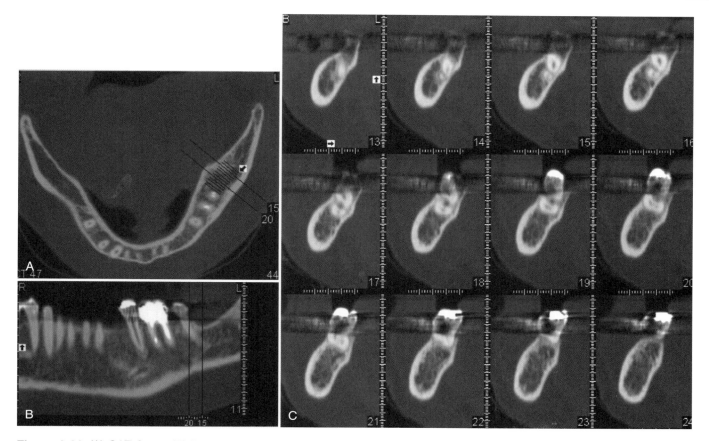

Figure 9.26 (A) CAT Scan. (B) Panoramic reformat. (C) Oblique (cross section) reformat.

(Figure 9.37) into the original loaf form with the incremental cut lines still visible. To make observations parallel to the surface but farther inside the stack of slices we can lift the edges away from the stack and explore the relationship of one slice to the next (Figure 9.38). A different perspective of the content in these slices can be generated by drawing a large knife perpendicular to the surface of the original stack and then separating the portions (Figure 9.39). In this way we can obtain a cross-sectional view of the same material, and we can measure inclusions if present, in this case olives (Figure 9.40).

Returning to the CAT scan format, if the sheets of data in voxel form are stacked together in a three-dimensional block, then different views could be derived by software that reformats the data in different planes using the same voxels. The block diagram in the picture (Figure 9.41) Depicts such a reformatting process done parallel to or at right angles to the original plane of image acquisition.

As noted, an axial CT scan is so called because it generates slices of information at right angles to the long axis of the patient's body, the vertebral column. The patient is positioned on a flat table, and the head is stabilized in line with the body.

Because the head is articulated and has multiple potential orientations relative to the "slicer," a separate reference plane needs to be chosen that allows reproducible positioning for sequential studies. For medical diagnosis, technicians commonly use the floor of the nose as a plane of reference for evaluation of the maxilla, whereas in the mandible, which has added possibility of movement, the reference plane is the base or lower border of the mandible. Scans that are done for dental implant treatment planning have a different orientation. The needs of a dental reconstruction are best served by images arranged perpendicular to the plane of occlusion because the reformats will be done at right angles to the original plane of acquisition. This requires a written order to the technician that specifies that "the dental scan should be taken parallel to the plane of occlusion" (Figure 9.41).

A CT scan does not discriminate between hard and soft tissue, and thus the acquired data set includes both. A typical slice of raw Hounsfield information is shown in Figure 9.42, which displays muscle, bone, air, and even denture plastic. The creation of a more refined image to evaluate either bone or soft tissue alone can be made by selective enhancement of one tissue or the other. This process is referred to as screening with a bone or soft tissue algorithm. The final

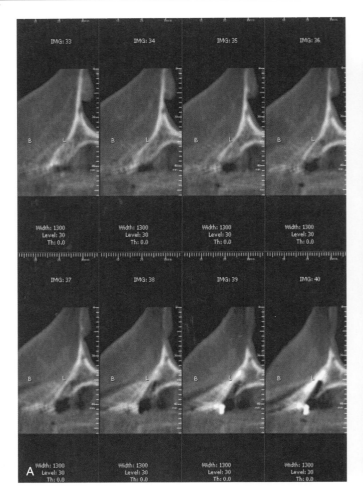

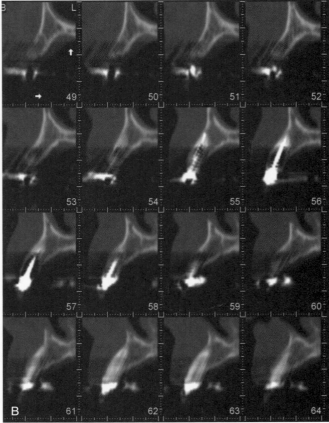

Figure 9.27 (A) Cone beam cuspid area. (B) Same patient: axial CT.

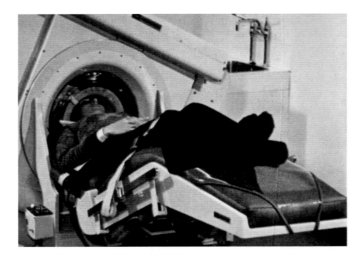

Figure 9.28 Dr. Hounsfield in original CAT scanner. Provided by Boston Imaging Associates.

product of this mathematical manipulation is a cleared or *reformated axial slice* (Figure 9.43).

Further processing of these clarified images can generate reformatted panoramic (mesial-distal) and oblique (buccal-lingual) images. To do this a new reference plane is needed that follows the specific curvature of the dental arch under review. The technician creates this reference line on one of the axial slices located near the middle of the acquired data set by application of an electronic pen (Figures 9.43–9.45). This reference line is subsequently incorporated into all the slices above and below. The computer can then display every pixel (voxel) that falls along this customized, curved reference plane and create a *reformatted panoramic slice* (Figure 9.46). Once this plane is available, a parallel series of panoramic planes can be generated at 1- to 2-mm distances from it in either the buccal or lingual direction. These panoramic reformats are quite different from the common dental panoramic

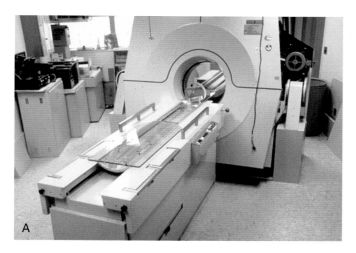
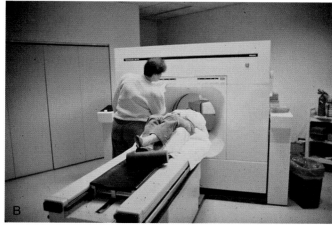

Figure 9.29 (A) Modern head scanners. (B) Note patient table moves into "slicer" at right angle to body axis. Provided by Boston Imaging Associates.

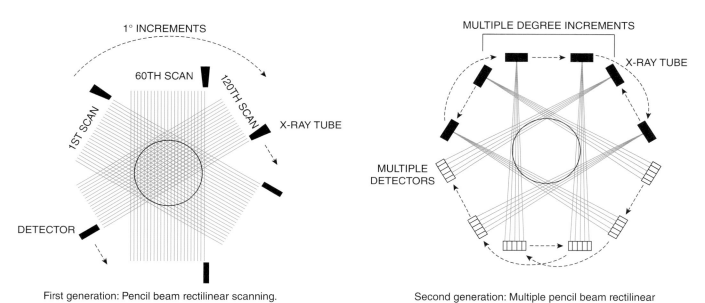

First generation: Pencil beam rectilinear scanning. 4½ to 5½ minutes.

Second generation: Multiple pencil beam rectilinear scanning. 20 seconds to 3½ minutes.

Figure 9.30 Modern scanners are faster than the noted scan times. Provided by Boston Imaging Associates.

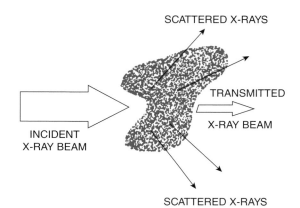

INCIDENT X-RAY BEAM

SCATTERED X-RAYS

TRANSMITTED X-RAY BEAM

SCATTERED X-RAYS

$$(\mu_1 + \mu_2 + \mu_3 + \cdots + \mu_n) = \frac{1}{w} \ln \frac{I_0}{I_n}$$

This equation shows that if the incident intensity I_0, the transmitted intensity I_n, and the incremental density segment length, w, are known, the <u>sum</u> of the attenuation coefficients $(\mu_1 + \mu_2 + \mu_3 + \cdots + \mu_n)$ along the path of the x-ray beam can be caluclated.

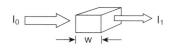

Figure 9.31 Sequence for calculation of Hounsfield numbers. Provided by Boston Imaging Associates.

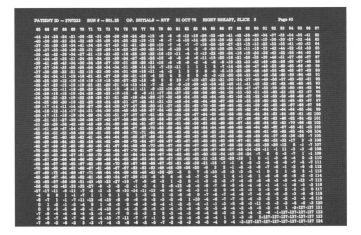

CT NUMBERS

A CT NUMBER IS A VALUE WHICH DE-SCRIBES THE DENSITY OF A GIVEN STRUC-TURE AS RELATED TO THE DENSITY OF WATER. AN ARBITRARY SCALE IS USED TO ASSIGN THESE CT NUMBERS AND WATER IS CONSIDERED TO BE ZERO.

Figure 9.32 Hounsfield numbers displayed on flat screen; note "picture." Provided by Boston Imaging Associates.

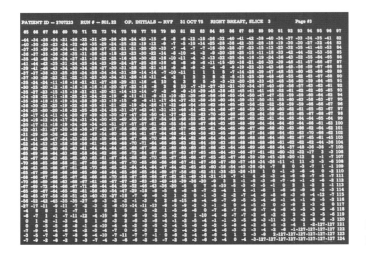

Figure 9.33 Magnified view of flat panel display seen in Figure 9.32. Provided by Boston Imaging Associates.

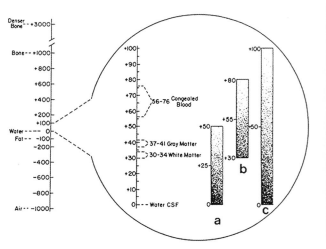

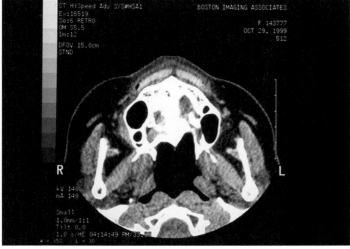

Figure 9.34 Compare spectrum to more refined shade next to "raw" axial scan. Provided by Boston Imaging Associates.

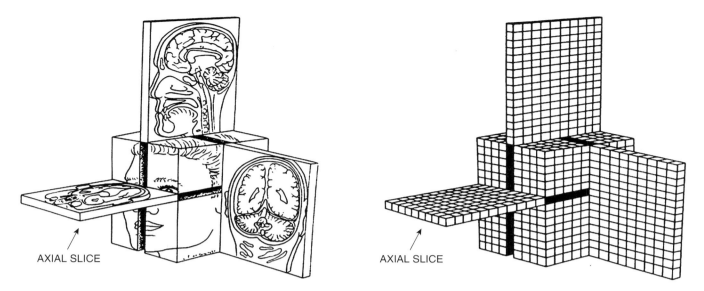

AXIAL SLICE   AXIAL SLICE

Figure 9.35 Geometry of computerized reconstruction. Provided by Boston Imaging Associates.

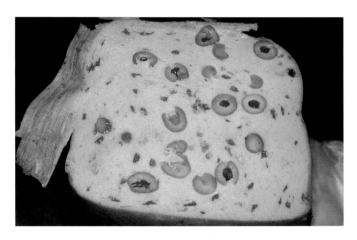

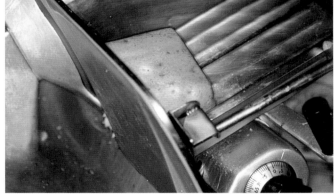

Figure 9.36 Common loaf slicer with olive loaf.

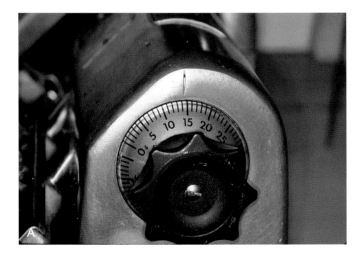

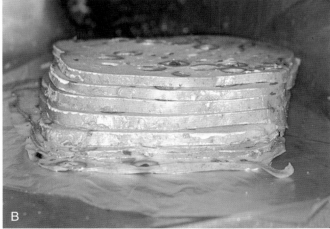

Figure 9.37 (A) Slice thickness selector dial. (B) Variation thickness of slices; thinner slices yield more information.

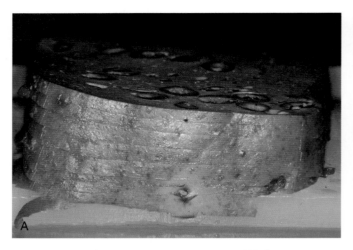
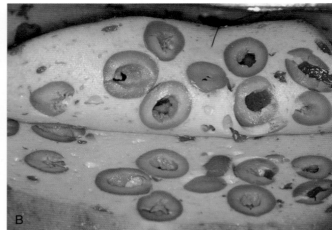

Figure 9.38 (A) Reconstructed olive loaf. (B) Comparison of "axial" slice information.

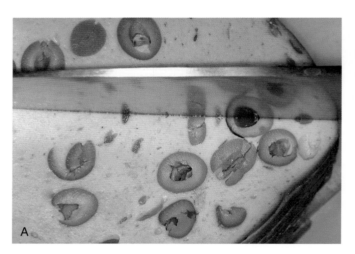
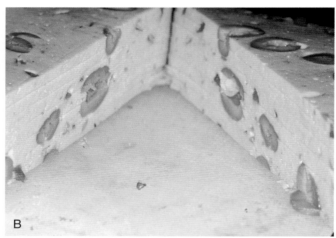

Figure 9.39 (A) Cutting at right angle to original plan of sectioning through the reconstructed loaf. (B) Reformatted cross-sectional or oblique slices.

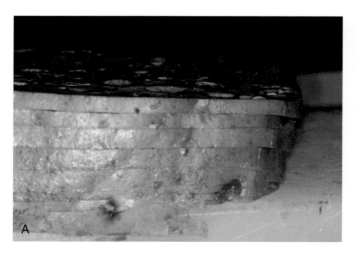
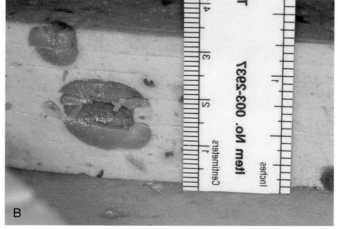

Figure 9.40 (A) "Reformatted" loaf. (B) Measurement of cross sections.

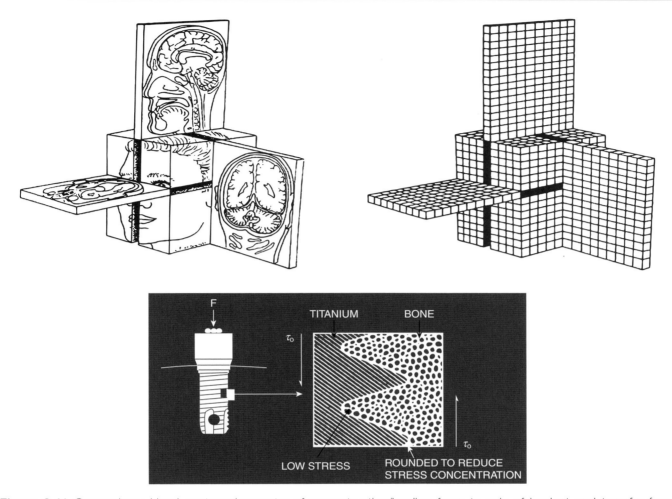

Figure 9.41 Comparison: Head anatomy/geometry of reconstruction/loading force to axis of implant and transfer force to bone.

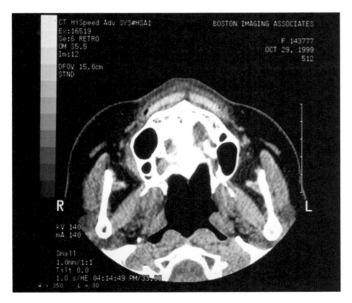

Figure 9.42 Raw CT axial slice—gray scale for soft and hard on left side.

tomographic technique, which averages the entire thickness of the examined structure while following a fixed external path around the patient. With the axial CAT scan, the panoramic view displayed is usually only a fraction of a millimeter in thickness and generates a clear mesio-distal cross-section along an internal plane that follows each unique arch form.

REFORMATTED OBLIQUE OR CROSS-SECTIONAL IMAGES

Once a panoramic plane is determined by superimposition of the center arch line on the restacked data, further images can be fabricated at right angles to both this curved plane and to the original stack of axial slices. This generates a third series of oblique or cross-sectional reformatted images in the desired buccal-lingual direction (Figures 9.47 and 9.48). The original axial slices can also be reconstructed into a three-dimensional model (Figure 9.49), and this could be used in the production of a computer-manufactured surgical template.

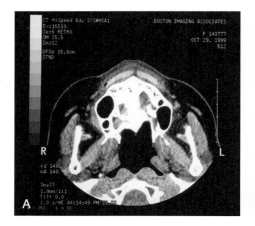
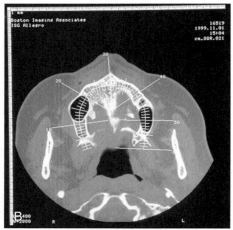

Figure 9.43 (A) Raw axial slice. (B) Reformatted axial slice through use of bone algorithm.

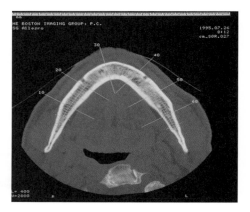

Figure 9.44 Cleared axial slice (patient x). Note mid-arch reference line with perpendicular reference numbers 10, 20, 30, etc.

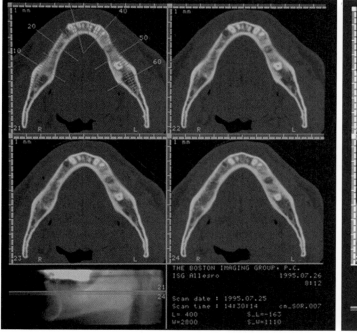
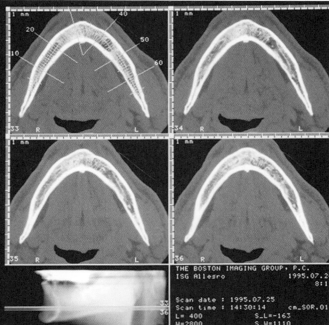

Figure 9.45 Serial reformatted axial slices (patient x).

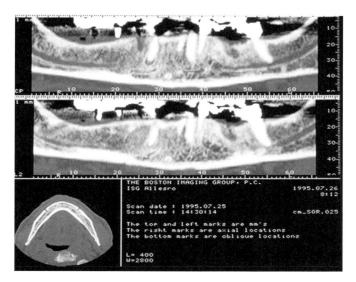

Figure 9.46 Cleared panoramic slices. Note the reference lines on axial image. Also note the periapical radiolucency below the cuspid on upper slice cut 27–28 (patient x).

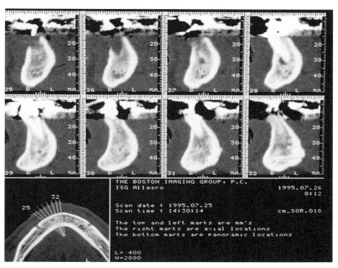

Figure 9.48 Cleared cross-sectional or oblique slices; note radiolucency cut #28 (patient x). See panoramic view in figure 9.45

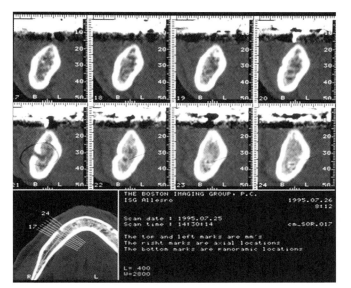

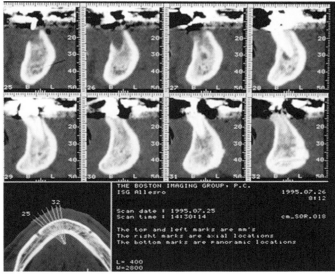

Figure 9.47 Serial reformatted cross-sectional slices (patient x); note mandibular canal, mental foramen, anterior loop; extraction socket and periapical areal not seen on either Panorex or regular periapical x-ray.

All of these reformats are done at 90 degrees or right angles to the original axial slices of information. From this pattern of reconstruction we can see that the alignment of the original slice (Figure 9.41) has implications for the reformats. It cannot be overstressed that the original reference scan must be ordered and aligned *parallel to the plane of occlusion.* Adherence to this order can be confirmed by checking the midsagittal reference supplied on the first sheet of the scan report (Figure 9.50). If this order was followed properly, then the reformatted cross-sectional images will be perpendicular to this and have the desired ideal relationship to loading. If anatomic planes such as the floor of the nose or base of the mandible are used by mistake, the reformatted images can still be used, but this requires a more difficult interpretation (Figure 9.51–9.53).

Newer axial scan techniques and cone beam scanners gather the original information in a slightly different format, but the technicians must start their analysis with a reference plane parallel to the plane of occlusion. They then must insert an

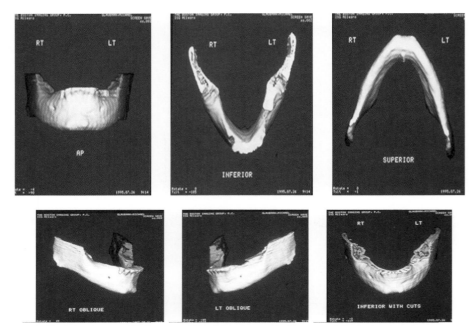

Figure 9.49 Reconstructed three-dimensional format from axial slices.

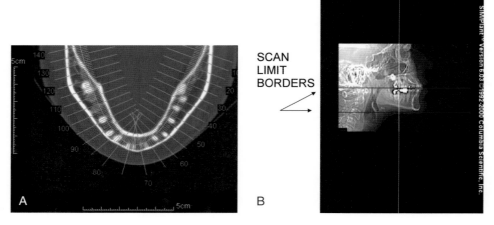

Figure 9.50 Reference slice. (A) Picked from middle slice between borders noted on right. (B) Reformat axial with no distortion, parallel to plane of occlusion. Note center of arch line superimposed on axial slice for reference. This line is used to generate panoramic and cross-sectional images.

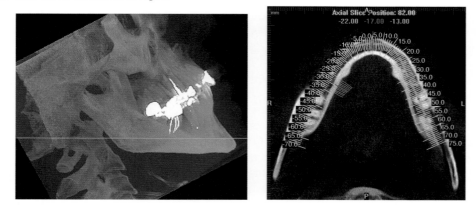

Figure 9.51 Effect of taking original axial scan parallel to base of mandible. Compare to 9.54 using different reference.

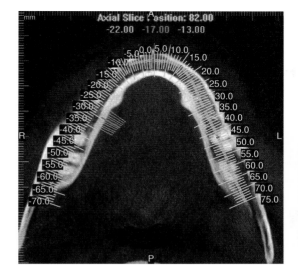

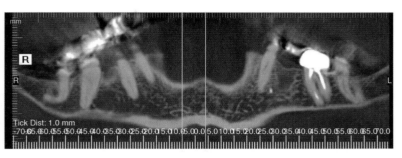

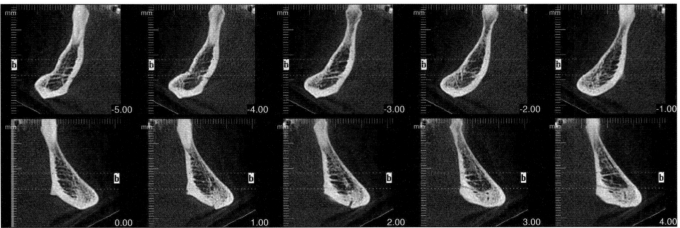

Figure 9.52 Effect on reformats when using base of mandible (compare Figure 9.55).

arch reference line to form the panoramic plane. Deviation from this alignment can display misleading relationships (Figures 9.51–9.56 compare result of different initial reference planes on reformats).

Computerized axial tomography analysis provides the best format for the surgeon's hunt for cortical structure, and searching for this enables an evaluation of limiting internal and external contours and vital gland, nerve, and vascular tissues areas. The addition of gutta-percha markers (see Figures 9.59, 9.64, and 9.65) or other contrast media to a template of the desired restoration can enhance the quality of information available for a specific analysis. The axial CAT scan allows visual dissection of internal compartments and is the most accurate assessment available for presurgical planning.

The following photos illustrate areas of anatomic interest.

LOCATION OF CORTICAL BONE IN THE MAXILLA

1. Buccal and palatal cortical plate (Figures 9.57–9.59)

2. Floor of nose (Figures 9.57–9.59, 9.72)

3. Floor of sinus (Figures 9.58, 9.59, 9.63, 9.66–9.68, 9.70–9.72)

4. Side of incisal canal (Figures 9.57, 9.67)

5. Socket walls (Figures 9.59)

LOCATION OF CORTICAL BONE IN THE MANDIBLE

1. Buccal and lingual plate (multiple)

2. Mandibular canal (Figures 9.45, 9.46, 9.53, 9.56, 9.60, 9.61, 9.64)

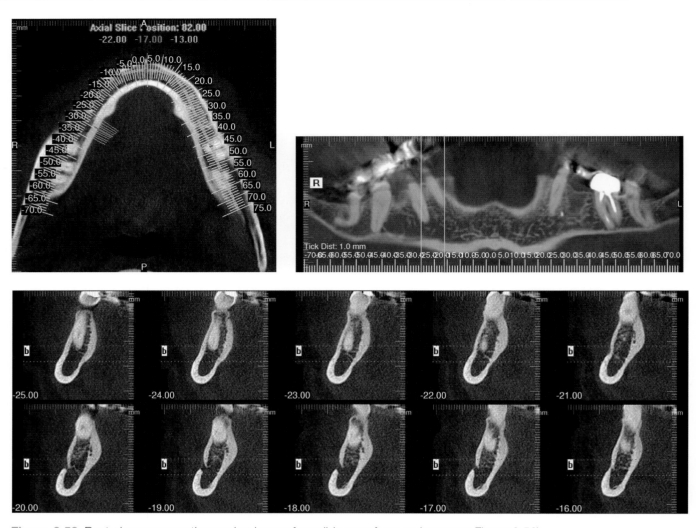

Figure 9.53 Posterior cross sections using base of manible as reference (compare Figure 9.56).

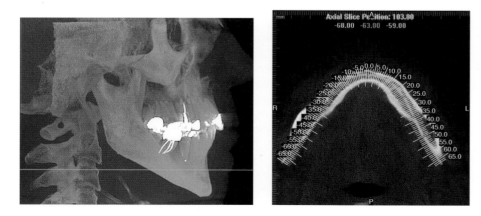

Figure 9.54 Reference plane for axials parallel to plane of occlusion. Compare to Figure 9.51 using different reference.

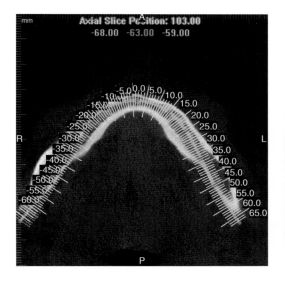

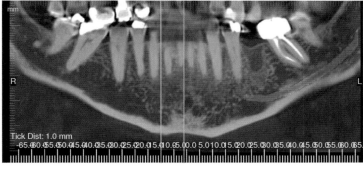

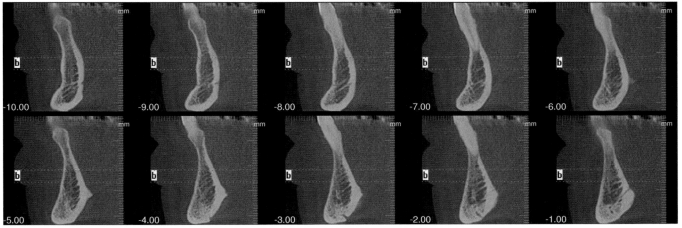

Figure 9.55 Reference plane used for reformat was parallel to plane of occlusion (compare to Figure 9.52).

3. Mental canal and foramen (Figures 9.44, 9.47, 9.48, 9.53, 9.56, 9.64)

4. Socket wall (Figures 9.47, 9.48)

LIMITING SURFACE CONTOURS

1. Incisal fossa, cuspid fossa (Figures 9.57, 9.59)

2. Mylohyoid attachment: submandibular gland concavity (Figures 9.53, 9.56, 9.61, 9.65)

3. Sublingual gland concavity (Figures 9.47, 9.48, 9.61)

4. Floor of sinus, floor of nose (Figures 9.57–9.59)

5. Incomplete socket (Figures 9.47, 9.48, 9.59)

6. Sinus septa, vessels (Figures 9.63, 9.73)

LIMITING CANALS

1. Mandibular canal (Figures 9.45, 9.46, 9.53, 9.56, 9.60, 9.61, 9.64, 9.65)

2. Mental canal and foramen (Figures 9.47, 9.48, 9.53, 9.56, 9.64)

3. Incisal foramen (Figures 9.57, 9.66, 9.67)

OTHER LIMITS AND AREAS OF INTEREST

1. Extensive alveolar resorption (Figures 9.64, 9.65, 9.72)

2. Extensive maxillary sinus (Figures 9.66, 9.67)

3. Extensive incisal canals (Figures 9.66, 9.67)

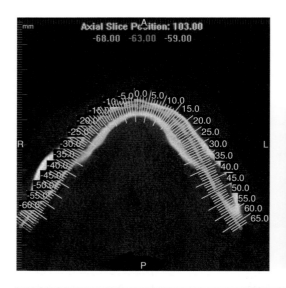

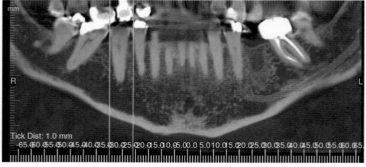

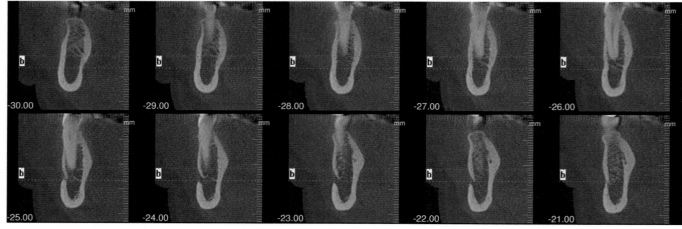

Figure 9.56 Reformats with plane reference parallel to plane of occlusion (compare to Figure 9.53).

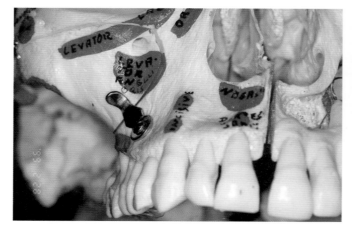

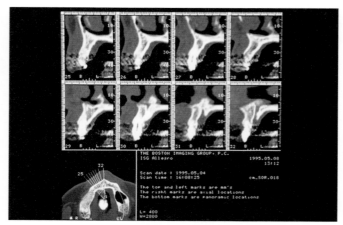

Figure 9.57 Compare dry skeleton to similar clinical areas.

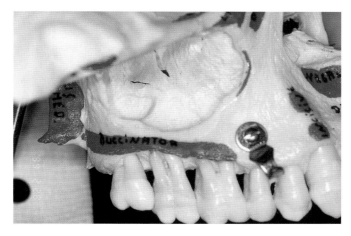

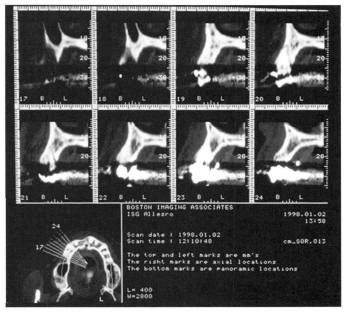

Figure 9.58 Maxillary sinus. See also Figure 9.59.

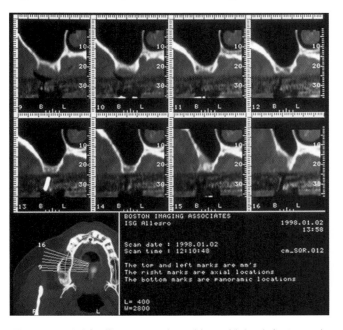

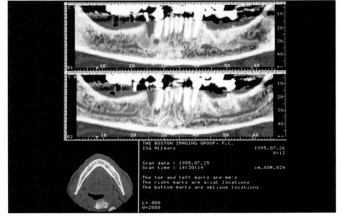

Figure 9.59 Maxillary posterior with multiple defects and anatomical deficiencies.

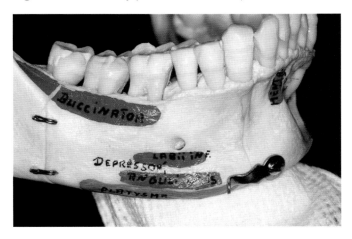

Figure 9.60 Mental foramen, concavities, and convexities. Find mandibular canal, extraction socket, periapical radiolucency.

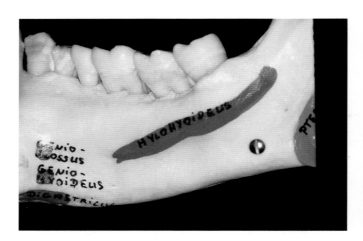

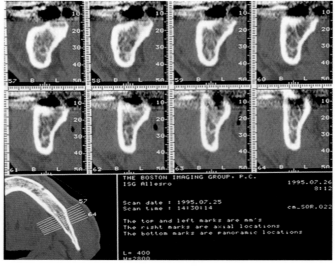

Figure 9.61 Note relationship of submandibular canal to mylohyoid attachment and to mandibular canal and potential axial placement direction of implant.

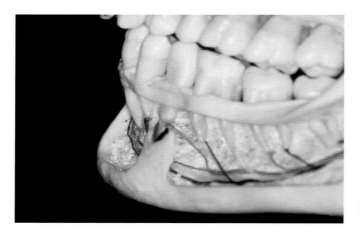

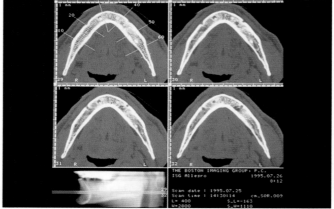

Figure 9.62 Serial axial reformatted slices.

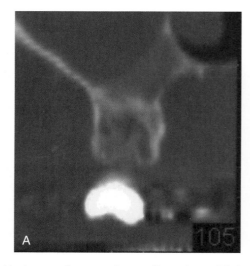

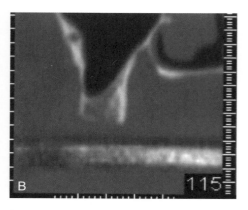

Figure 9.63 (A) Underwood's septa in maxillary sinus. (B) Arteriole in buccal wall of maxillary sinus needing sinus lift.

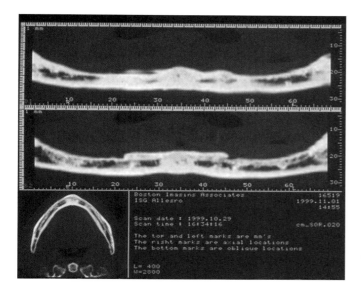
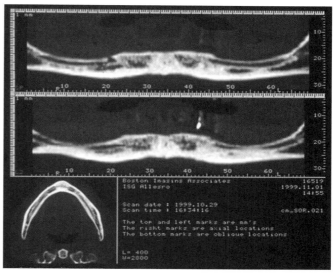

Figure 9.64 Mandibular severe resorption. Note mandibular canal on crestal surface with mental foramen opening upward (cut 20 and 45).

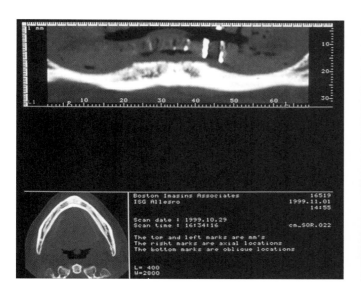
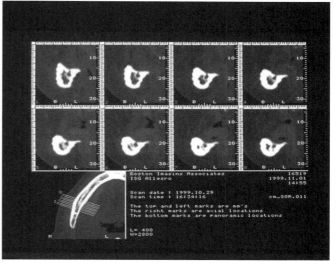

Figure 9.65 Cross-referenced axial, panoramic, and cross-sectional reformatted images.

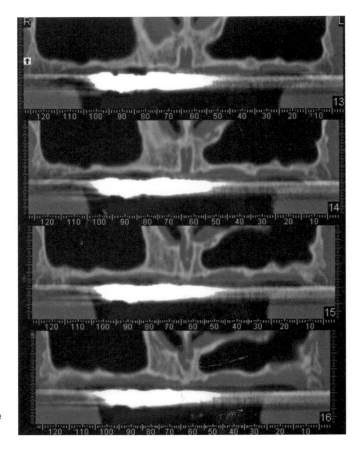

Figure 9.66 Extreme variation in maxillary sinus and incisive foramen.

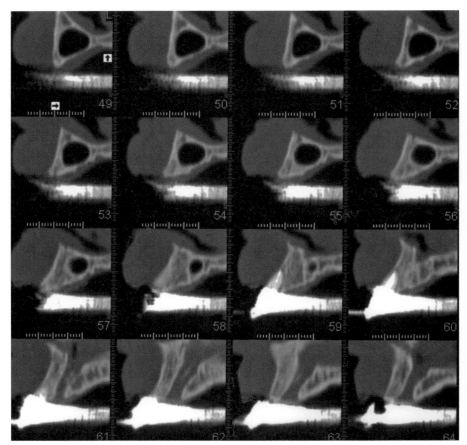

Figure 9.67 Cross-sectional reformats of Figure 9.66 showing 1.0 mm of bone between antrum and incisal canal.

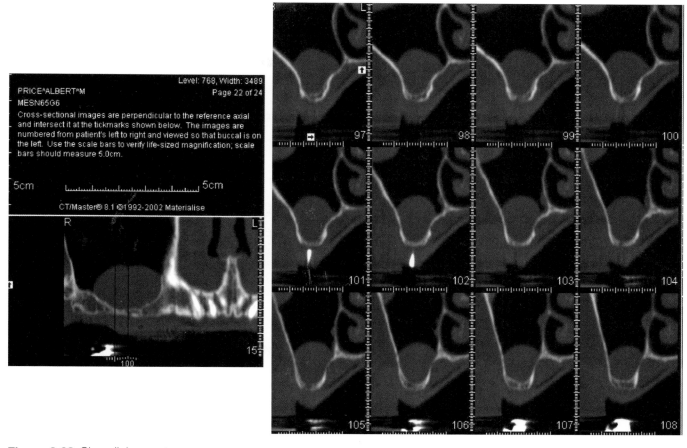

Figure 9.68 Sinus lining cyst.

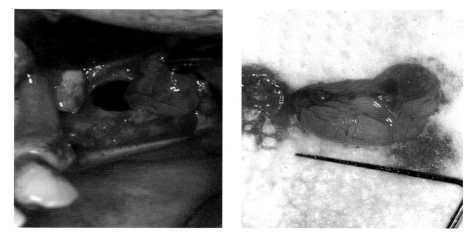

Figure 9.69 Cyst removed from patient in Figure 9.68.

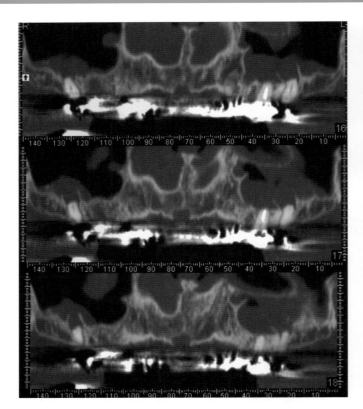

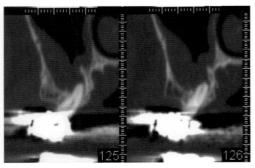

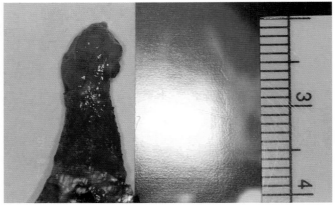

Figure 9.70 Multiple periapical leakage below sinus mucosal lining seen in CAT scan panoramic reformats; not detected on Panorex.

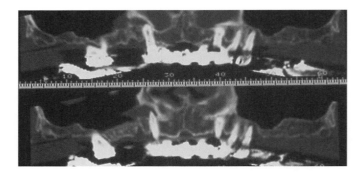

Figure 9.71 Endodontic abscess on right cuspid draining into antral mucosa was not seen on Panorex film or periapical of same area.

4. Possible donor sites for cortical bone:

    A. Chin (Figures 9.45–9.48)

    B. Ramus (Figures 9.26, 9.45)

5. Pathology

    A. Abscess in mandible (Figures 9.45, 9.46, 9.48)

    B. Abscess in maxilla (Figures 9.70, 9.71)

    C. Cyst in sinus (Figures 9.68, 9.69)

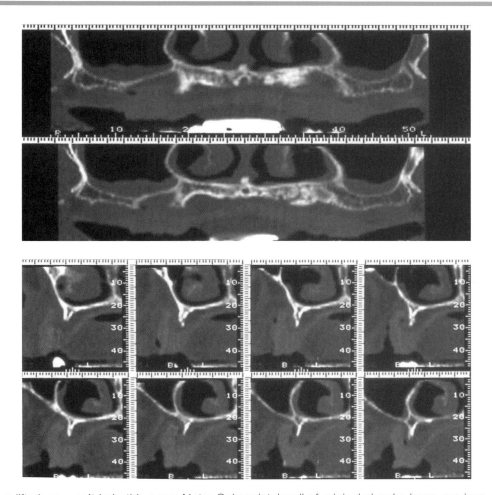

Figure 9.72 Sinus lift alone won't help this case. Note: Only palatal wall of original alveolar bone survives. It is necessary to view three dimensions possible with CAT scan reformats.

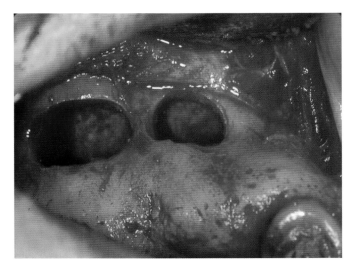

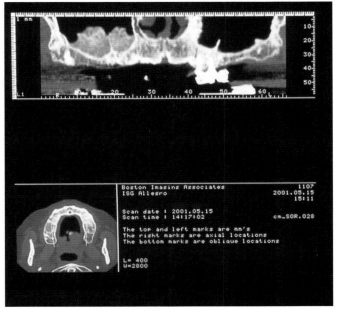

Figure 9.73 Note 15–20 mm septa negotiated with two lateral windows with aid of preoperative CAT scan. See the postoperative scan of the graft on left.

REFERENCES

Ash MM Jr. 1993. *Wheeler's Dental Anatomy, Physiology and Occlusion*, 7th ed. Philadelphia: WB Saunders.

Bartold PM, et al. 1998. *Biology of the Periodontal Connective Tissues*. Chicago: Quintessence Books.

Branemark PI, et al. 1985. *Tissue-Integrated Prostheses*. Chicago: Quintessence Books.

Caewood J, et al. 1991. Reconstructive preprosthetic surgery. *J Oral Maxillofac Surg*. 20:75–82.

Dawson PE. 2007. *Functional Occlusion*. St. Louis: Mosby.

Goldman HM, Cohen DW. 1968. *Periodontal Therapy*. 4th ed. St. Louis: CV Mosby.

Kierzenbaum AI. 2007. *Histology and Cell Biology: An Introduction to Pathology*, 2nd ed. Philadelphia: Mosby.

Misch CE. *Contemporary Implant Dentistry*. Philadelphia: Mosby.

Norton MR. 1997. An in vitro evaluation of the strength of an internal conical interface compared to a butt joint interface in implant design. *Clinical Oral Implants Research*. 8:290–98.

Price A. 2007. "The Wound-healing Process." In Dibart, S. *Practical Advanced Periodontal Surgery*. Ames, Iowa: Blackwell Munksgaard.

Price A, Su MF. 2007. "Dental Implant Placement Including the Use of Short Implants." In Dibart S. *Practical Advanced Periodontal Surgery*. Ames, Iowa: Blackwell Munksgaard.

Price AM. 1974. *Comparison of the Microvascular Disruption and Regeneration Following Full, Partial, and Modified Partial Thickness Flaps in the Alveolar Mucosa of* Macaca mulatta. D.Sc.D. Thesis, Boston University.

Rangert Bo, et al. 1989. Forces and moments on Branemark implants. *Int J Oral Maxillofac Implants*. 4:241–47.

Sonick M et al. 1994. A comparison of the accuracy of periapical, panoramic, and computerized tomographic radiographs in locating the mandibular canal. *Int J Oral Maxillofac Implants*. 9:455–60.

Chapter 10 Immediate Implants: Controversy or Risk Assessment?

Albert M. Price, DMD, DSc

Branemark's (1985) original protocol for placement and loading of endosseous implants was associated with a limited experimental design: the placement of multiple implants in anterior edentulous areas with severe alveolar bone loss to support a hybrid prosthesis. Techniques soon evolved for single tooth replacement, posterior sites, grafted sites, and even immediate implant placement. Lazarra (1989) was among the first to document that an implant might be placed into a fresh extraction socket, and since then multiple reports have confirmed long-term retention of immediate implants is possible. Consideration of immediate placement presents an added challenge in the surgical decision-making process with the potential reward of a more compressed restorative time line. The treatment planning for this technique requires review of issues familiar to any endosseous implant surgery: achieving primary stability, knowledge of the rate of bone formation and remodeling, and planning for the longer term biological, biomechanical, and aesthetic stability of the final restoration.

Biological stability under ideal conditions requires at least 1 mm of vital bone on all sides of a single implant and 2–3 mm of bone between adjacent implants and/or teeth. The principal concern is to preserve adequate vascular supply to the bone. Biomechanical stability is secured by placement of the implant platform in the center of the load-bearing surface (the occlusal table) and placement of its long axis as close as possible to a 90-degree angle relative to the plane of occlusion. This minimizes lateral stress and maximizes compressive loading of the crown-abutment-implant-bone complex (Figure 10.1). Aesthetic concerns require that the implant platform be centered on and slightly smaller than the emergence profile of the tooth form to be replaced and that the platform be placed at a suitable vertical level to allow a transition from the round head of the implant to the varied profiles of the natural tooth (Branemark et al. 1985; Ash 1993; private patient files; Figures 10.1, 10.2; see also 10.44)

Immediate and long-term biomechanical stabilization in edentulous sites requires maximum engagement of the available mineralized component of the bone at a specific site. The bone present at that site should be vital or should have the capacity to convert to vitality because osseointegration depends on interaction with live bone. Because the mineralized microarchitecture (cortical bone and trabecular arrangement) varies with each location, a continuous tactile feedback sensitivity is necessary at the time of surgery to maximize the bone's contribution to this stability (see also Chapter 9 in this text). Socket sites are defined by different microarchitecture parameters from that of the mature edentulous site, with the socket offering little stability and available cortical bone often limited to the apical one-third of the site. It is imperative to be conversant with individual site variation and to separate consideration of single-rooted teeth from multirooted teeth. (*Wheeler's* text (1993) is an excellent source for reviewing root dimensions and therefore visualization of the socket dimension) (see Figures 10.2–10.8).

Bone formation rates in socket-healing studies suggest that a minimum of 3–4 months are required before new trabeculae are mineralized enough to support minimal loads and that a 6-month wait is necessary before bone is sufficiently mineralized to withstand full functional loading. (See variation in grafted versus ungrafted sites in Figures 10.9 and 10.10; private patient files).

SOCKET SITE ANATOMY

In the maxillary anterior, the socket profile is often a single-rooted tooth placed near the buccal plate with the socket-tooth profile often penetrating the buccal of the alveolar profile (Ash 1993). This natural tooth location often results in a "washboard" effect to palpation of the buccal anatomy (Figure 10.14). The facial bone is stretched thin over the roots, and it is not uncommon to find less than 0.5 mm of bone on the buccal wall of the residual socket (Ash 1993; private patient files; Figures 10.3, 10.4, 10.11–10.13). Because the implant's biological need requires at least 1 mm of bone over the buccal surface, this requires positioning the osteotomy closer to the center of the alveolar profile. In addition, the lateral incisor site has an apical depression on the buccal (private patient files; Figures 10.14, 10.15). Given the average socket depth of 8–13 mm for incisors and bicuspids

Practical Osseous Surgery in Periodontics and Implant Dentistry, First Edition. Edited by Serge Dibart, Jean-Pierre Dibart.
© 2011 John Wiley & Sons, Inc. Published 2011 by John Wiley & Sons, Inc.

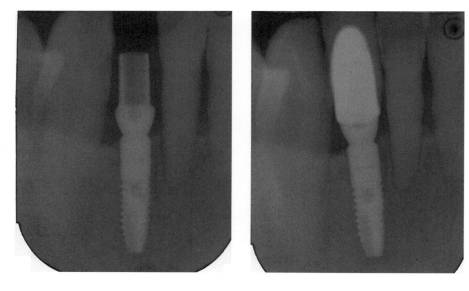

Figure 10.1 Implant placed at right angle to occlusal plane. Appropriately sized.

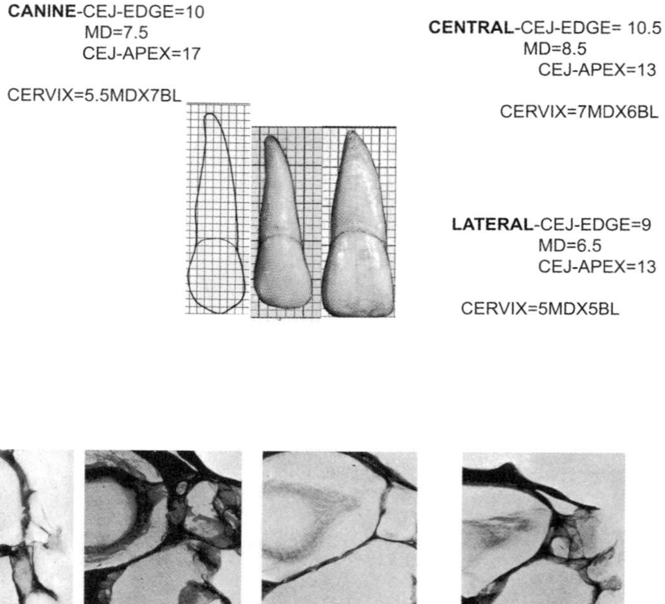

CANINE-CEJ-EDGE=10
MD=7.5
CEJ-APEX=17

CERVIX=5.5MDX7BL

CENTRAL-CEJ-EDGE= 10.5
MD=8.5
CEJ-APEX=13

CERVIX=7MDX6BL

Figure 10.2 Mean measures of tooth dimension. Abstracted from Ash, MM Jr. 1993. *Wheeler's Dental Anatomy, Physiology and Occlusion*, 7th ed. Philadelphia: WB Saunders.

LATERAL-CEJ-EDGE=9
MD=6.5
CEJ-APEX=13

CERVIX=5MDX5BL

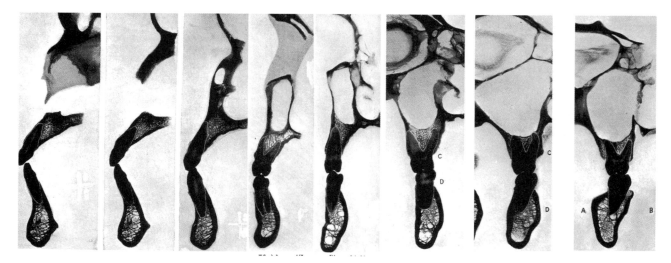

Figure 10.3 Location of roots relative to alveolar housing.

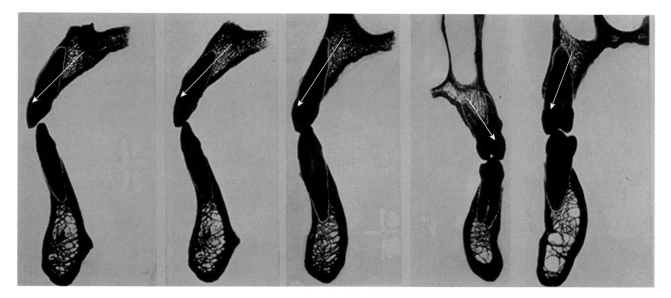

Figure 10.4 Tooth position and angulation within alveolar bone. Note: The root position buccal results in thin buccal bone. Arrows denote midline of alveolous.

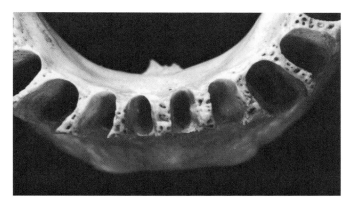

Figure 10.5 Mandibular incisors-sockets. From Ash, MM Jr. 1993. *Wheeler's Dental Anatomy, Physiology and Occlusion*, 7th ed. Philadelphia: WB Saunders.

MAND. CANINE -CEJ-EDGE= 11
MD= 7
CEJ-APEX= 16

CERVICAL= 5.5MDX7BL

MAND. CENTRAL -CEJ-EDGE=9
MD=5
CEJ-APEX=12.5

CERVICAL-3.5MDX5.3BL

MAND. LAT CEJ-EDGE=9.5
MD=5
CEJ-APEX=14

CERVICAL=4MDX5.8BL

Figure 10.6 Composite of mean measures of human teeth. Adapted from Ash, MM Jr. 1993. *Wheeler's Dental Anatomy, Physiology and Occlusion*, 7th ed. Philadelphia: WB Saunders.

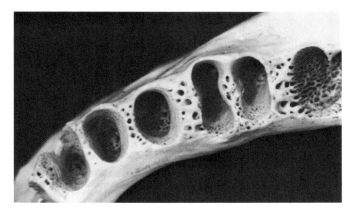

Figure 10.7 Sockets mandibular bicuspids/molars.

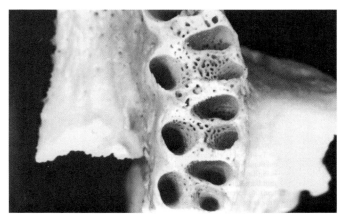

Figure 10.8 Sockets maxillary molars.

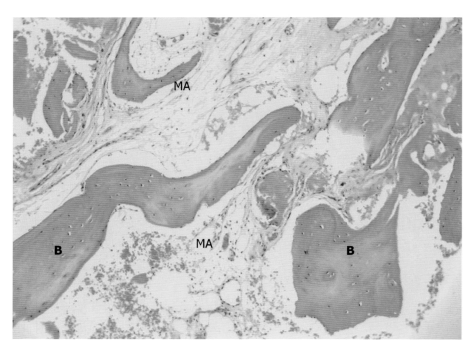

Figure 10.9 97-3-2 (6-month extraction site—no graft) Note the premolar site—thinner trabeculae alternate with a mixed fibrous-fatty marrow. (From Price and Van Dyke 2003).

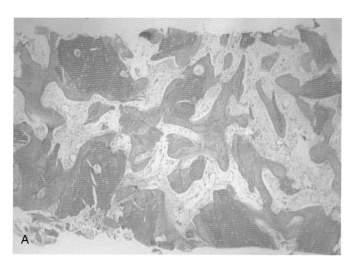
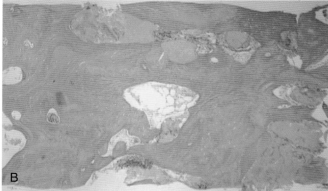

Figure 10.10 (A) #14 socket graft: Decalcified freeze-dried bone allograft (DFDBA): 5 months. (B) #5 socket graft: PUROS: 6 months. (From Histology and Cores: Caterina Venuleo, 2007.)

(15–16 mm for the cuspid) and the void presented by the socket, it is necessary to place the osteotomy against and into the palatal aspect of the socket and use a 13- to 16-mm implant to gain anchorage. This requires placement at a more protrusive angle. In the maxillary arch from central incisor to second bicuspid, the projection of the geometric center of the alveolar profile tends to parallel the palatal slope and is projected at the buccal cervical line of the natural tooth crown (private patient files; Figure 10.12). The placement of the maxillary lateral incisor requires an even more acute angle due to the incisal fossa. To compensate for the potential of buccal exposure of the "knee" presented by the subsequent abutment-implant interface, the implant needs to be driven further subcrestally and apically. The first bicuspids in the maxillary arch often have thin buccal plates and a bifurcated root (Ash 1993; private patient files; Figures 10.3, 10.4,

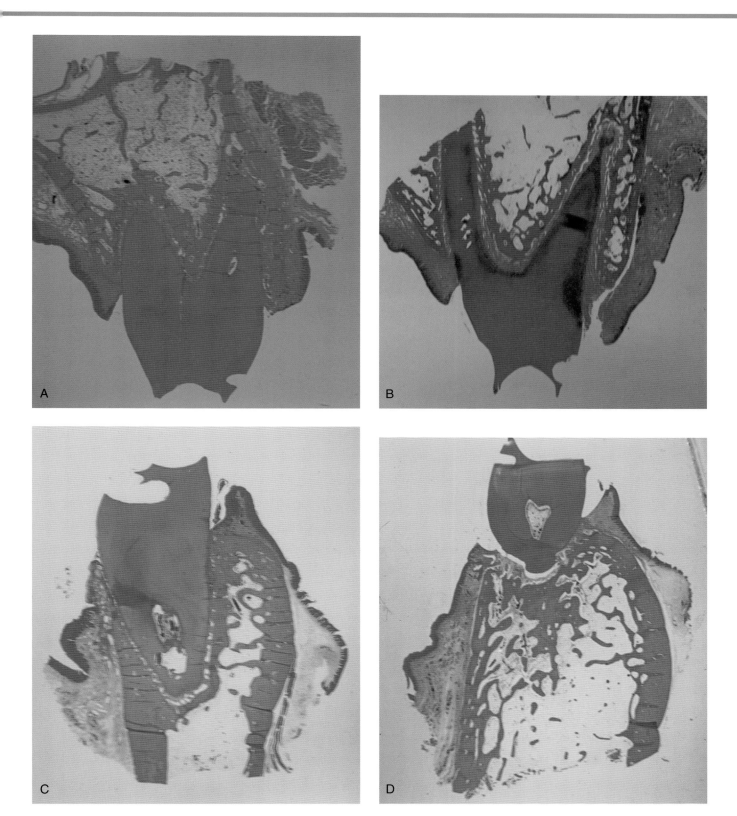

Figure 10.11 (A) Maxillary first bicuspid. (B) Maxillary first molar. (C) Mandibular first bicuspid. (D) Mandibular first molar furcation area.

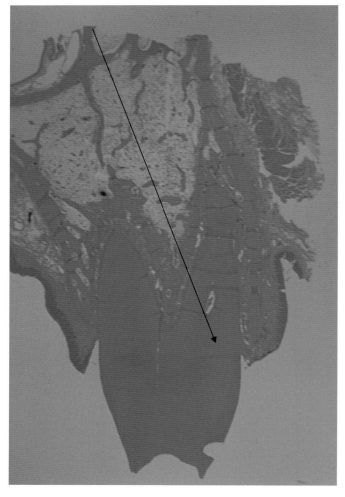

Figure 10.12 Alveolar housing projection midline maxillary first bicuspid.

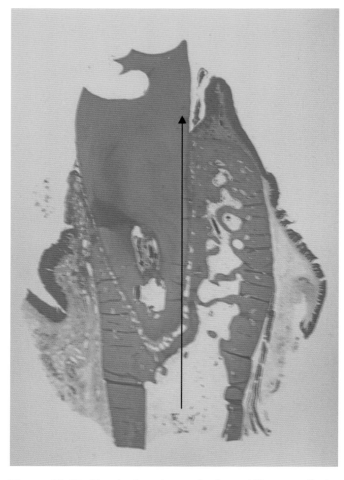

Figure 10.13 Alveolar housing projection midline mandibular first bicuspid.

10.11A, 10.12), which is further complicated by the cuspid root tipping into the site and the proximity of a buccal depression comparable to the lateral incisor, the cuspid fossa. The osteotomy for an immediate implant in this site often favors the palatal root socket and is impacted by the complex angulations of the adjacent cuspid, which forces the axis of the osteotomy to the palatal and distal.

The maxillary first molar may have intact furcal bone (Ash 1993; private patient files; Figures 10.8, 10.11B), but the maxillary sinus sometimes extends into the furcation area (private patient files; Figure 10.16). The socket walls are farther apart (7–10 mm), and sinus proximity often precludes apical extension of the osteotomy (Figures 10.16, 10.17). All of these descriptions assume that the tooth loss was from fracture or caries, with no periodontal disease–

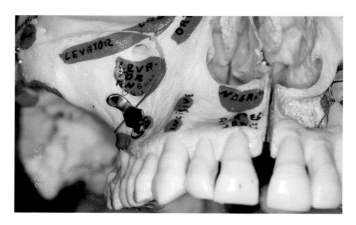

Figure 10.14 Malar process, cuspid eminence, incisal fossa.

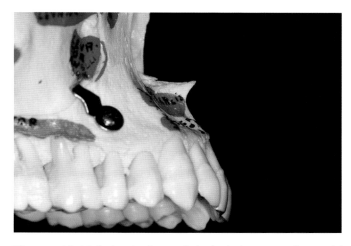

Figure 10.15 Lateral view of incisal fossa and cuspid eminence.

related bone loss or defects related to extraction trauma that would affect the postextraction socket shape.

In the mandibular arch, similar variations exist, with buccal-lingual dimensions in the anterior segment being smaller and more cortical. (Ash 1993; Figures 10.4, 10.5). The mandibular incisor's mesio-distal dimensions (5–5.5 mm) create proximity problems for the use of implants greater than 2.5 mm in diameter (Figures 10.1, 10.5). Angulations of the alveolar housing in the mandibular anterior are more centered, and the projection of the geometric center line tends to be through the buccal cusp tip (Ash 1993; Figures 10.3, 10.4). The cuspid and the first and second bicuspid are set very close to thin buccal plates, whereas most have heavy lingual cortical anatomy that is too far to the lingual to be useful (Figures 10.11C, 10.13). The first bicuspid center line tends to project through the lingual cusp tip (private patient files; Figure 10.13).

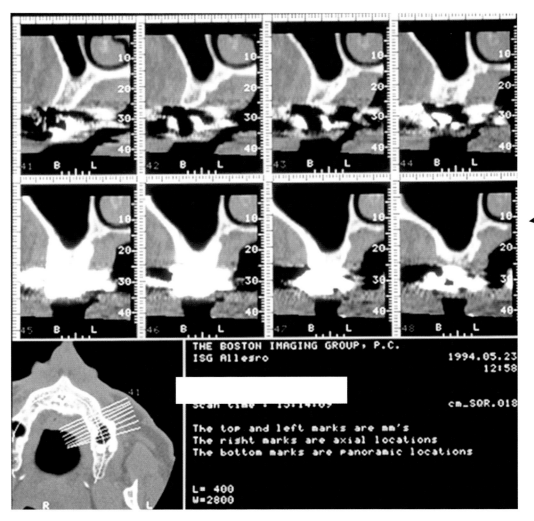

Maxillary sinus extension between first molar roots

Figure 10.16 Cross section reformats visualized by computed tomography (CT).

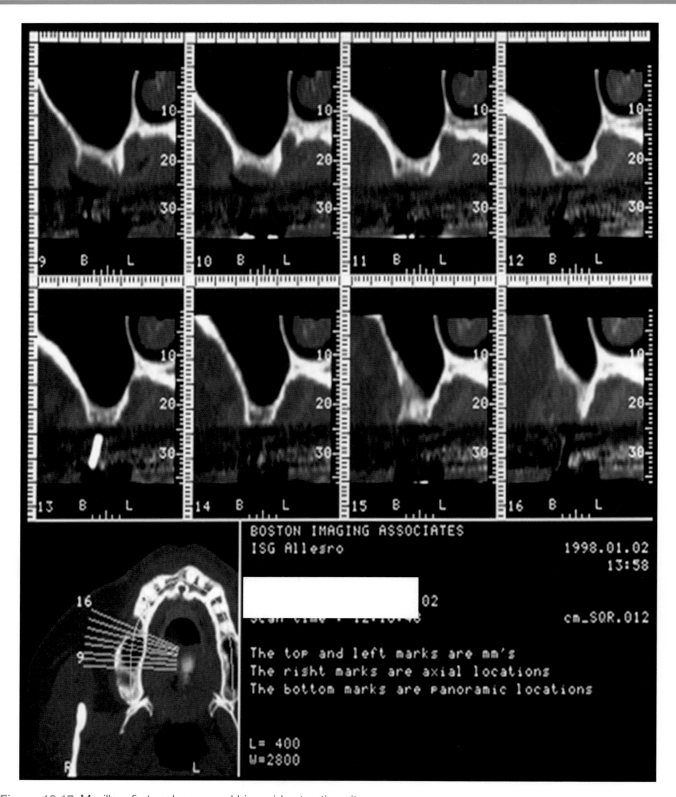

Figure 10.17 Maxillary first molar, second bicuspid extraction sites.

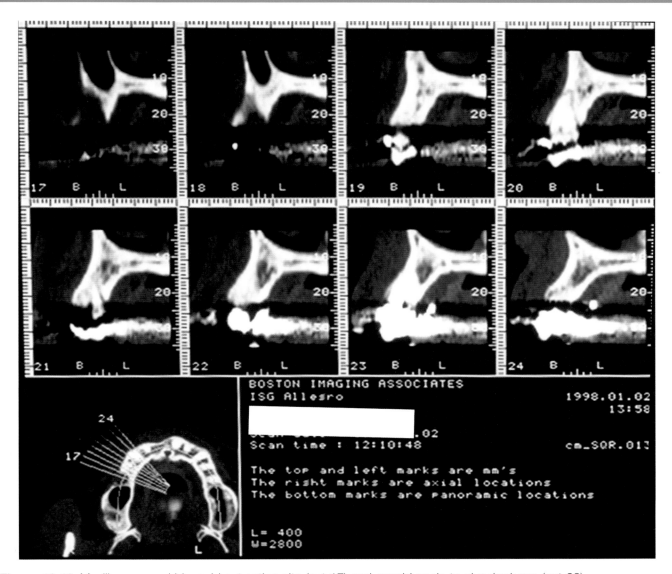

Figure 10.18 Maxillary second bicuspid extraction site (cut 17) and cuspid angle to alveolar bone (cut 23).

The mandibular molars are larger at the neck and may have useful furcation bone (Ash 1993; private patient files; Figures 10.7, 10.11D), unless periodontal disturbance has occurred.

Because there is minimal crestal engagement in the immediate implant socket to create "bicortical stabilization," (Branemark et al. 1985) tapered implants, which achieve stability by lateral compression (Price 2007), are more suited to immediate placement. The consensus among clinicians is that there is a need to allow at least 1.5–2.0 mm of space between the inner aspect of the socket wall on the buccal and the implant head to allow for some resorption during healing. Often, the residual buccal contour is thin and diminished from recession or has fractured during the trauma of extraction (private patient files; Figures 10.14, 10.15, 10.17, 10.18).

As noted in the earlier chapter on computed tomography (CT) analysis (Chapter 9), the biomechanics of implant components are best served if compression is the dominant loading effect. Because the most stable bone in the socket site is on the palatal-lingual and apical zones, the greatest biomechanical compromise of immediate implantation is a long-term increase in lateral stress. When the support platform of the implant is palatal relative to the occlusal table, there is an added cantilever effect. If apical displacement is necessary, there is an increased crown/root ratio, and if increased angulation is necessary, there is an increase in rotational forces and the potential for later aesthetic compromise related to potential exposure of the abutment-implant interface.

RISK ASSESSMENT EXAMPLES

The following cases present examples of the risk assessment involved (private patient files).

1. 70 year-old White Female with History of Endodontic Treatment, Periapical Surgical Procecure, and Recent Fistula on Buccal #10

During extraction, the root tip was elevated through the buccal plate, into the vestibular mucosa. The root tip was retrieved through a small mucosal incision. An implant was placed to the palatal with stability, and a temporary was placed. The immediate implant restoration was loose at 2 weeks, and the entire implant restoration was removed. Subsequent site augmentation revealed a weak, poorly mineralized buccal plate, which was removed. After site augmentation with particulate bone and a confining membrane, and after waiting for 4 months, a new implant was placed and successfully restored in a two-stage procedure. (Figures 10.19–10.23).

Posttreatment Review

The history of multiple endo procedures and infections should have dictated a delayed approach. Root tip displacement was sign of bone weakness.

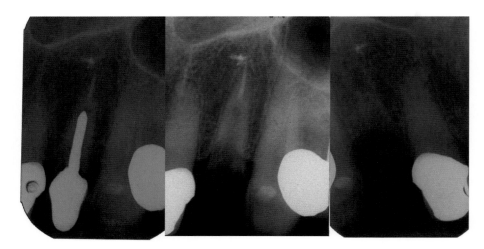

Figure 10.19 Site #10 at various time periods.

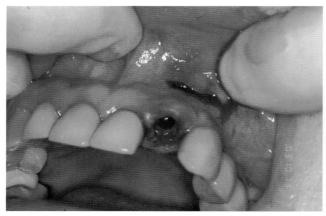
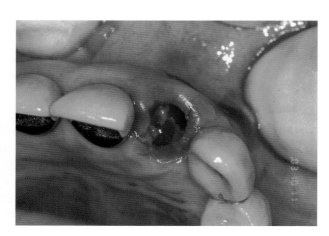

Figure 10.20 Patient 1: Extraction site #10.

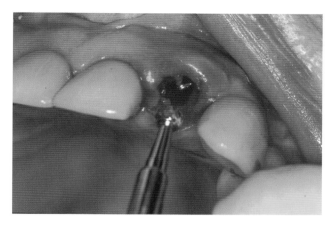

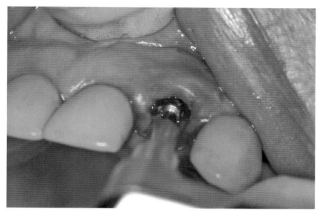

Figure 10.21 Patient 1: Use of large round bur to initiate osteotomy in palatal wall of socket.

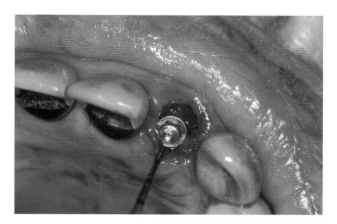

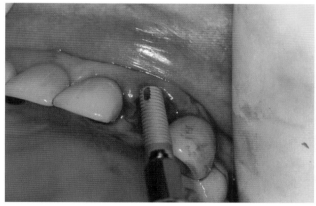

Figure 10.22 Patient 1: Check direction, insert implant. Note palatal position of guide.

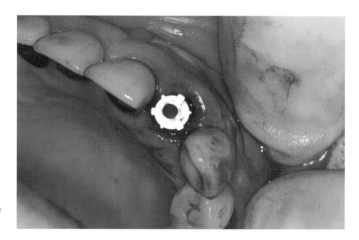

Figure 10.23 Impression transfer for final crown. Note buccal inclination.

2. 60 Year-old Black Male, Fractured Tooth #9, Which Had Also Extruded, Was Extracted and Resulted in a Short Narrow Socket Form

Good basal bone was present for primary stability. A processed temporary fabricated on immediate transfer for optimal tissue shaping was placed with minimal contact, and final restoration was delayed for 6 months. (Figures 10.24–10.30)

Posttreatment Review

Alterations in the bone related to change in tooth extrusion were favorable and increased the possibility of a positive outcome.

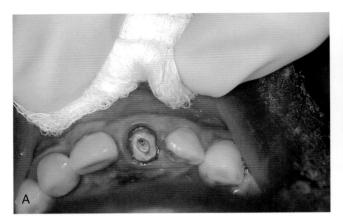
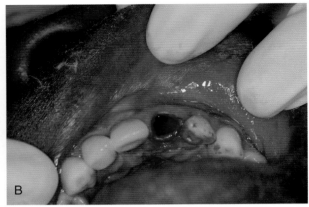

Figure 10.24 Site #9. (A) Fractured tooth. (B) Extraction socket.

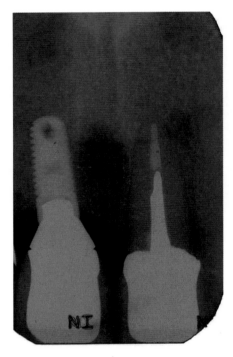
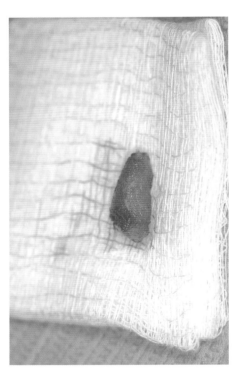

Figure 10.25 Patient 2: PA before fracture root tip.

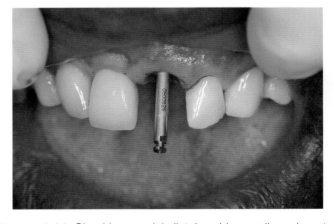
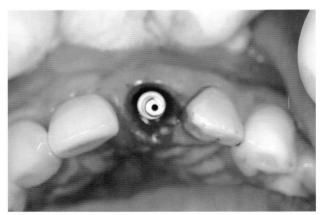

Figure 10.26 Checking mesial-distal and bucco-lingual centering.

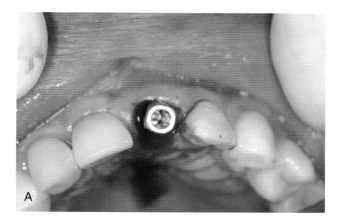

Figure 10.27 (A) Mount direction. (B) Cover screw.

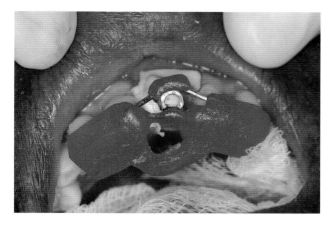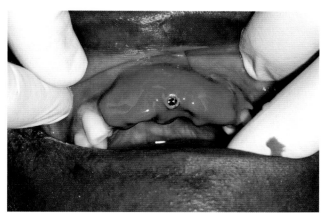

Figure 10.28 Immediate impression index.

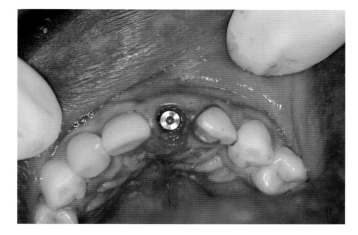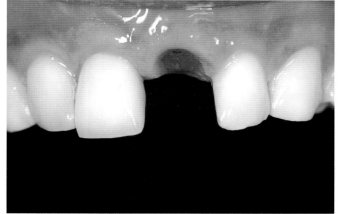

Figure 10.29 Cover screw in place, occlusal view.

Figure 10.30 Cover screw in place, buccal view.

3. 15-year-old White Female with Acute Infection at #9 Site had Immediate Implant Placed by Dentist

At abutment phase and after the temporary was placed, the patient was referred for "repair with a gingival graft." Clinical examination revealed the buccal profile of implant and crown protruded beyond normal adjacent contours and that 7–8 mm of buccal threads were exposed through bone. Soft tissue cover on the buccal was mucosal in nature and very thin. Periapical radiograph showed reasonable mesio-distal placement but overly large root form implant. CT reformats showed a 15-mm implant through the nasal floor (Figure 10.41B) and within the previous socket (which itself was outside the normal alveolar housing). The implant (Figure 10.41A) was too large and too close to the crest to allow development of an appropriate emergence profile. Treatment required removal of the previous implant and a two-phase graft procedure to recover soft and hard tissue mass, followed by replacement with a 4 × 13 mm implant placed slightly apical to crest to allow emergence of profile aesthetics. (Figures 10.31–10.44)

Posttreatment Review

Several errors in judgment were made that increased the risk of failure. Acute infection at time of extraction led to poor soft tissue healing. Inappropriate sizing led to poor restorative outcome. Failure to engage and penetrate the palatal wall of the socket led to buccal displacement placement and subsequent loss of buccal plate and recession.

Experience in delayed placement has shown that an extraction socket can be grafted and, after waiting 3 months, allows predictable implant placement in optimal three-dimensional positions and angulation. After a further conservative 3-month wait, the abutment and then final restoration can be placed with optimal control of aesthetics. It is difficult to justify the potential compromises and risks inherent in immediate placement unless there is some change in the local anatomy that makes it favorable (Case 2). There are cases where the socket is shortened (by extrusion or resorption) or can be obliterated

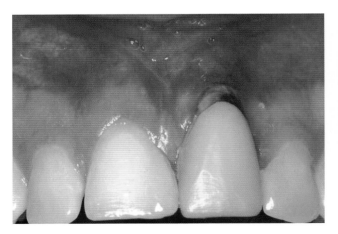

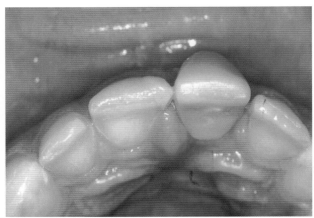

Figure 10.31 Immediate implant #9. 15-year-old white female with temporary in place after 6 months' healing. Patient referred from another practice for gingival graft.

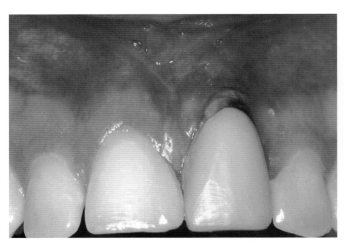

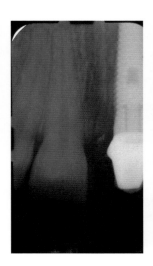

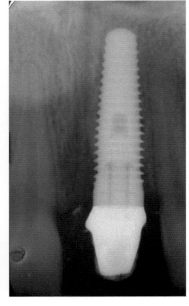

Figure 10.32 The picture shows recession on tooth #9 (the maxillary left central). The recession was related to poor placement of an oversized implant which resulted in 7- to 8-mm dehiscence on the buccal.

Figure 10.33 Periapical radiograph of original implant.

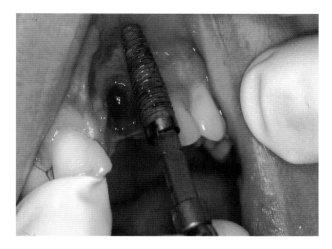

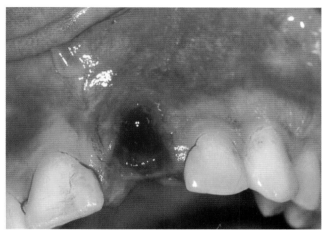

Figure 10.34 Implant removal.

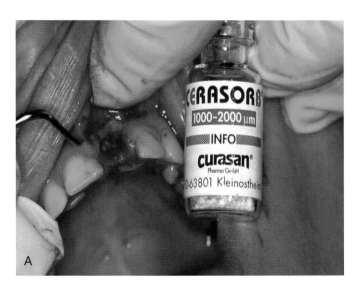

A

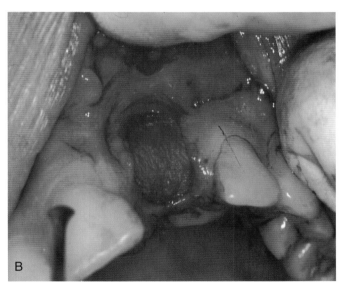

B

Figure 10.35 Tri-calcium phosphate (TCP). (A) Graft in place. (B) Five-month collagen membrane.

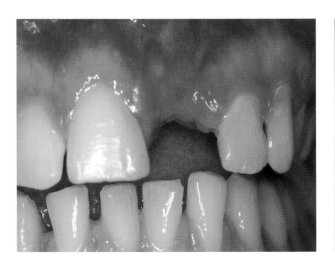

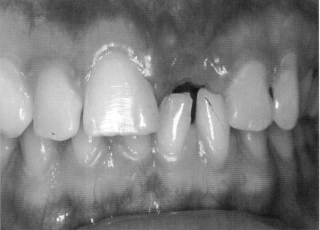

Figure 10.36 Four months post-TCP graft—soft tissue regenerated.

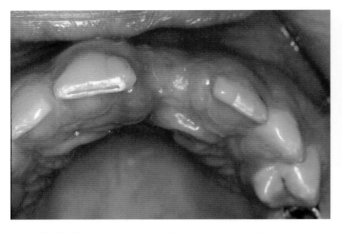
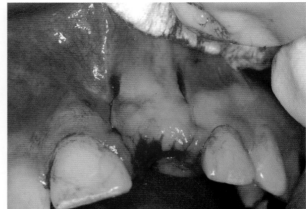

Figure 10.37 Occlusal view soft tissue regeneration.

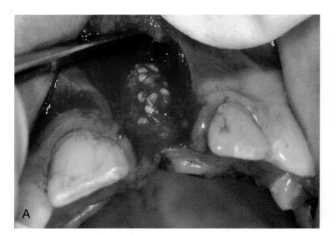
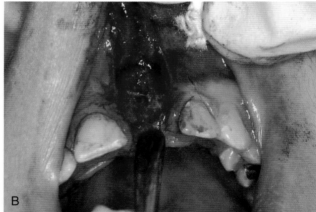

Figure 10.38 (A) Expose TCP graft at 2 months, fibrous healing. (B) Remove top graft.

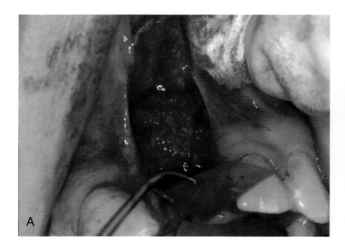
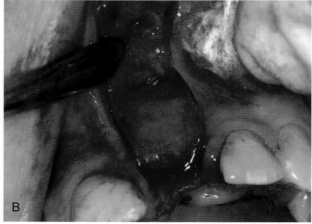

Figure 10.39 (A) Replace TCP with irradiated vertebral bone. (B) Cover with laminar bone.

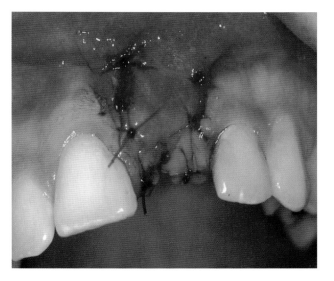
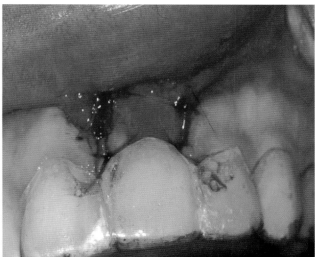

Figure 10.40 Suture for primary closure.

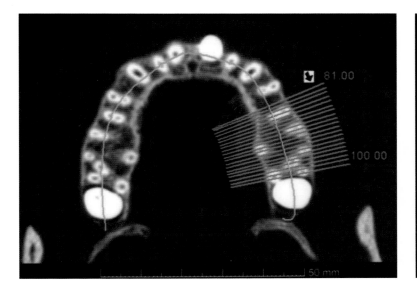
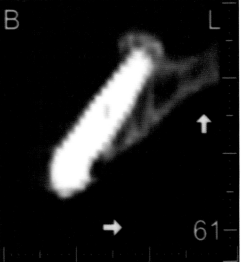

Figure 10.41 Note difference in root diameter #8 natural tooth root vs. #9 Implant

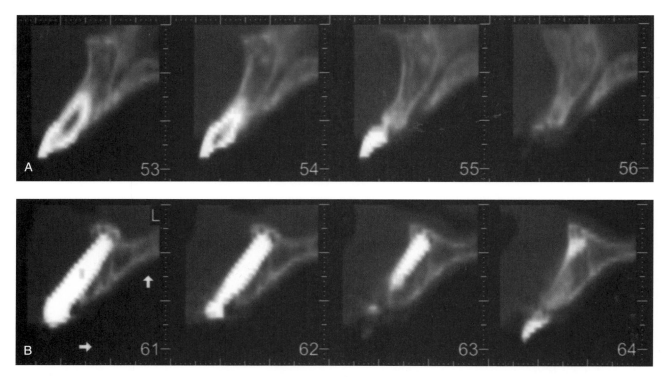

Figure 10.42 (A) #8 Natural tooth profile and location in alveolar housing. (B) #9 Oversized implant and location within alveolar housing.

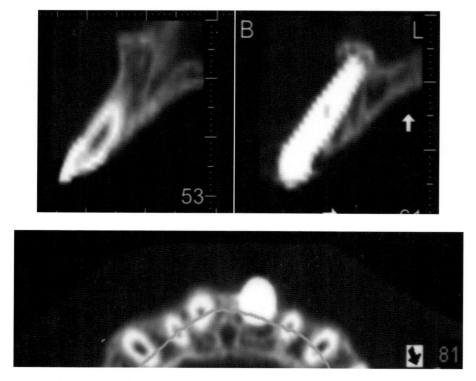

Figure 10.43 Comparison of natural tooth profile to original implant.

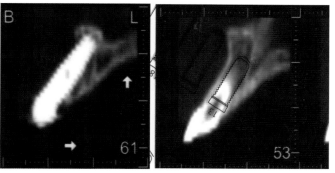

APICAL TIP
IN FLOOR
INFRINGES
ON INCISAL
FORAMEN
TOO CLOSE
TO BUCCAL
PLATE

COMPARISON ORIGINAL IMPLANT TO REPLACEMENT IMPLANT

5X15MM   4.3MMX13

Figure 10.44 If cervical diameter of tooth is 6–7 mm and fills the crestal profile, then 1 mm bone required on buccal and palatal dictates 4- to 4.5-mm implant.

by the osteotomy (maxillary lateral with minimal incisal fossa above, peg lateral or mandibular lateral, or small first bicuspid). If the risk can be minimized, then an immediate implant is a good choice. If it is calculated that the risk is more than a 5% increase in failure, then the surgeon is obligated to err on the side of caution and choose the more predictable delayed approach.

REFERENCES

Ash MM Jr. 1993. *Wheeler's Dental Anatomy, Physiology and Occlusion*, 7th ed. Philadelphia: WB Saunders.

Branemark PI, et al. 1985. *Tissue-Integrated Prostheses*. Chicago: Quintessence Books.

Brunswig JD. 1988. Biomaterials and biomechanics in dental implant design. *Int J Oral Max Impl*. 3:85–97.

Lazzara R. 1989. Immediate implant placement into surgical extraction sites: Surgical and restorative advantage. *Int J Perio Restor Dent*. 9:332–43.

Price A. 2007. The Wound-healing Process. In Dibart S. *Practical Advanced Periodontal Surgery*. Ames, Iowa: Blackwell Munksgaard.

Price A, Su MF. 2007. Dental Implant Placement Including the Use of Short Implants. In Dibart S. *Practical Advanced Periodontal Surgery*. Ames, Iowa: Blackwell Munksgaard.

Price A, Van Dyke T. 2003. Poster presentation at the International Association of Dental Research (IADR), Goteborg, Sweden.

Chapter 11 Atraumatic Piezosurgical Extractions: A Solution for Bone Preservation

Yves Macia, DDS, Francis Louise, DDS

HISTORICAL REVIEW

Pioneering work using ultrasonic devices for bone surgery began more than 30 years ago with Horton et al. (1975), shortly followed by Aro et al. (1981). Other practitioners, such as Vercellotti (2005), subsequently widened the field of application for piezosurgical instruments, and they developed considerably to extend their use to all types of buccal bone surgery. Improved control of powers and frequencies came hand in hand with new generations of tips, increasingly better adapted to clinical requirements. Today's powers and frequencies (between 28 and 36 kHz) are optimal and are electronically controlled to adapt to different types of tissues encountered, allowing the practitioner to cut delicately and precisely. With piezosurgery, the timeworn image of oral surgeons with their hand pieces and bone scissors gives way to that of artists with paintbrushes.

Although preservation of bone tissue is one of the most important issues in modern dentistry, traumatic extractions still account for much of the bone losses that preclude implants and are simply no longer acceptable in aesthetic terms. In all complicated extraction cases, the Piezotome proves its worth as the instrument best adapted to limiting the destruction of bone tissue.

PIEZOSURGERY COMPARED WITH STANDARD TECHNIQUE

The action of piezoelectrical tips has still not been clearly established, but it is probably applied to the three tissue structures concerned—bone, ligament, and tooth—with varying degrees of efficiency. The practitioner can easily direct this action, however, by exercising a light pressure toward the tooth rather than the bone. Piezoelectrical tips operate more effectively on hard tissue than on soft, where their efficiency diminishes considerably (Louise and Macia 2009). Indeed, soft tissues are generally pushed back rather than sectioned. Because of this, literally caught between a rock and a hard place—the bone and the cementum—and unable to escape the vibratory action of the tip, the ligament

is mechanically destructured. By applying light pressure toward the tooth, the practitioner allows the tip to glide over the bone and focus its action on the tooth, thus preserving the precious bone tissue.

One of the major advantages of tips is their shape. Combined with the oscillatory movement imparted by the ceramic pellets in the hand piece, this design allows the surgeon to use both the tip and the edges of these ultrasonic scalpels (Figure 11.1.) Long and slim, they can be slipped into spaces where not even a small-diameter drill could be used without collateral damage (Figure 11.2). In order to preserve bone, these inserts must follow the root as closely as possible, whatever its face and whatever the angular formation of the tooth. To facilitate this contact, the cutting faces of tips are now produced with different angulations to meet all situations (Figures 11.3–11.9).

A trench up to 8 or 9 mm deep is cut around the tooth. This point of access allows the practitioner to slide a thin manual instrument down between the root and the bone. Because the long, narrow nature of the trench gives the instrument the necessary grip, only a slight rotational movement is required to create mobility and allow the avulsion of the tooth. The microvibrations transmitted by the tip gripped in this narrow sheath will oscillate toward the hardest tissue—the tooth itself—and thus help dissociate it from the bone.

In order to observe the mechanical effect of the piezoelectrical tips on both bone and tooth, we used ultrasonic tips on a dried human jawbone (Figures 11.10–11.22). With neither organic matter nor hydration, both tissues were very hard, noncompressible, and thus highly reactive to ultrasound. A straight tip was used for the lingual side, with an angled tip to the right and another angled insert to the left for all four angles. They were introduced to a depth of 5–6 mm, slightly angled toward the tooth. So as not to destroy the fine cortical bone, the buccal side was barely opened. This compact vestibular bone is often very fine and must be protected from instruments during extractions. Once the encircling trench was completed, the tooth was easily

Practical Osseous Surgery in Periodontics and Implant Dentistry, First Edition. Edited by Serge Dibart, Jean-Pierre Dibart.

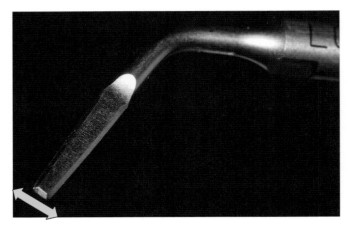

Figure 11.1 Long and slim (working head 9mm, thickness 0.5mm), the Satelec extraction tip is easily slipped between root and bone, facilitating access toward fractured roots (the double yellow arrow matches the tip motion).

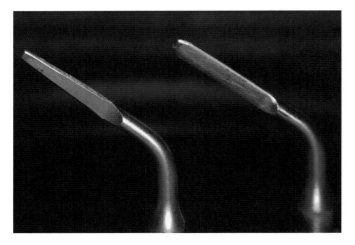

Figure 11.2 With their longitudinal oscillation, these (Satelec) tips can be used both along their edges and at the tip. Vibration amplitude is between 30 and 60μm. The working head is 9mm long and only 0.5mm thick.

extracted. We noted that except for a little chip on the vestibular rim, the socket was almost wholly preserved, notwithstanding the fragility of such dry, brittle bone. The crest of the socket was slightly enlarged to a height of around 1–2mm and to a width corresponding to the thickness of the inserts (0.5mm). This very minimal bone loss is highly favorable in support of the concept of immediate extraction/implant. Examination of the extracted tooth showed that, in order to preserve the bone, the trench had cut into the dental tissue. Sizeable marks, observed on the proximal and lingual sides, bore witness to the highly effective action of the ultrasonic tips. The pressure applied toward the tooth should thus be moderated to avoid weakening the root and running the risk of a fracture during the avulsion.

Piezoelectrical tips do have an abrasive effect, however slight, on bone as a hard tissue. This is thus an inconvenience with respect to standard techniques, which do not destroy bone if successfully applied in moderately difficult extraction cases. In situations were action on the bone is necessary to extract the tooth, however, piezoelectrical tips are better suited, for the osteotomy is very delicate, easily controlled, and considerably less aggressive for the bony tissue.

In a study on dogs, Vercellotti et al. (2005) compared bone cicatrisation following osteotomy with diamond burs, carbide burs, and piezoelectrical tips. The rate of postoperative wound healing was compared at 14, 28, and 56 days. In comparison with baseline measurements, they noted that at 14 days the sites operated on with diamond or carbide burs had lost bone, whereas those treated with piezoelectrical inserts had gained bone. By day 28, all three surgical sites demonstrated increased bone level. By day 56, on the other hand, those sites treated with the diamond or carbide burs showed bone loss, whereas the piezosurgical sites evidenced bone gain. The authors concluded that osseous repair and remodeling were more favorable with piezosurgery than with standard burs when surgical osteotomy and osteoplasty procedures were performed. Thus, in this animal model, osseous cicatrisation is continuous and quantitatively better with piezosurgery. If the same applies for humans, piezosurgical operations would seem highly indicated for immediate extraction/implant procedures.

In a histomorphometric evaluation, Berengo and colleagues (2006) compared different methods of harvesting bone sections. Using nine methods, ten bone harvests were taken from the retromolar bone in the course of extractions of embedded wisdom teeth. The histological preparations were examined with microphotography and histomorphometric analysis to evaluate particle size, percentages of vital bone, and numbers of osteocytes per unit of surface area. The study indicated that whereas harvested bone was 100% nonvital, with a complete absence of osteocytes, in those specimens harvested with burs, the percentage of nonvital bone was intermediate, with a low number of cells, in the specimens harvested using piezosurgery.

These studies show that when piezosurgical instruments are used for osteotomies rather than burs, osseous cicatrisation is more extensive and of better quality. Where osteotomy is indicated, piezoelectrical tips should be preferred, notably in cases where the extraction is followed by an implant.

INDICATIONS

The piezoelectric ultrasonic generator should not be used systematically for extractions. It should correspond to precise indications calling for the advantages it offers in situations

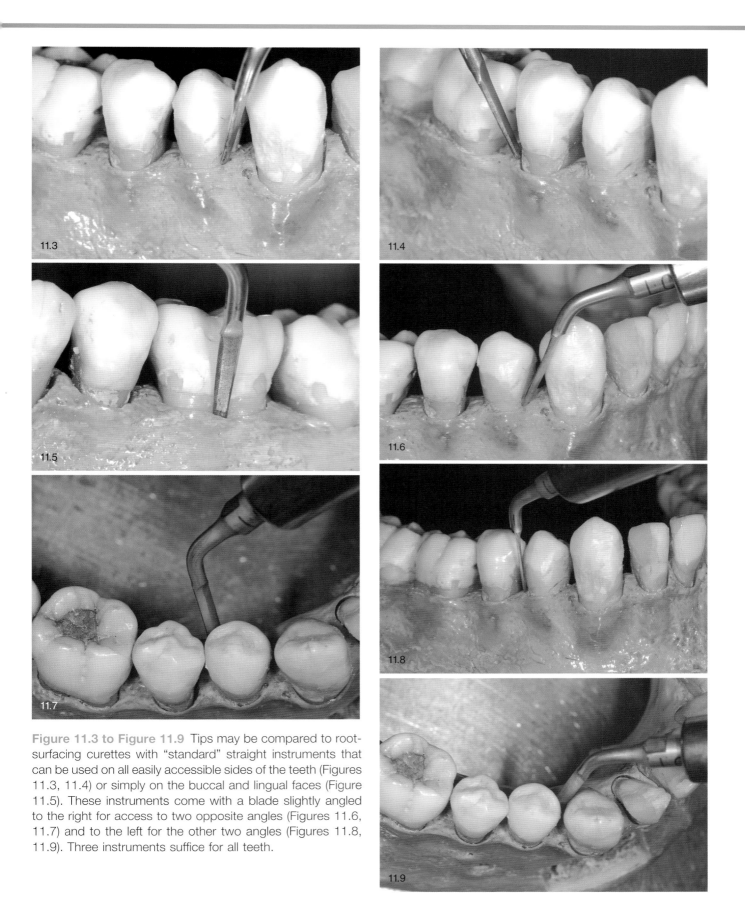

Figure 11.3 to Figure 11.9 Tips may be compared to root-surfacing curettes with "standard" straight instruments that can be used on all easily accessible sides of the teeth (Figures 11.3, 11.4) or simply on the buccal and lingual faces (Figure 11.5). These instruments come with a blade slightly angled to the right for access to two opposite angles (Figures 11.6, 11.7) and to the left for the other two angles (Figures 11.8, 11.9). Three instruments suffice for all teeth.

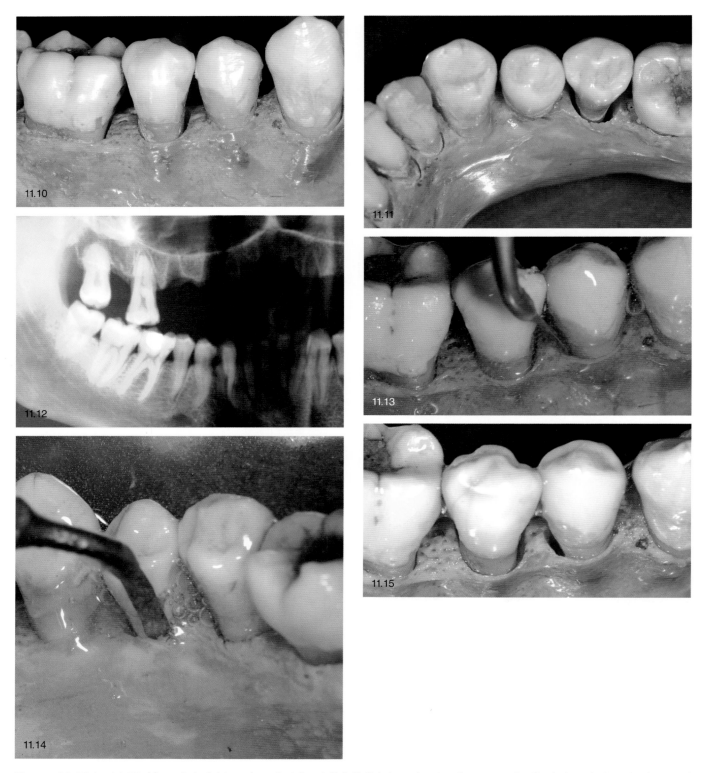

Figure 11.10 to 11.22 Use of straight and angled tips LC 2 R & L to extract a first premolar firmly bonded to the bone of a dry skull (Figures 11.10–11.14). By tilting the tip slightly (Figure 11.15), the cleavage zone is cut into the tooth itself. A trench is cut right round the tooth, except for the buccal side (Figure 11.16). Once the tooth is loosened, it is withdrawn (Figure 11.17), showing that the ultrasonic action was focused essentially on the root (Figure 11.18), safeguarding the alveolar bone socket. The only remaining traces are a slight buccal nick (yellow arrow) and a small surrounding trench of 1 to 2 mm (red arrow) (Figures 11.19–11.22).

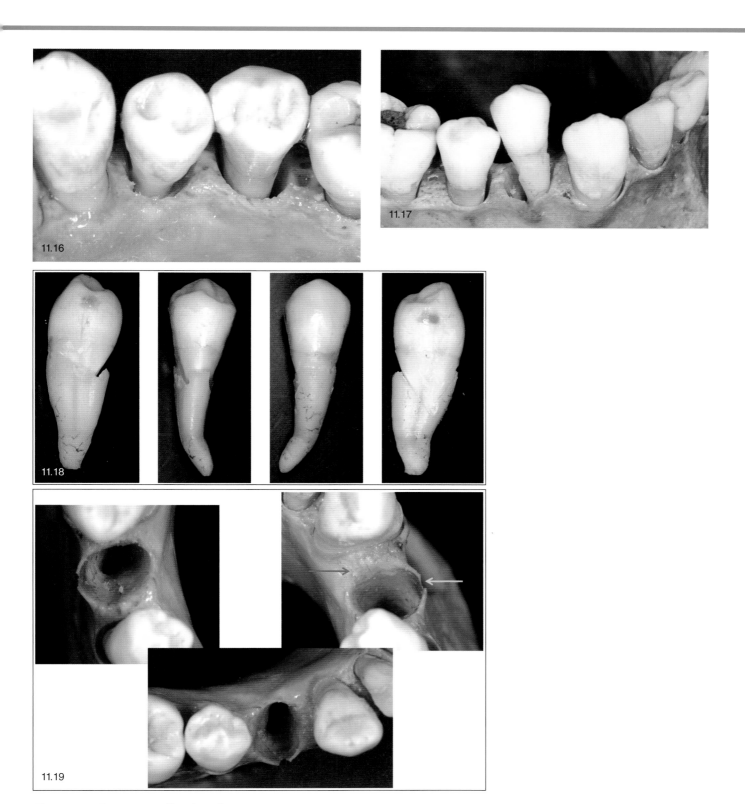

Figure 11.10 to 11.22 *Continued*

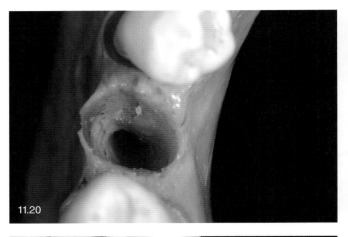

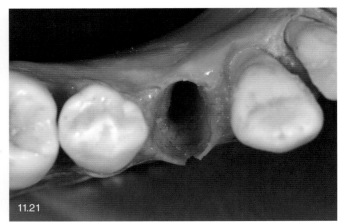

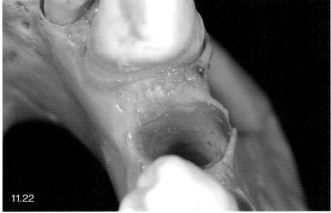

Figure 11.10 to 11.22 *Continued*

where conservation of alveolar bone is essential or in certain difficult extraction cases. The three main reasons justifying recourse to piezosurgery are (1) unavoidable osteotomy, (2) unavoidable sectioning of a tooth, and (3) problematic access.

Unavoidable Osteotomy

To free an impacted or ankylosed tooth, ultrasonic surgery minimizes bone loss and preserves bone vitality.

An impacted tooth situation is illustrated by a patient whose loose milk canine had to be extracted and replaced with an implant (Figures 11.23–11.35). The scan showed a deeply impacted canine whose extraction was necessary to make way for an implant. After opening a full-thickness flap in the palate, an osteotomy was undertaken to free the crown of the tooth. Care was taken during the osteotomy to avoid the roots of the lateral incisor and of the first premolar and to conserve as much bone as possible for an immediate implant. Most of the osteotomy was performed with a tip originally designed to collect bone chips (Satelec BS6), which handled the spadework rapidly and remained inactive when in contact with the tooth. A more delicate phase was then undertaken

with a diamond tip (Satelec SL2) to free the crown of the tooth and the top of the root. Before separating the crown from the root, it is useful to loosen the tooth slightly with a small elevator to facilitate the subsequent avulsion of the root. The canine was sectioned diagonally with the odontotomy insert (Satelec Ninja), penetration being controlled by graduations every 3 mm. The two sections of the tooth were then easily withdrawn. Bone deterioration being kept to a minimum, it was possible to install an implant (Nobel Ti Unit 4x13) immediately after the avulsion of the milk tooth. Bone insufficiencies around one side of the fixture were filled with biomaterials (Bio-Oss). Since the implant was securely screwed into the bone (32 N/cm²), a temporary implant-supported tooth was created to complete the session.

Ankylosed or impacted in dense bone, certain teeth resist all attempts to loosen them. In such cases, the tooth can easily fracture at root level, especially if weakened by decay or deprived of elasticity through previous devitalization. Recourse to a rotary instrument around the root or to alveolectomy generally results in considerable and often definitive bone loss. For Dahlin et al. (1989), peri-implantory postsurgical crestal bone loss regenerates naturally if it does not exceed

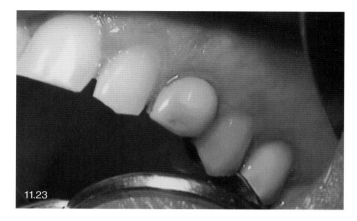

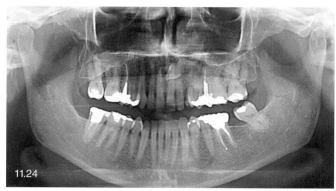

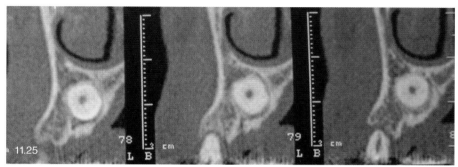

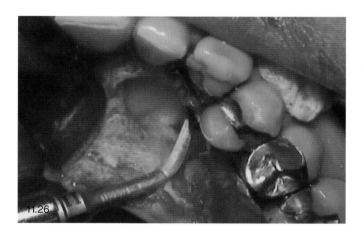

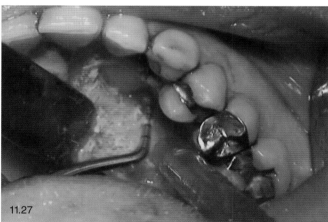

Figure 11.23 to Figure 11.33 Extraction of an impacted canine. The milk canine is present and mobile (Figure 11.23), but the position of the impacted tooth keeps us from placing an implant (Figures 11.24, 11.25). The bone clearing is performed with two tips, BS6 and SL2 (Satelec[T]) (Figures 11.26, 11.27) to free the crown of the tooth. The crown is separate from the root by odontotomy tip (Ninja[T]) (Figure 11.28). Thus crown and root can be easily withdrawn (Figures 11.29–31). The remaining bone is adequate for an immediate implant placement (Nobel Ti Unit 4x13) (Figure 11.32). Bone insufficiencies are filled with biomaterials (Bio-Oss). Since the implant was securely screwed into the bone (32 N/cm^2), the implant is loaded by a temporary (Figure 11.33).

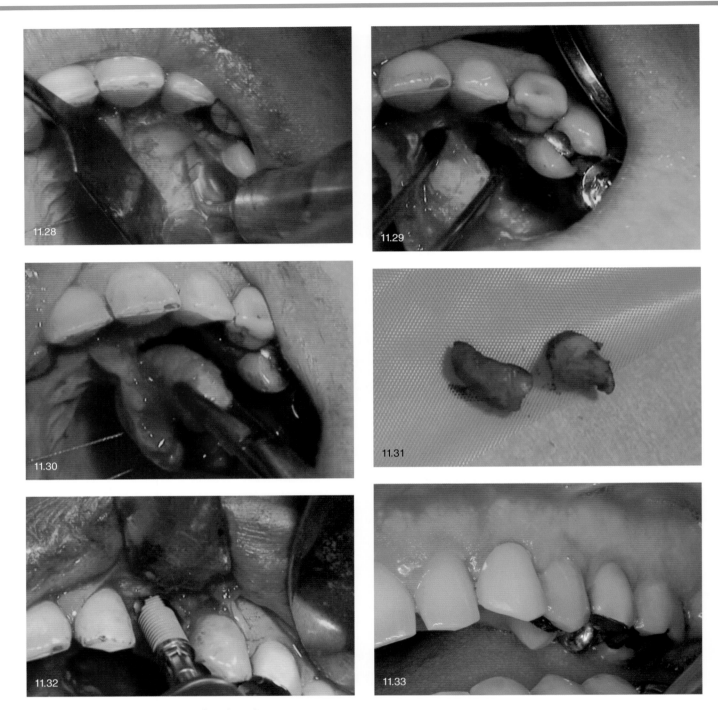

Figure 11.23 to Figure 11.33 *Continued*

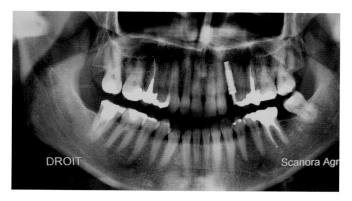

Figure 11.34 Panoramic radiograph showing the implant fixture replacing tooth #11.

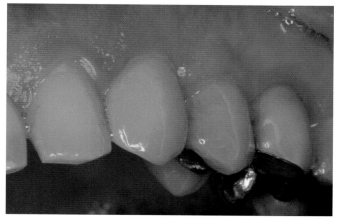

Figure 11.35 Final restoration of tooth # 11.

a certain size, the "critical size defect." For Covani et al. (2007), this peripheral space must be less than 2 mm. It is also important to preserve the continuity of the bone surrounding the implant and notably not to lose the buccal bony table in an alveolectomy. In cases where an implant is envisaged, it is thus preferable to use piezoelectrical tips rather than rotary instruments to limit and to direct the bone loss around the implant site. Use of piezoelectrical tips allows practitioners to select the faces on which to focus their action and those they wish to protect during the extraction. The bone covering the buccal sides is often fine, for example, and in such cases practitioners may decide to use tips only on the proximal and lingual sides, thereby protecting the buccal cortex.

This ankylosed case (Figures 11.36–11.47) illustrates the attempted extraction of a maxillary incisor that resulted in a fracture at the level of the alveolar rim. The tooth presented a buccal crack that led to the onset of bone loss. In order to contain this loss, and because implants were envisaged, we decided to use piezoelectrical tips and to preserve the buccal face. After using different tips to a depth of 5–6 mm, a trench of about 0.5 mm was created around the root to allow a fine elevator to be applied, facilitating luxation of the tooth without bone loss.

The piezoelectric method can also be used to remove an implant. It offers the same advantages as it does for extractions, that is, preservation of bone and protection of delicate cavity walls. Use of a reverse-torque instrument to remove an osteointegrated implant involves the risk of an uncontrollable bone fracture, especially in cases where the surrounding bone is delicate. Similarly, use of a trephine presents the serious disadvantages of (1) an oversized hole with respect to the diameter of the implant and (2) a peripheral cut all around the implant with no means of preserving any cavity wall that may be too fine. Using the implant as a support, the

tip cuts a cleavage zone of 0.5 mm to allow access for a fine instrument to loosen the implant. These situations, which formerly led to major tissue loss requiring a subsequent bone graft, can now be handled piezosurgically with the attendant advantages of minimal bone loss and four cavity walls that can regenerate themselves once filled with bone substitute (Figures 11.48–11.54).

Sectioning of a Tooth

Use of fine-cutting tips allows precise sectioning of dental tissue without modification of surrounding structures. These tips can be used both for root amputations and for cases where the tooth has to be sectioned to allow its extraction (Figures 11.55–11.64).

It may be noted that not all manufacturers of piezosurgical equipment supply these tips.

Problematic Access

Piezosurgical extraction instruments are generally slim and long (see Figure 11.1), designed to slip along the ligament between the roots and the bone and allowing them access to awkward sites such as an apex at the bottom of an alveolar socket.

The extraction of a root under a bridge poses problems of access, illustrated in the treatment of this patient with a recent full bridge with caries at the level of the first upper left premolar (Figures 11.65–11.79). The patient wished to keep her bridge and requested an extraction with the least possible aesthetic impact. A full-thickness flap was raised without releasing incisions. To separate the crown from the root, we used a tip capable of sectioning dental tissue (Satelec Ninja). The design of this tip, notably its slimness and the fact that only its toothed sides are active (the flat sides remain passive), enabled us to perform a perfectly controlled

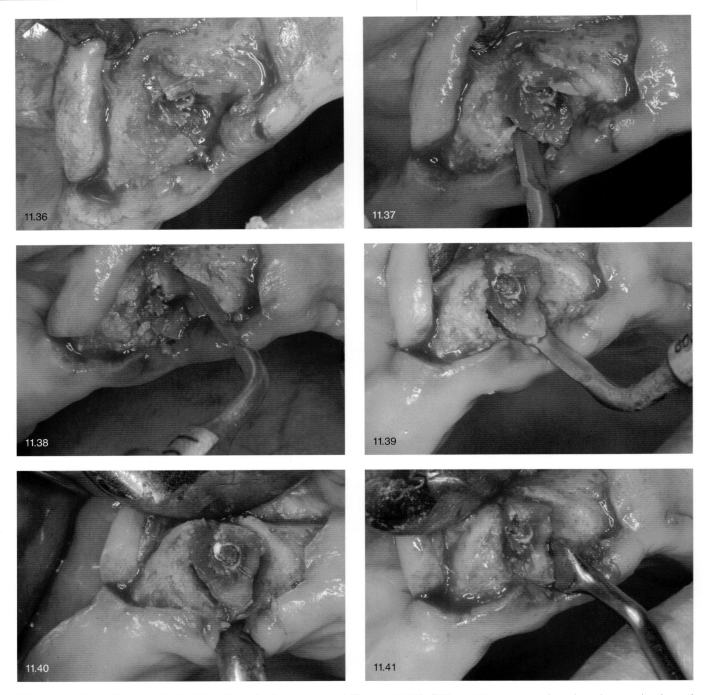

Figure 11.36 to Figure 11.46 Extraction of a fractured root (Figure 11.36). Different tips are used against the proximals and palatal sides (Figures 11.37–11.39). An encircling trench is realized around the root except, the buccal side of the tooth (Figure 11.40), allowing a thin instrument to slide in for an easy avulsion (Figures 11.41, 11.42). The bone socket is well preserved (Figure 11.43). Ten days later the soft and hard tissues show an optimal healing (Figure 11.44) for the placement of an implant (Figure 11.45). The little buccal bone insufficiencies are filled by the collected bone from the drilling (Figure 11.46).

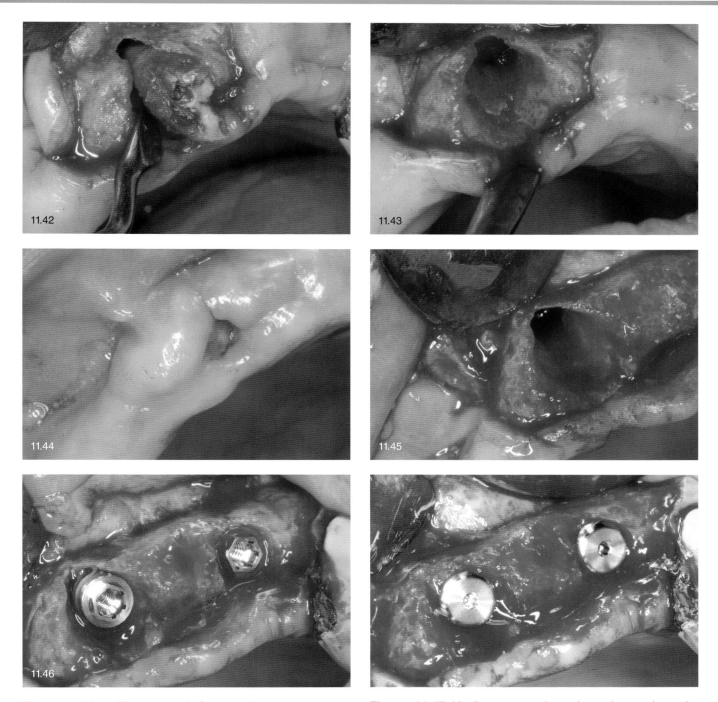

11.42

11.43

11.44

11.45

11.46

Figure 11.36 to Figure 11.46 *Continued*

Figure 11.47 Healing screws have been inserted on the implants.

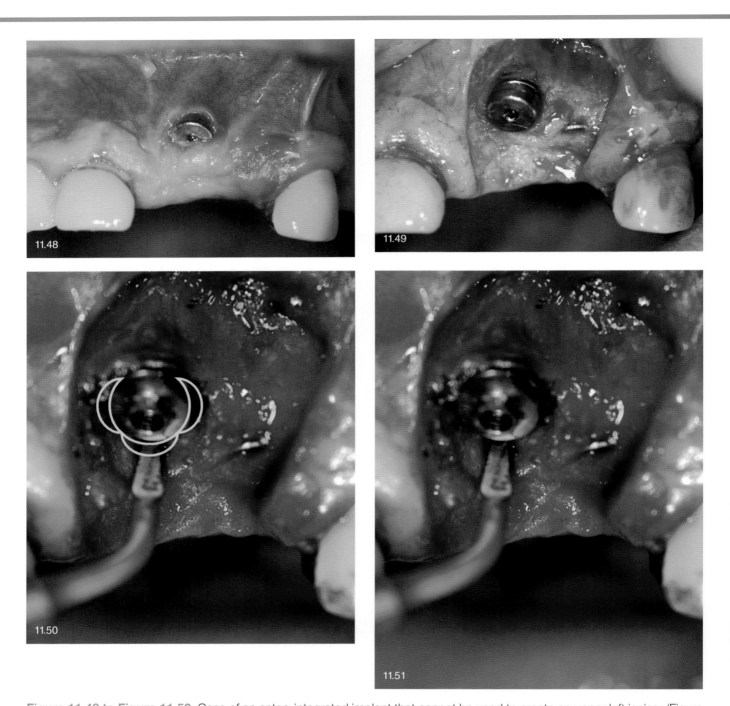

Figure 11.48 to Figure 11.52 Case of an osteo-integrated implant that cannot be used to create an upper left incisor (Figure 11.48). It must be removed, without too much bone loss, for the installation of a new implant. A full thickness flap is raised, but the buccal cavity wall appears very delicate (Figure 11.49). To avoid destruction of the buccal plate, the tip is employed through the proximal and palatine sides only (Figure 11.50). This enables the implant to be removed easily, without serious bone destruction. The defect is then filled with biomaterials (Bio-Oss) (Figures 11.51, 11.52).

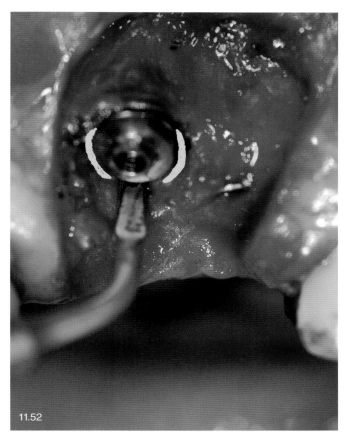

11.52

Figure 11.48 to Figure 11.52 *Continued*

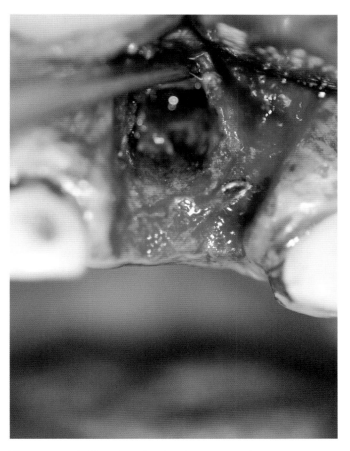

Figure 11.53 The site after implant removal.

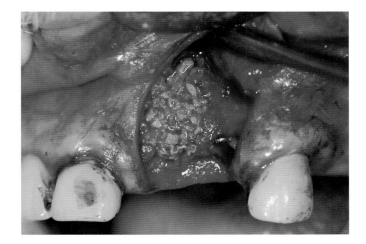

Figure 11.54 Implant removal site grafted with biomaterial.

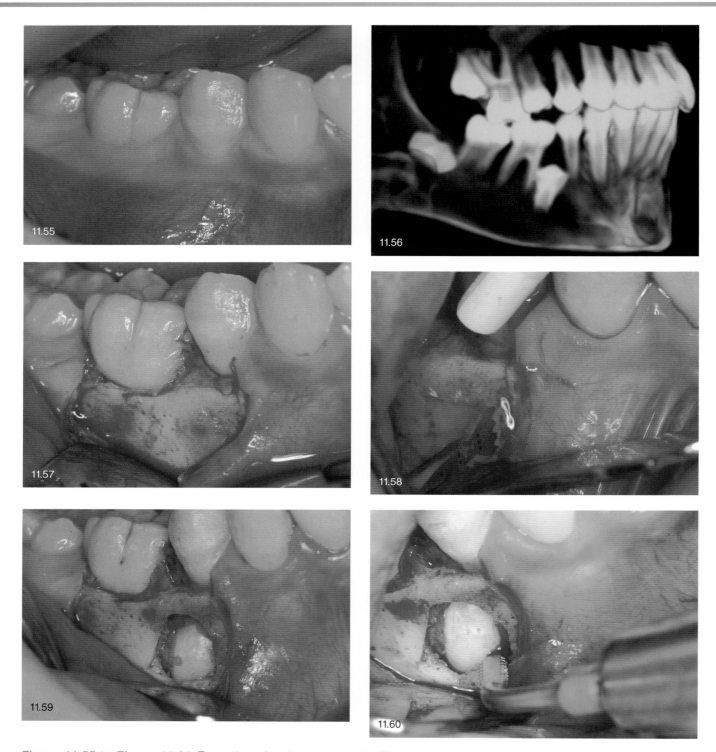

Figure 11.55 to Figure 11.64 Extraction of a obstructed tooth. The second premolar has to be extracted for orthodontic reasons, but the lack of space between the surrounded teeth created the need for a bony access (Figures 11.55, 11.56). After rising a full-thickness flap, a bone window is realized to reach the tooth (Figures 11.57–11.59). Root and crown are separated (Satelec Ninja) to facilitate the withdrawing of each part (Figures 11.60–11.64).

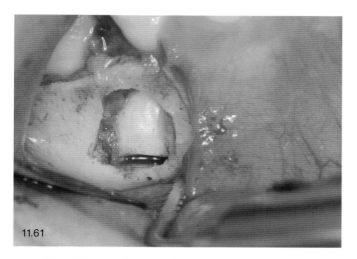

11.61

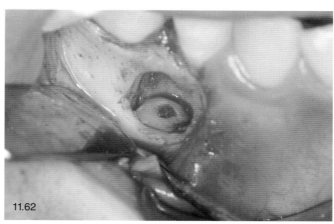

11.62

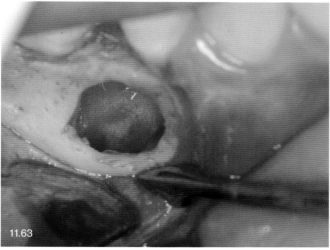

11.63

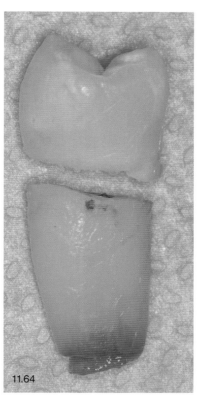

11.64

Figure 11.55 to Figure 11.64 *Continued*

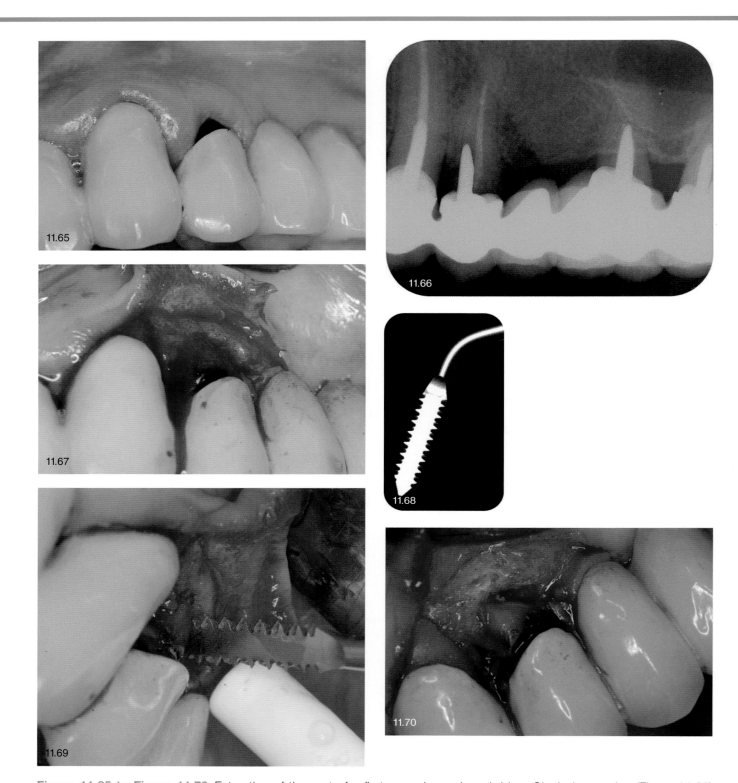

Figure 11.65 to Figure 11.79 Extraction of the root of a first premolar under a bridge. Gingival recession (Figure 11.65) and an x-ray (Figure 11.66) indicate juxta-osseous decay in a bridge pillar tooth. A full-thickness flap is raised (Figure 11.67). A Ninja odontotomy tip (Figure 11.68) is used to section the root diagonally, using the bony rim for support (Figure 11.69). This diagonal cut allows the two parts to be withdrawn more easily and avoids the metal pivot (Figure 11.70). Standard extraction tips (Satelec LC2) are then used along the proximal sides (Figure 11.71) to cut little trenches (Figure 11.72) and allow a small elevator to be inserted (Figure 11.73). Once loosened, the root is extracted with college pliers (Figures 11.74–11.78). The alveolar socket remains wholly preserved (Figure 11.79).

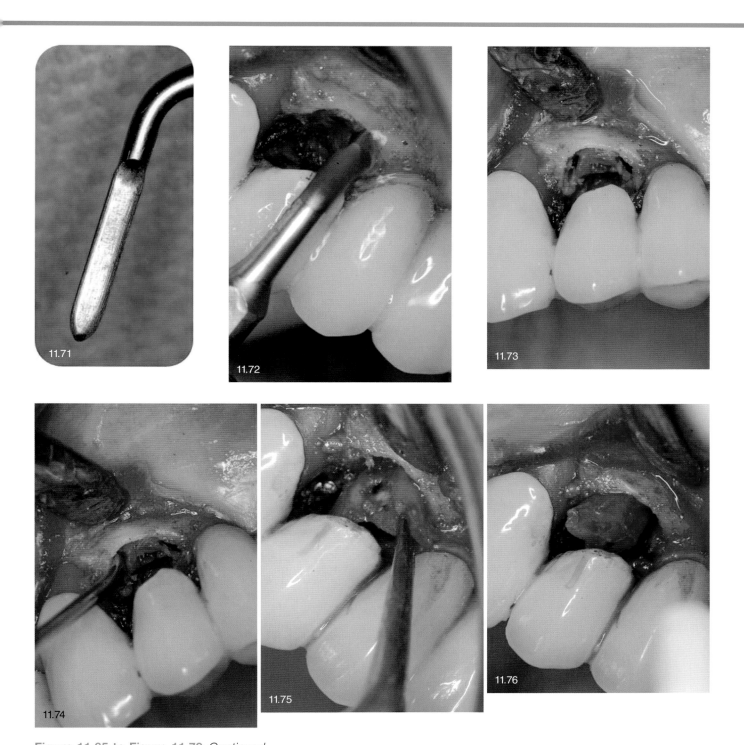

Figure 11.65 to Figure 11.79 *Continued*

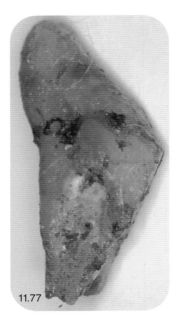
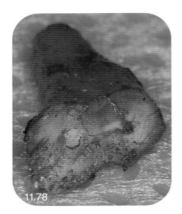
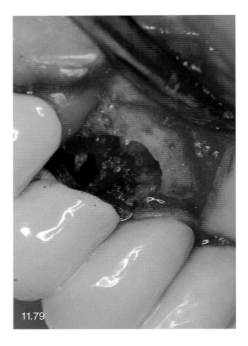

11.77

11.78

11.79

Figure 11.65 to Figure 11.79 *Continued*

odontotomy. These specific features enabled us to brace the flat side of the instrument against the bony rim while we sectioned the root crosswise. The cut was made diagonally to pass over the metal pivot and to facilitate removal of the two parts. When the root was clearly visible after withdrawal of the crown section, standard extraction tips were brought into action along the proximal sides to create a narrow trench, into which a small excavator was introduced to loosen the tooth. Extracted with college pliers, the root showed that the alveolar walls had been totally and perfectly preserved.

REFERENCES

Aro H, Kallioniemi H, Aho AJ, et al. 1981. Ultrasonic device in bone cutting. A histological and scanning electron microscopical study. *Acta Orthop Scand*. 52:5–10.

Berengo M, Bacci C, Sartori M, et al. 2006. Histomorphometric evaluation of bone grafts harvested by different methods. *Minerva stomatologica*. 55:189–98.

Covani U, Cornelini R, Barone A. 2007. Vertical crestal bone changes around implants placed into fresh extraction sockets. *J Periodontol*. 78:810–15.

Dahlin C, Sennerby L, Lekholm U, et al. 1989. Generation of new bone around titanium implants using a membrane technique: an experimental study in rabbits. *Int J Oral Maxillofac Implants*. 4:19–25.

Horton JE, Tarpley TM, Wood LD. 1975. The healing of surgical defect in alveolar bone produced with ultrasonic instrumentation, chisel and rotary bur. *Oral Surg Oral Med Oral Patho*. 39:536–46.

Louise F, Macia Y. 2009. Can piezoelectric surgery change daily dental practice? *Australasian Dental Practice*. 3:140–144.

Vercellotti T, Nevins ML, Kim DM, et al. 2005. Osseous response following resective therapy with piezosurgery. *Int J Periodont Restor Dent*. 25:543–49.

Chapter 12 The Minimally Invasive Maxillary Sinus Surgery

Part 1: Serge Dibart, DMD, Yun Po Zhang, PhD, DDS (hon), Mingfang Su, DMD, MSc
Part 2: Yves Macia, DDS, Francis Louise, DDS
Part 3: Serge Dibart, DMD, Yun Po Zhang, PhD, DDS (hon), Mingfang Su, DMD, MSc

Part 1: The Atraumatic Partial or Full "Balloon" Sinus Lift Using the Subantral Membrane Elevator with or without Concomitant Implant Placement

HISTORICAL REVIEW AND ANATOMICAL REMINDER

The posterior region of a toothless maxilla has certain peculiarities that, for many years, limited the possibilities of placing implants. The first obstacle is the low mineralization rate for this bone, an unfavorable factor for basic implant stability (type 3 or 4 in the classification proposed by Lekholm and Zarb 1985). The second obstacle, all too frequently encountered, is the insufficient quantity of available bone. This paucity is caused by dual resorption, both centripetal through periodontal disease or postextraction loss of function and centrifugal through sinus pneumatization.

To correct this centrifugal resorption, various techniques have been described to move and fill the sinus floor and wall. They range from invasive (external or lateral approach) to minimally invasive (internal approach using osteotomes, "balloon" elevation, and piezoelectric Intralift). They all have advantages and disadvantages.

THE EXTERNAL OR LATERAL APPROACH

The lateral approach to treating sinus pathologies was described by Caldwell in the United States in 1893 and by Luc in France 4 years later. Still known as the Caldwell-Luc procedure, this approach is practiced at the level of the canine fossa, a depression of variable depth above the premolars. This osteotomy allows not only curettage of infection but also irrigation, drainage, and observation of the sinus. Despite an increasing tendency toward nasal endoscopy today, the old surgical approach is still employed in parallel with or as an alternative to the endoscopic solution because of the optimal visual access it offers to the maxillary sinus (Chobillon and Jankowski 2004).

In cases where the sinus floor needs to be raised, however, an opening at the level of the canine fossa does not present many advantages. This is a zone where the suborbital nerve surfaces twice, in company with two other intraossary nerves (the anterior superior and intermediary alveolar nerves). Any lesion of the neurofibers contained in the upper third of this floor may give rise to mucogingival allodynia and, in some cases, neuropathic pain (Geha and Carpentier 2006). Moreover, since an osteotomy at the level of the canine fossa is limited by the front wall of the sinus, the opening may be too constricted to allow instruments access to the cavity. As a final consideration, the lowest point of the sinus is generally at the level of the first molar, and this is usually the site that requires raising. It is generally acknowledged that the optimal site for a side opening of the sinus is perpendicular with the first molar.

Although this zone is more practical for the surgeon and much safer from a neurological standpoint, it should be borne in mind that a rich vascular system exists at the level of the lateral wall of the sinus. Two branches of the maxillary artery vascularize this wall: the posterior superior alveolar artery and the infraorbital artery. Each divides into an intraosseous branch in the side wall and an extraosseous branch that vascularizes the periosteum in the molar region. These intraosseous branches anastomose with each other to form a vascular loop known as the alveolar antral artery (Figure 12.1). This is the most voluminous and the most regular of the arteries vascularizing the sinus, contained in the thickness of the lateral wall, either in a bony channel or in a trough that may be recessed into the inside face of the wall or under the sinus membrane. For Geha and Carpentier (2006), this artery is always intraosseous, opposite the first molar, at the base of the zygomatic process and most commonly under the sinus mucous membrane at the level of the canine fossa. Let

Practical Osseous Surgery in Periodontics and Implant Dentistry, First Edition. Edited by Serge Dibart, Jean-Pierre Dibart.
© 2011 John Wiley & Sons, Inc. Published 2011 by John Wiley & Sons, Inc.

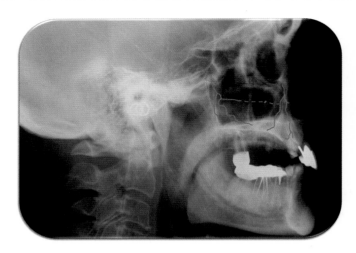

Figure 12.1 The intraossary branches of the posterior superior alveolar artery and the infraorbital artery anastomose with one other to form the antral artery.

Table 12.1. The advantages, disadvantages, and possible complications associated with the lateral window approach.

Advantages	Disadvantages	Possible Complications
• Clear view of the sinus • Independent of preexisting amount of bone • Large volumes of bone can be grafted	• CAT scan mandatory • Invasive procedure • Implants may or may not be placed at the time of the procedure	• Membrane perforation • Bleeding • Septae • Incision line opening • Infection

us now look at The advantages, disadvantages, and possible complications associated with the lateral window approach (see Table 12.1).

Possible Complications

1. *Schneiderian membrane perforation:* This membrane perforation is the most common complication. It can occur in 11%–56% of the cases. It usually happens at the time of window preparation (especially if rotary instruments are used for membrane access) or at the time of manual instrumentation during membrane elevation. It is interesting to note that the rate drops to 7% with piezoelectric surgery (Wallace and Froum 2007). The unfortunate outcome of a perforation is the lack of containment of the graft material as well as its contamination and possible infection. The action to take in such a case usually depends on the size of the tear and the experience of the surgeon. One approach is to repair the tear by "folding" the Schneiderian membrane "upward" onto itself, using a col-

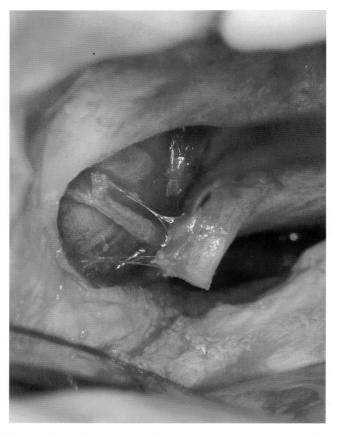

Figure 12.2 The alveolar antral artery in submucous position at the level of the first molar.

lagen membrane, and continuing the surgery; the other approach is to abort the procedure, wait 2–3 months, and start again. Waiting will have the advantage of allowing the surgeon to work with a thicker and less friable membrane (scar tissue) at the later date (Barone et al. 2005; Testori et al. 2008; Wallace and Froum 2007).

2. *Bleeding:* The infra-orbital artery and the posterior superior dental artery form an intraosseous anastomosis in the lateral wall of the maxillary sinus. In 20% of the cases, this vascular structure will be present low enough (15–16 mm from the alveolar crest) that it will interfere with the position of the bony window during surgery. This is particularly true in cases of severely atrophic ridges where the probability of transecting the vessel is high. A very elegant way to circumvent this issue is to use piezoelectric surgery, which will allow a dissection of the artery by "peeling" the maxillary bone away and avoiding a hemorrhage (Figure 12.2; Elian et al. 2005; Mardinger et al. 2007).

3. *Presence of septae:* Septae have been first described by Underwood in 1910, hence their name "Underwood's septa." They are present in about 26% of the cases and are predominant in the middle region of the sinus (50% of

the time). They complicate the surgical procedure as they may contribute to membrane perforation. It is of paramount importance to study closely the preoperative computed tomography (CT) scan before undertaking a sinus lift procedure in order to know the exact location and extent of the septae (Kim et al. 2006; Velasquez-Plata et al. 2002).

4. *Incision line opening:* Incision opening is usually the result of poor suturing and/or lack of control of the immediate postoperative edema by using corticosteroids. It may result in exposure of the collagen membrane and contamination of the graft material.

5. *Infection:* This will usually follow an opening of the incision line or could be the result of a surgery done on a sinus with an existing nondiagnosed pathology.

THE INTERNAL APPROACH

At the annual meeting of the Alabama Implant Study Group in 1977, Tatum described the crestal approach to the sinus. In this technique, a large-size trephine is employed to a depth of around 2 mm short of the bony floor of the sinus. A large osteotome is then used to fracture the floor (Tatum 1977). In a regular sequence, successive loads of bone graft materials are inserted into the osteotomy site and pushed to displace the Schneider membrane. This technique was further described by Summers in 1994. He first used drills to prepare the implant site to within 2 mm of the sinus floor. The drill hole was then packed with bone substitute material and/or recov-

Table 12.2. The advantages, disadvantages, and possible complications of the internal osteotome-facilitated approach.

Advantages	Disadvantages	Possible Complications
• Less invasive procedure • Markedly less patient discomfort • Better patient acceptance	• CT scan recommended • Technically demanding (blind technique) • Limited bone grafting (Toller 2004) • Usually used for one or two teeth	• Membrane perforation (Nkenke et al. 2002) • Paroxysmal positional vertigo (PPV) (Di Girolamo et al. 2005.)

Nkenke et al. 2002; Rosen et al. 1999; Di Girolamo et al. 2005.

ered bone. This material, together with the subsinus portion of bone and the Schneider membrane, were then progressively pushed back into the sinus with osteotomes lightly tapped with a surgical mallet. The operation was renewed several times with progressively larger osteotomes, and each time the access hole to the sinus was packed with material. In addition to the sinus bone gain, this technique also compacts the area around the implant site, thereby increasing basic stability. To be successfully paired with simultaneous implant placement this technique requires at least 5 mm of original bone. Toffler (2004) reports 26.7% implant failure when residual bone height was 4 mm or less and 5.1% failure when 5 mm or more. Let us look at the advantages, disadvantages and possible complications of the internal osteotome-facilitated approach (Table 12.2).

Part 2: IntraLift Technique

Over recent years, piezoelectrical surgery has continually gained ground over standard bone surgery. As part of this process, 2007 marked the appearance of insert kits designed to raise the sinus floor by the crestal approach. These inserts were developed by the scientific group of Troedhan, Kurrek & Wainwright (TKW) and the Acteon Group in France. The resulting technique is called the IntraLift, and the tips used are TKW1, TKW2, TKW3, TKW4, and TKW5.

The IntraLift is thus a technique for raising the sinus floor via the crestal approach, using ultrasonic tips to first pierce an access hole to the sinus floor and then to hydrodynamically push back the Schneider membrane.

INDICATIONS

Unlike the Summers technique, the IntraLift procedure does not automatically call for immediate installation of the implant.

Thus, the required minimum height of 5 mm is no longer necessary for securing this installation. Indeed, the authors mention the possibility of employing their technique with crestal heights below 3 mm. This means that the technique can be adopted, with immediate or deferred insertion of the implant, to raise and fill precise sections of the sinus membrane.

One of the major advantages of this technique resides in the fact that, by avoiding an osteotomy of the lateral wall, it precludes any of the complications associated with this approach and notably any rupture of the alveolar antral artery in cases where it follows an intraossary course. In view of the absence of vessels in the alveolar crest and the limited vascularization of the sinus membrane, all risk of hemorrhage is avoided with the IntraLift procedure.

In cases where the site requiring filling is narrow and bordered by teeth, the lateral approach entails the danger of damage

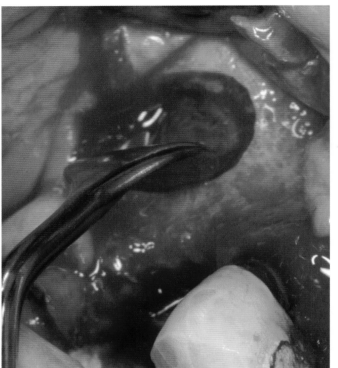

Figure 12.3 Too narrow a window can curtail use of instruments (7-mm sinus curette) inside the sinus.

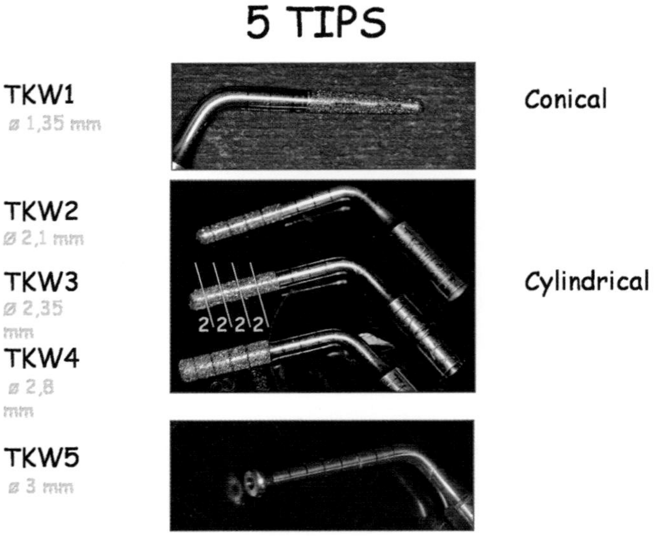

5 TIPS

TKW1
ø 1,35 mm

TKW2
ø 2,1 mm

TKW3
ø 2,35 mm

TKW4
ø 2,8 mm

TKW5
ø 3 mm

Conical

Cylindrical

Figure 12.4 Tips in the IntraLift kit. The first conical tip is used for access to the sinus. The three cylindrical tips enlarge the hole to 2.8 mm. The "trumpet" tip jets water to hydrodynamically push back the Schneider membrane. All these tips feature 2-mm graduations.

to their roots. This being so, the window is generally very small, offering poor visibility and only limited access for instruments (Figure 12.3). When detaching the Schneider membrane, these instruments run the risk of sectioning the neurovascular bundles at the apex of neighboring teeth if they emerge into the sinus.

Thus, the IntraLift technique is indicated in those cases in which the toothless gap is limited, access drilling presents no risk for the roots of neighboring teeth and the detachment of the sinus membrane is achieved by hydrodynamic action rather than through use of potentially aggressive and cutting instruments.

TECHNIQUE

The IntraLift technique follows a precise protocol established by the inventors, Wainwright et al. (2007), and the firm Satelec, which markets the IntraLift kit. Although the user may introduce certain adaptations, depending on situations, the recommendations concerning the sequence of instruments and the adjustment of the ultrasonic generator (Piezotome) must be followed scrupulously.

Wainwright et al. (2007) recommend use of a biopsy punch to reach the crestal bone. The punched gingiva is bedded in

sterile sodium chloride and sutured upon completion of surgery. As resorbed alveolar ridge crests frequently lack keratinized gingival tissue, it seems simpler and safer to practice a crestal incision without a vertical release incision. Indeed, limited detachment of the mucous membrane simplifies postoperative recovery.

The IntraLift technique as such may be summarized as three steps in which five tips of increasing diameter are employed successively (Figure 12.4). The first of these steps is the access to the sinus floor. If the residual bone height is less than 3 mm, the conic TKW1 tip (1.25 mm) is used to reach the membrane. It is important to measure the bone height carefully beforehand and to reduce the pressure on the graduated (every 2 mm) tip when approaching the sinus floor. Although ultrasonic diamond-coated tips present no danger for soft tissue, excess pressure applied to cut through the cortical bone layer of the sinus floor may tear the Schneider membrane. A blunt instrument should be used to check that the floor has been pierced and that the membrane is undamaged. Visual examination remains problematic in these cases and it is prudent to check, by touch, that the membrane remains undamaged after use of each diamond-tipped instrument. If, on the other hand, the residual bone height is greater than 3 mm, the drilling should be begun with a 2-mm pilot drill and stopped 2 mm short of the sinus floor. From there, the membrane is easily accessible with the TKW1 tip.

The second step is the gradual enlargement of the drilling hole and entails successive use of tips TKW2 (2.1 mm), TKW3 (2.35 mm), and TKW4 (2.8 mm). These cylindrical tips are also graduated every 2 mm to allow the practitioner to control their penetration, notably when approaching the sinus membrane. The greater the diameter, the greater the resistance encountered, and it is often advisable to impart a slight rotary movement to facilitate penetration.

The final diameter of the well should be 2.8 mm, but according to the manufacturer, friction caused by the diamond-coated tip increases this diameter to 3 mm (+/− 0.1 mm). All these diamond-coated tips require full power and substantial irrigation to counteract any rise in temperature caused by friction. The Piezotome is thus set at full power (mode 1 of the four modes available), and the irrigation is adjusted to 80 mL/min.

The third step is the raising of the sinus membrane. Tip TKW5 is inserted to within 2 mm of the Schneider membrane and then activated (on mode 2 or 3) in 5-second bursts with an irrigation set initially at 40 mL/min and increased progressively to 50 mL/min and then to 60 mL/min for the following sequences. In theory, the membrane is thus pushed back hydrodynamically. Between each sequence, it is important to check the membrane for possible damage and to measure the progress achieved. To do so, the practitioner should employ a large-diameter graduated probe with a rounded end (Nobel Biocare depth probe; Figure 12.5). Because of the risk of its perforating the mucous membrane, a periodontal probe is not recommended. The probe enables the prac-

titioner to check the firmness and elasticity of the membrane (which supposes that it has not been torn) and to measure the distance achieved between the membrane and the rim of the bony crest. The Valsalva maneuver may also be used to check that the membrane is undamaged. In this case, for fear that this might aggravate any small perforation, the patient is requested not to exhale too strongly.

It may be noted that any lateral movement of the instrument during the widening sequences may either over-enlarge the diameter or give the hole an oval shape. This in turn would create a hiatus between tip TKW5 and the walls of the hole, which might result in water leakage or a drop in hydraulic pressure. Thus, one of the keys to the success of the rest of the procedure lies in the correct preparation of the access hole to the membrane.

Prior to filling with alloplastic or autogenous augmentation material, Wainwright et al. (2007) advise insertion of a collagen sponge or resorbable membrane to hold the material in place in case of perforation or quite simply as a buffer before osseous filling. They employ the TKW5 as a plug to fill the new subantral cavity with graft material via the osteotomy. To ensure that the augmentation material is distributed homogeneously, the trumpet (TKW5) is employed in low-level mode (level 4) and the irrigation is adjusted to 40–50 mL/min, alternating every 3 seconds. Practitioners are warned that in cases where an implant is inserted in the same operation, highly compacted filling material may lead to uncontrollable tearing of the Schneider membrane through pressure applied when screwing the implant into place. This being the case, and in view of the favorable bone regeneration conditions generally encountered in sinuses, care should be taken not to overfill the site, notably when an implant is inserted immediately.

The IntraLift procedure is illustrated here in clinical terms with a patient who required an implant to replace tooth #12. The CT scan indicated the presence of the antral artery in the bone wall bordering the implant site (Figure 12.6). In addition, the patient regularly took platelet antiaggregants (Kardegic). Thus, any lateral opening of the sinus involved a serious risk of hemorrhage. Moreover, the proximity of the front wall of the sinus and the roots of adjacent teeth considerably complicated the cutting of a bone window. The height of the residual bone was measured at 7.5 mm and the site thus required filling, via the crestal approach, for the installation of a suitably sized implant.

A crestal incision (without a vertical release incision) allowed access to the alveolar crest and a round bur was then used to pass through the cortical bone (Figures 12.7–12.9). The TKW1 tip was employed to give access to the sinus floor (Figure 12.10). A round-ended probe (Nobel Biocare depth probe) was used to check the depth of the drilling and to

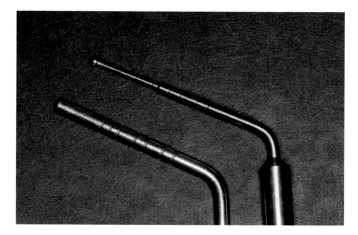

Figure 12.5 Graduated depth probes (Nobel Biocare) with blunt ends are used to check the sinus membrane for damage without risk of perforation and to measure the available height between this mucous membrane and the crest rim.

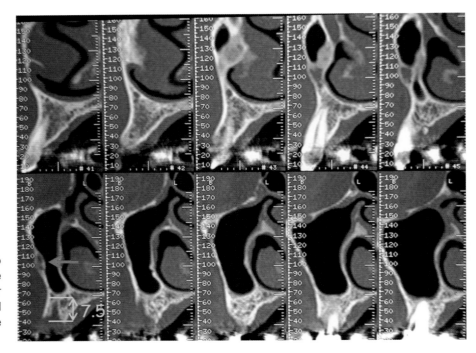

Figure 12.6 An IntraLift performed to replace tooth #12 with immediate installation of the implant. The scanner printout showed the voluminous antral artery in the lateral wall and an available bone height of 7.5 mm.

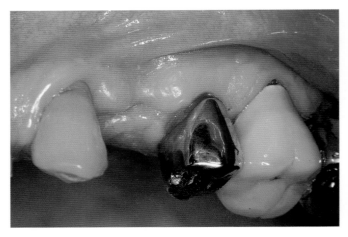

Figure 12.7 There is limited space between two teeth, which makes the lateral approach problematic.

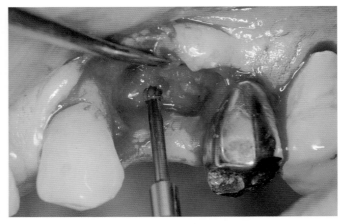

Figure 12.9 The bone was marked with a round bur.

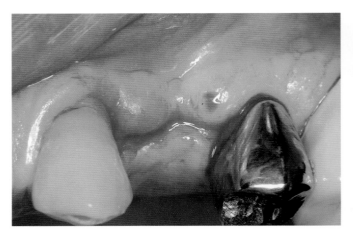

Figure 12.8 A crestal incision was made, without a vertical release incision.

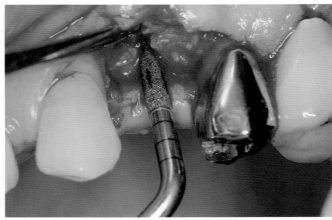

Figure 12.10 Tip TKW1 is used in the osteotomy.

verify that the membrane remained undamaged (Figure 12.11). This access cavity was enlarged by successive use of tips TKW2, TKW3, and TKW4 to obtain a diameter of between 2.8 and 3 mm (Figures 12.12–12.15). Then, used in 5-second bursts, the TKW5 pushed back the membrane (Figure 12.16).

The new submembrane cavity was then measured and the elasticity of the membrane verified with a large-diameter probe (Figure 12.17). A bone graft (Bio-Oss) was inserted in sufficient quantities to fill the space, care being taken not to create tension under the sinus membrane by overfilling (Figures 12.18, 12.19). After insertion of the implant (Figure 12.20), the site was closed (Figure 12.21) and a cicatrisation period of 6 months was observed with regular radiographic verifications (Figures 12.22, 12.23). The scant amount of material inserted facilitated observation of the ossification. The final prosthetic crown was inserted 6 months after surgery (Figure 12.24) and evaluated 1 year later (Figure 12.25).

Advantages and Results

As previously mentioned, the IntraLift technique offers the considerable advantages of being relatively nonaggressive and noninvasive for surrounding tissue (arteries, nerves, and roots of neighboring teeth). With regard to a standard lateral approach, it has the additional advantage of improved postoperative recovery, probably because of the reduced

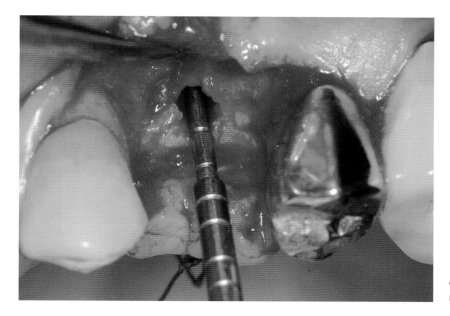

Figure 12.11 A blunt probe was used to check that the sinus membrane remained undamaged.

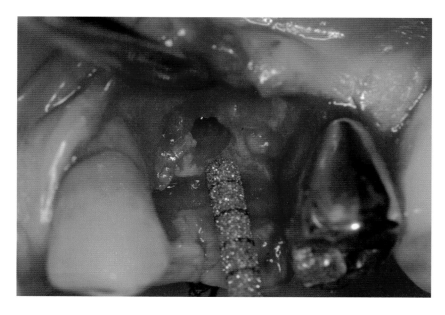

Figure 12.12 Tip TKW2 entering the osteotomy site.

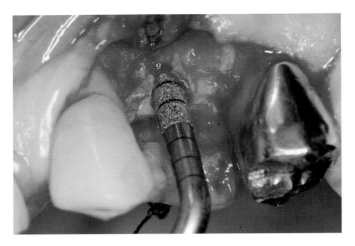

Figure 12.13 Tip TKW2 used to enlarge the osteotomy.

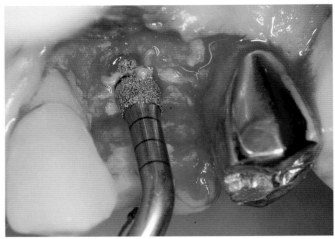

Figure 12.14 Tip TKW3 used to enlarge the osteotomy.

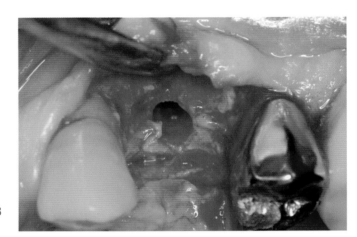

Figure 12.15 An osteotomy with a diameter between 2.8 and 3 mm was created, providing a perfect fit for tip TKW5.

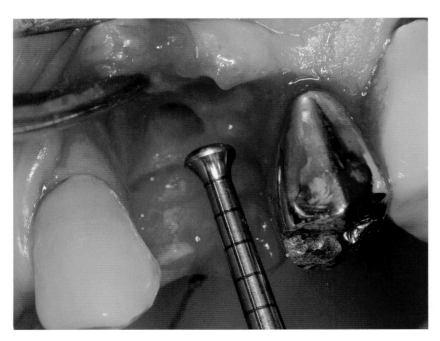

Figure 12.16 Tip TKW5 inserted into the osteotomy.

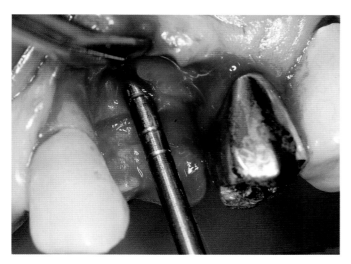

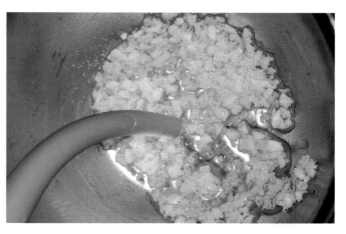

Figure 12.17 Following the hydrodynamic action of tip TKW5, the submembrane cavity was measured and the mucous membrane checked for damage.

Figure 12.18 The bone graft (Bio-Oss)is hydrated.

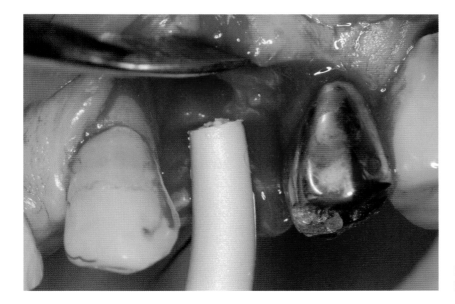

Figure 12.19 The bone graft in the syringe is inserted and lightly compacted.

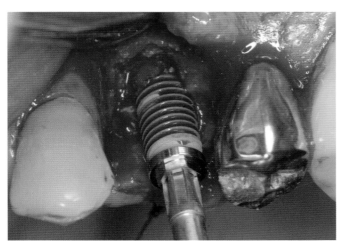

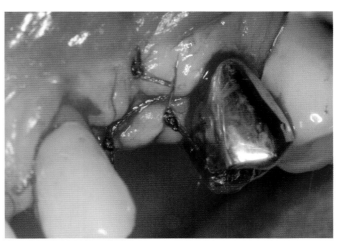

Figure12.20 The implant was installed (MK3® 4 × 11.5 Nobel Biocare).

Figure 12.21 The site was closed with three sutures.

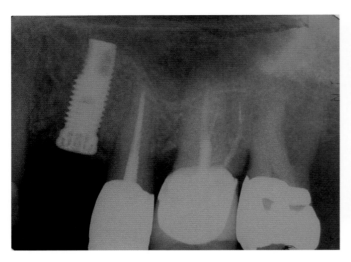

Figure 12.22 An immediate radiograph did not show the 4- to 5-mm gain in bone.

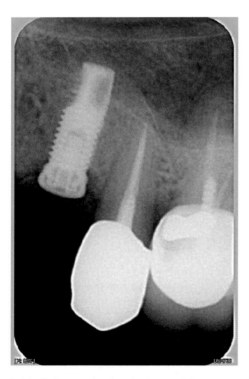

Figure 12.23 A 6-month check showed bone densification in the space lifted in the form of a periapical dome.

opening of soft tissue and the limited size of the osteotomy.

The inventors of the technique stress the fact that it includes the advantages of Summers's technique—few postoperative complications—while avoiding its disadvantages—the threat of an uncontrolled rupture caused by the osteotome and a restricted area of submucosal augmentation. When the

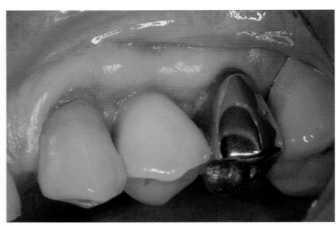

Figure 12.24 Final prosthetic crown inserted at 6 months.

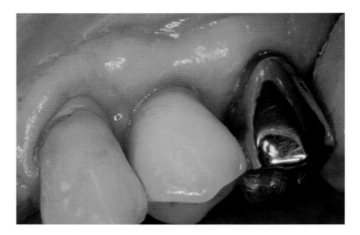

Figure 12.25 Final prosthesis was checked at 1 year.

IntraLift is used to detach the membrane of an egg from the shell, we note a homogeneous detachment in the shape of a dome induced by the water spreading under the membrane (Figures 12.26, 12.27). The detachment of the Schneider membrane thus seems wider and less aggressive than is the case with osteotomes.

The resulting submembrane cavity can thus be of considerable size, and its dome shape allows sufficient peripheral bone gain to afford the implant good stability. It is nevertheless difficult to affirm that the perforation rate for the sinus membrane remains low with this technique; we have no visual verification of the detachment achieved and of any possible damage to the membrane. For this reason, it is important to check this by touch between each change of tip. This is also why Wainwright et al (2007) insert a collagen sponge or a resorbable membrane into the bottom of the cavity before filling it.

We note that although results for sinus-filling surgery are satisfactory, whatever the technique and material used, this

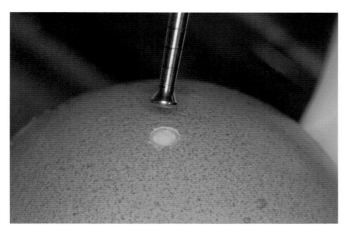

Figure 12.26 In this simulation of how the Schneider membrane is pushed back, an egg shell is first pierced with instruments TKW1–4 before tip TKW 5 is used.

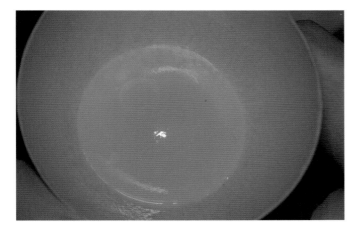

Figure 12.27 The membrane is detached atraumatically in a dome form.

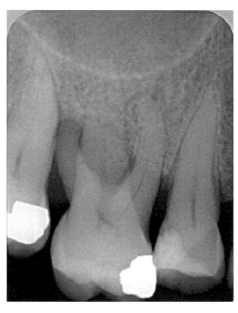

Figure 12.28 For periodontal reasons, the first molar has to be extracted.

is because sinus elevations may be assimilated with a guided bone regeneration procedure performed in optimal conditions. Indeed, once the regeneration cavity has been created and the membrane is correctly held in position, the site must simply have reasonable osteogenic potential for bone regeneration to take place naturally, with little or even no filling material (Figures 12.28–12.31).

The conservation of the lateral crestal wall offers the advantage of further improving the osteogenicity by creating a closed filling site, entirely surrounded by bony walls. Although, contrary to broad, flat sinuses, those that are anfractuous or built with many separating partitions have high cicatrisation potential; these partitions, with their strong adherence, may represent an obstacle for the tips and for detachment of the membrane. It is therefore important to study the anatomy of the sinus floor beforehand using the scanner to pinpoint the

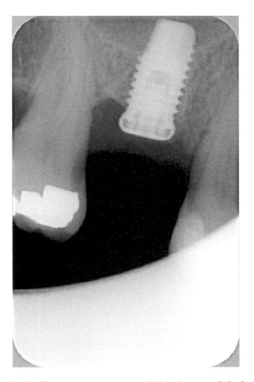

Figure 12.29 The site shows available bone of 6–8 mm. An 11.5 × 5 mm implant (MK3, Nobel Biocare) is installed once the Schneider membrane has been pushed back, without biomaterial filling.

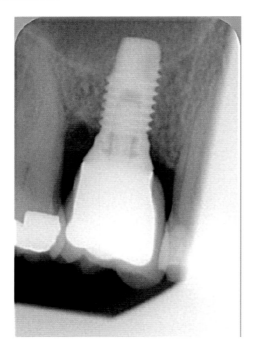

Figure 12.30 The implant is restored at 6 months.

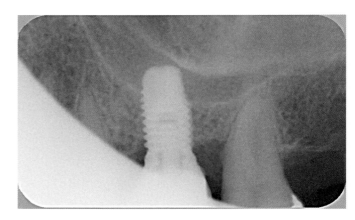

Figure 12.31 At 3 years, neo-ossification is visible around the apical part of the implant, and a new sinus floor may be seen. Contrary to a site filled with biomaterial, the resulting bone formation is not dome shaped.

most suitable site for the trepanation hole between the partitions. This preparation greatly influences the predictability of the result.

As a final word, an enlarged database and additional studies are required to confirm the effectiveness of this technique.

Part 3: Balloon Sinus Elevation

In 2007, Kfir et al. described an innovative technique: the minimally invasive antral membrane balloon elevation (MIAMBE), followed by bone augmentation and implant placement. It combined the use of an inflatable balloon (Figure 12.32) to elevate the Schneider membrane atraumatically in areas of severe maxillary atrophy (crestal bone ≤ 3 mm) and the placement of a bone graft comparable in volume to what can be achieved with a lateral window approach. The major advantage of this procedure is the possibility of grafting large volumes of bone from a small crestal opening, making it a possible alternative to the lateral window technique.

TECHNIQUE

After local anesthesia has been completed, a crestal incision is made and a full-thickness flap is reflected in order to expose the underlying bone. An osteotomy is made on the alveolar crest at the site of (future) implant placement (Figure 12.33). This osteotomy of about 3–4 mm in diameter (depending on the size of the implant to be placed) will stop short of the sinus floor (about 0.5 mm). This osteotomy can be done using various diameter implant burs or a trephine bur. The sinus floor is in-fractured gently using an osteotome and gentle mallet taping.

The balloon is tested in the operating room prior to insertion, according to the manufacturer guidelines. If a large volume of bone graft is necessary, the use of a straight subantral membrane elevator that inflates up to 4 cc is recommended, otherwise a micro-mini elevator (maximum inflation of 2 cc) will do. Once the balloon is inserted in the cavity (Figure 12.34), it is inflated very gently. At this point, one can do a visual check of the balloon into the sinus cavity, using a radio-opaque liquid and a radiograph (Figure 12.35). The manufacturer's recommendations are as follows: 1 cc of inflation will give a vertical height of 6 mm after grafting 1 cc of bone. Thus, if the residual alveolar bone height is 3 mm and the plan is to place a 10-mm-long implant, an inflation of 1.5 cc with the same volume of graft will give an additional height of 9 mm of bone. Once the membrane is elevated to the desired height, the balloon is gently deflated and removed from the cavity. The Valsalva maneuver is performed to evaluate membrane integrity, and bone is grafted into the sinus (Figure 12.36). If there is not enough residual alveolar bone to ensure primary stability of the implant, the placement is postponed for a later date and the flaps sutured back in place (Figure 12.37). Otherwise, implants are placed simultaneously.

Conclusions

This is a relatively new procedure, with limited longitudinal data. The results of a multicenter study (Kfir 2009) shows a 95% implant survival rate at 6–9 months. It is an atraumatic, minimally invasive surgery that generates minimal discomfort.

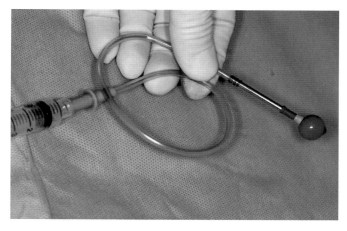

Figure 12.32 Subantral membrane elevator also known as the "balloon" (Osseous Technologies of America, Huntington Beach, CA).

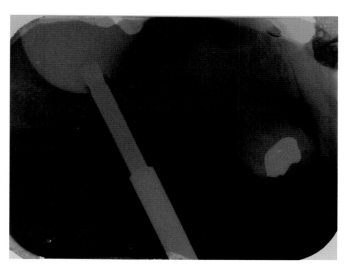

Figure 12.35 Radiograph of the partially inflated balloon in the sinus cavity.

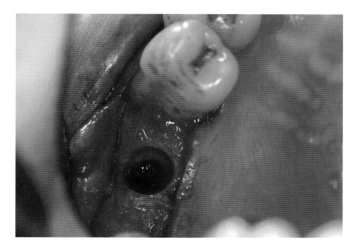

Figure 12.33 Osteotomy accessing the sinus cavity.

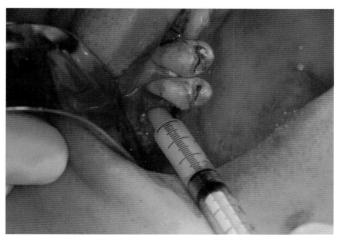

Figure 12.36 Bone is grafted into the sinus after the elevation of the Schneider membrane.

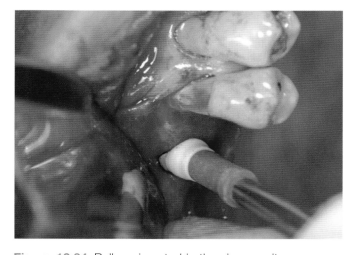

Figure 12.34 Balloon inserted in the sinus cavity.

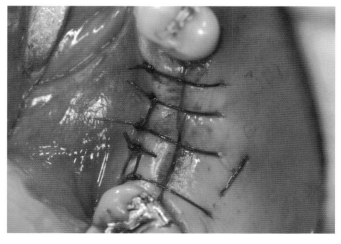

Figure 12.37 The site is sutured.

It is nonetheless technically demanding (as it remains a "blind" procedure), and the risks for membrane perforation are very real. The utilization of an endoscope in the sinus, during and after balloon elevation could reduce this eventuality.

REFERENCES

Barone A, Crespi R, Aldini NN, et al. 2005. Maxillary sinus augmentation: Histologic and histomorphometric analysis. *Int J Oral Maxillofac Implants.* 20:519–25.

Buser D. 1997. Long term evaluation of non submerged ITI implants. Part 1. 8 years life table analysis of a prospective multicenter study with 2359 implants. *Clin Oral Implant Res.* 8:161–72.

Caldwell GW. 1893. Diseases of the accessory sinuses of the nose and an infrared method of treatment of suppuration of the maxillary antrum. *NY Med J*, 58:526–28.

Chobillon MA, Jankowski R. 2004. What are the advantages of the endoscopic canine fossa approach in treating maxillary sinus aspergillomas? *Rhinology.* 42:230–5.

Di Girolamo M, Napolitano B, Arullani CA, et al. 2005. Paroxysmal positional vertigo as a complication of osteotome sinus floor elevation. *Eur Arch Otorhinolaryngol.* 262:631–33. Epub 2005 Feb 27.

Elian N, Wallace S, Cho SC, et al. 2005. Distribution of the maxillary artery as it relates to sinus floor augmentation. *Int J Oral Maxillofac Implants.* 20:784–87.

Geha N, Carpentier P. 2006. Les boucles artérielles du sinus maxillaire. *Journal de Parodontologie & d'Implantologie Orale.* 25:127–40.

Kfir E, Kfir V, Eliav E, et al. 2007. Minimally invasive antral membrane balloon elevation: Report of 36 procedures. *J Periodontol.* 78:2032–35.

Kfir E, Goldstein M, Yerushalmi I, et al. 2009. Minimally invasive antral membrane balloon elevation. Results of a multicenter registry. *Clin Implant Dent Relat Res.* 11:e83–91.

Kim MJ, Jung UW, Kim CS, et al. 2006. Maxillary sinus septa: Prevalence, height, location, and morphology. A reformatted computed tomography scan analysis. *J Periodontol.* 77:903–908.

Lekholm U, Zarb GA. 1985. Patient selection and preparation. In: Branemark PI, Zarb GA, Albrektsson T, eds. *Tissue-Integrated Prostheses: Osseointegration in Clinical Dentistry.* Chicago: Quintessence Publishing Co., pp. 199–209.

Luc H. 1897. Une nouvelle méthode opératoire pour la cure radicale et rapide de l'empyème chirurgique de sinus maxillaire. *Arch Int Larynol Otol Rhino.* 10:273–85.

Mardinger O, Abba M, Hirshberg A, et al. 2007. Prevalence, diameter and course of the maxillary intraosseous vascular canal with relation to sinus augmentation procedure: A radiographic study. *Int J Oral Maxillofac Surg.* 36:735–38. Epub 2007 Jul 12.

Nkenke E, Schlegel A, Schultze-Mosgau S, et al. 2002. The endoscopically controlled osteotome sinus floor elevation: A preliminary prospective study. *Int J Oral Maxillofac Implants.* 17:557–66.

Rosen PS, Summers R, Mellado JR, et al. 1999. The bone-added osteotome sinus floor elevation technique: Multicenter retrospective report of consecutively treated patients. *Int J Oral Maxillofac Implants.* 14:853–58.

Summers RB. 1994. A new concept in maxillary implant surgery: The osteotome technique. *Compendium.* 15:152, 154–156, 158, 162.

Tatum OH. 1977. Maxillary Sinus Grafting for Endosseous Implants. Presented at the Annual Meeting at the Alabama Implant Study Group, April, 1977, Birmingham, AL.

Testori T, Wallace SS, Del Fabbro M, et al. 2008. Repair of large sinus membrane perforations using stabilized collagen barrier membranes: Surgical techniques with histologic and radiographic evidence of success. *Int J Periodontics Restorative Dent.* 28:9–17.

Toffler M. 2004. Osteotome-mediated sinus floor elevation: A clinical report. *Int J Oral Maxillofac Implants.* 19:266–73.

Wainwright MA, Troedhan A, Kurrek A. 2007. The Intralift: A new minimal invasive ultrasonic technique for sinus grafting procedures. *Implants.* 3:30–34.

Wallace SS, Mazor Z, Froum SJ, et al. 2007. Schneiderian membrane perforation rate during sinus elevation using piezosurgery: Clinical results of 100 consecutive cases. *Int J Periodontics Restorative Dent.* 27:413–19.

Chapter 13 The Narrow Ridge in the Maxilla and the Mandible and Its Correction: Ridge Splitting Using Piezoelectric Surgery and Grafting with or without Simultaneous Implant Placement

Rima Abdallah, BDS, CAGS, DSc, Serge Dibart, DMD

INTRODUCTION

Patients requiring dental implant treatment usually require ridge augmentation prior due to the resorptive process of the edentulous ridge following tooth loss. Several methods of augmentation have been reported in the literature, including particulate graft, block graft, distraction osteogenesis, and ridge-splitting technique, also known as the edentulous ridge expansion.

The edentulous ridge expansion (ERE) technique aims at creating a sagittal osteotomy of the edentulous ridge using instruments such as chisels or piezoelectric inserts between the two cortical plates to expand the ridge width and consequently allow for the placement of implants at the same visit or at a later stage.

The ERE technique is not a method for augmenting the ridge vertically; therefore, the presence of enough vertical height for implant placement is a requirement. Also, a minimum of 3 mm of bone width, including at least 1 mm of cancellous bone, is desired in order to insert a bone chisel between cortical plates and consequently expand the cortical bones. It has been shown that when using the piezoelectric inserts this procedure can be attempted in ridges with less than 3 mm bone width. A pyramidal form ridge with a wider base is the ideal indication for this technique because it will prevent the risk of buccal plate fracture. This approach can help in decreasing the treatment time where the implant is placed in the same visit; it also will correct the buccal concavity that is caused by the ridge resorption.

DEFINITION

Ridge splitting is a procedure for augmenting implant sites with a reduced bucco-lingual thickness (Seibert class I), by repositioning the buccal cortical plate.

The ridge-splitting technique aims at the creation of a new implant bed by longitudinal osteotomy of the alveolar bone.

The buccal cortex is repositioned laterally by greenstick fracture, and the space between the buccal and the lingual cortical plates is filled with autologus, allogenic, or alloplastic graft material.

Classification

There are two types of ridge splitting:

1. One-stage (ridge split with immediate implant placement)
2. Two-stage (ridge split plus graft, followed by implant placement at a later date)

HISTORY

Tatum (1986) first described a technique to expand the cortical wall in cases with inadequate bucco-lingual thickness of bone using various sizes of channel formers (Figure 13.1).

The edentulous ridge expansion was then reintroduced in 1990 by Bruschi and Scipioni. The technique consists of splitting the vestibular and buccal cortical plates (Scipioni et al. 1994) and further opening the space with Summers's osteotomes (Summers 1994).

INDICATIONS

Indications for use of ridge splitting include:

1. Sufficient vertical bone height
2. Horizontal defect/narrow ridges (wide apically)
3. Presence of cancellous bone between the cortical plates

See Figures 13.2 and 13.3.

Practical Osseous Surgery in Periodontics and Implant Dentistry, First Edition. Edited by Serge Dibart, Jean-Pierre Dibart.
© 2011 John Wiley & Sons, Inc. Published 2011 by John Wiley & Sons, Inc.

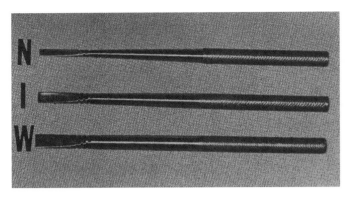

Figure 13.1 Bone splitting chisels (W, wide; I, intermediate; N, narrow).

CONTRAINDICATIONS

Contraindications for use of ridge splitting (Figure 13.4) include:

1. Ridge width less than 3 mm
2. Vertical ridge deficiency
3. Overangulated maxillary edentulous ridge
4. Single site in the mandible

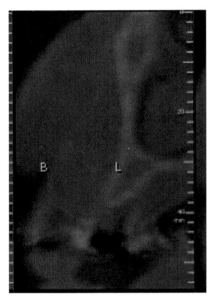
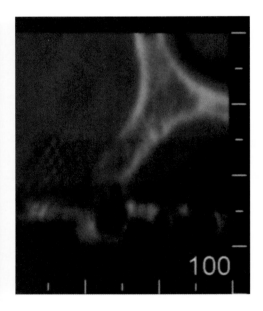

Figure 13.2 CT scan of two different type of ridges. The ridge on the left side is of triangular shape (base wider than coronal portion) and amenable to splitting. The ridge on the right side is parallel and not amenable to splitting.

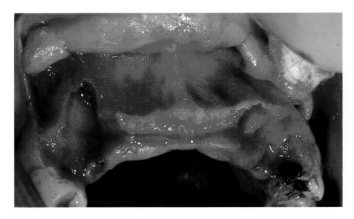

Figure 13.3 Clinical picture of a ridge that is narrow and "parallel", thus not a good candidate for splitting.

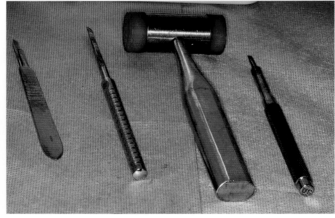

Figure 13.4 Scalpel, bone chisels, and mallet used in ridge splitting.

TECHNIQUES

Splitting is classically performed with the following:

1. *Chisel and mallet* (Tatum 1986; Bruschi and Scipioni 1990; Coatoam and Mariotti 2003; Basa et al. 2004).

2. *Oscillating saws* (Zijderveld et al. 2004; Figure 13.5).

3. *Extension crest device* (Chiapasco et al. 2006).

4. *Ultrasonic/piezosurgery* (Vercelotti 2000).

The use of bone chisel traumatizes and stresses the patient.

Fine-tuning of the splitting can be difficult when the crest is dense, especially in the mandible.

Rotating and oscillating instruments are time effective and less stressful for the patient. For the surgeon, however, the risk of encroaching the gingiva, the lips, or the tongue limits the accessibility and complicates the procedure.

Ultrasonically moved knives have the ability to cut hard tissues, such as teeth and bone (Figure 13.6).

In contrast, soft tissues such as gingiva, blood vessels, nerves, and sinus membranes are preserved from injury because they vibrate with the tip.

Segmental ridge-split with ultrasonic bone saw (USBS) is predictable and does not lead to bone overheating or bone injury.

Advantages

There are several advantages for using splitting techniques:

- Discards the need for onlay graft (hip, maxillary tuberosity, chin, or the external oblique ridge)

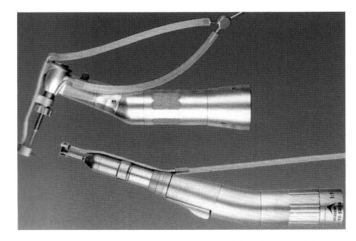

Figure 13.5 Oscillating bone saw used for ridge splitting.

- Avoids the use of a secondary surgical site that exhibits postoperative morbidity associated with bone harvesting

- Shortens the treatment due to immediate implant placement

- Reduces healing time

- Avoids palatally placed implants

- Avoids concave emergence profile

Disadvantages

There are also disadvantages to using splitting techniques:

- Fracture of the buccal plate

- Resorption of the buccal plate

- Possible surgical complications

- Benign paroxysmal positional vertigo

Buccal plate fracture may occur during (1) ridge expansion with chisels/osteotomes, (2) implant site preparation with drills, and (3) implant insertion (Figures 13.7, 13.8).

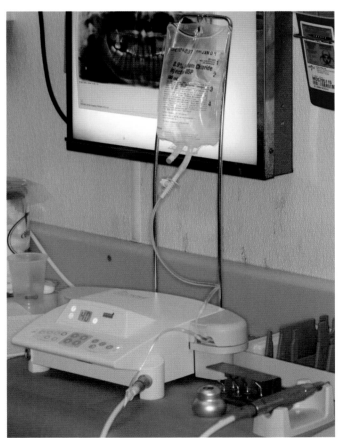

Figure 13.6 Piezotome (Satelec, Acteongroup, Merignac, France). Piezoelectric knife used for ridge splitting.

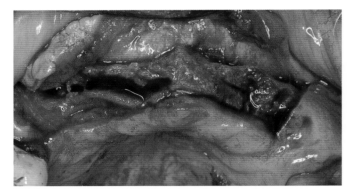

Figure 13.7 Buccal plate fracture in the front maxilla.

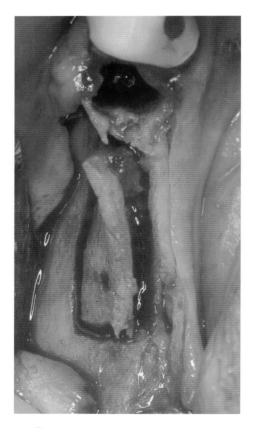

Figure 13.8 Buccal plate fracture in mandible.

THE USE OF DIFFERENT FLAP TECHNIQUES

Three types of flaps can be used in association with the edentulous ridge expansion technique: the full-thickness mucoperiostael flap, the partial-thickness flap, and the osteoperiosteal flap. The presence of osseointegration is not the only criteria of success in ridge-split cases; we need to maintain marginal bone stability and avoid buccal bone resorption or creation of fenestrations, which leads to the long-term success of the implants. It has been shown that the muco-

periosteal flap maintains the blood supply to the expanded area and stabilizes the displaced buccal plate of bone. Alveolar expansion, when done using either a partial-thickness flap or the minimally exposed osteoperiosteal flap approach, appears to consistently lead to sustainable alveolar width and osseointegration according to Jenson, Ellis and Glick (2009). Full mucoperiosteal flap approaches are less predictable with regard to buccal plate bone loss and resorption. The use of a full-thickness flap helps to avoid excessive bleeding, resulting in better visualization of the operating sites and better handling of the surgical steps. In cases where there is thin connective tissue, the partial-thickness flap procedure becomes extremely difficult, and the remaining tissue over the alveolar bone is too thin to protect the bone adequately. The osteoperiosteal flap is more technique sensitive, as it leads to the blind placement of implants and the failure to be able to visualize the entire length of the alveolar crest, which might lead to improper placement and positioning of the implants.

SURGICAL STEPS

Ridge Split without Implant Placement (Two Stages)

The evaluation of the preoperative computed tomography (CT) scan shows a bony structure that is favorable to splitting, but that will not allow simultaneous implant placement (Figure 13.9).

Local anesthesia is achieved by infiltrating xylocaine 2% containing 1:100,000 epinephrine. A midcrestal incision is made, and full-thickness flaps are reflected. If this technique is used in the maxilla, then the first bony cut could be done using a Rib-Back Bard-Parker blade (Figure 13.10). Subsequently, the crestal bone incision and the anterior and posterior bone-releasing incisions are completed with a surgical tungsten carbide bone cutter to create a trapezoidal-shape osteotomy. A bony chisel is then inserted in the initial crestal incision using a mallet and a light tapping force. The bone chisel is then gently "wiggled" bucco-lingually to enlarge the width of the osteotomy by gently displacing the buccal bony plate (Figure 13.11). This can be done in the maxilla quite easily as the bone is less dense than in the mandible. Once that opening between the two cortices (buccal and palatal) has been created, a bone graft is placed (Figure 13.12) and covered with a membrane (Figure 13.13). A periosteal release is necessary prior to closing the flaps by primary intention (Figure 13.14).

Ridge Split with Implant Placement Using the Osteotome Technique (One Stage)

After CT scan evaluation (Figures 13.15, 13.16), local anesthesia is achieved by infiltrating xylocaine 2% containing

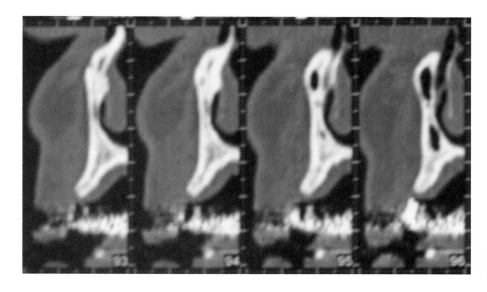

Figure 13.9 Preoperative CT scan prior to two-stage ridge splitting.

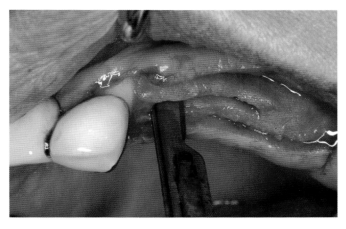

Figure 13.10 Crestal bony incision using a #15 blade and mallet.

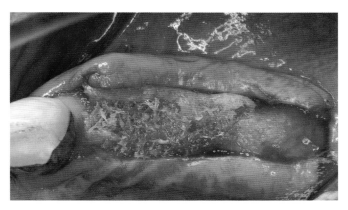

Figure 13.12 Intercortical bone grafting.

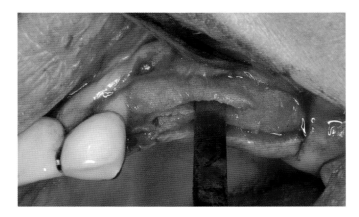

Figure 13.11 Deepening of the crestal bony incision using a bone chisel and mallet.

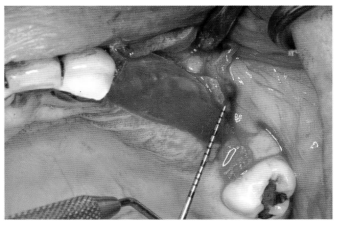

Figure 13.13 Membrane placed over the bone graft.

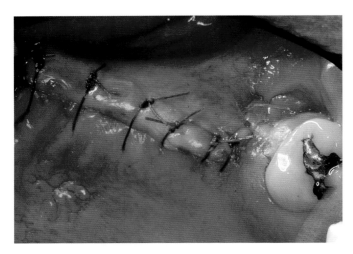

Figure 13.14 flaps sutured together (single interrupted sutures).

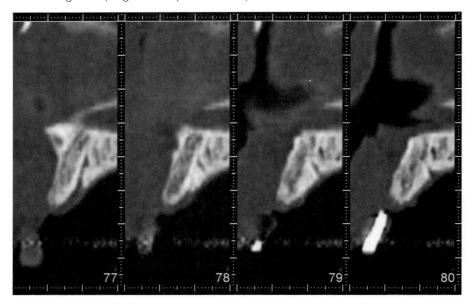

Figure 13.15 Preoperative CT scan prior to one stage ridge splitting and implant placement (#9).

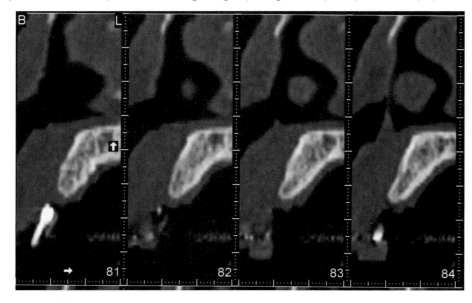

Figure 13.16 Preoperative CT scan prior to one-stage ridge splitting and implant placement (#9) (osteotome technique).

1:100,000 epinephrine around teeth #8 and 10 (Figures 13.17, 13.18). A soft-tissue incision is made to create a total-thickness flap approximately 5 mm palatal from the crest of the ridge and extended at least 6 mm anterior and posterior to the area where fracture of the bone crest is planned (Figure 13.19). An anterior and a posterior releasing incision should be done, then a labial mucoperiosteal flap reflected, exposing the alveolar ridge and about 5 mm of the buccal cortex (Figure 13.20); the periosteum should then be dissected to produce a split-thickness flap. Different flap designs can be used as explained previously, depending on the surgeon's preference. If this technique is used in the maxilla, then the first cut should be done using a Rib-Back Bard-Parker blade (Figures 13.21, 13.22). Because of the cortical nature of the mandibular ridge, the bone incision in the mandible should be made over the crest by first using a round diamond bur with diameter 0.8 mm and profuse irrigation to mark a dotted line;

subsequently, the crestal bone incision and the anterior and posterior bone-releasing incisions are completed with a surgical tungsten carbide bone cutter to create a trapezoidal shape osteotomy.

The first osteotome is usually introduced into the ridge to approximately 10 mm and placed between the labial and palatal plates and between the adjacent teeth to indicate the direction of the proposed osteotomy (Figures 13.23, 13.24). After the initial separation with the first osteotome, the surgeon can proceed to the other osteotomes using a light tapping force with the mallet to progressively separate the cortical plates by increasing the depth and width of the osteotomy.

When the cortical plates are separated, the bone site for the implants is prepared in such a way as to obtain a rigid primary

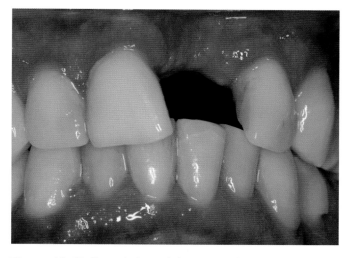

Figure 13.17 Buccal view of the space that needs implant-supported crown (#9).

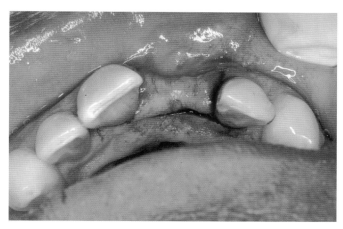

Figure 13.19 The soft tissue crestal incision is carried slightly palatally, and two releasing incisions are made mesially and distally.

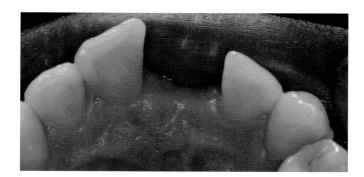

Figure 13.18 Occlusal view of the ridge.

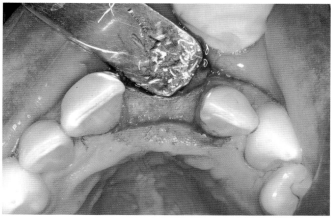

Figure 13.20 The full-thickness flap is raised and the bony ridge is exposed.

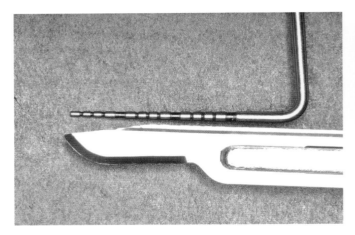

Figure 13.21 Bard-Parker Rib-Back carbon steel surgical blade #15.

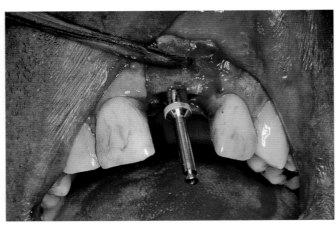

Figure 13.24 The direction indicator is in place to check for proper implant placement.

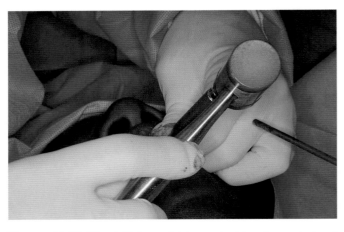

Figure 13.22 The initial crestal bony incision is carried out with the blade and mallet.

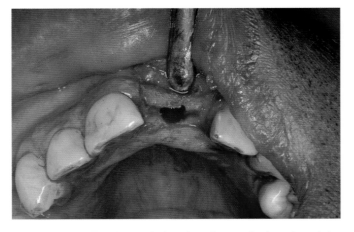

Figure 13.23 The buccal plate has been displaced and the osteotome inserted to create the implant osteotomy.

fixation that is considered fundamental to the success of the procedure. The primary stability is obtained with the precise preparation of the apical part of the implant site. Where the bone distraction is not done, the use of a root form implant and not a parallel implant increases the initial stability, as the apical portion of the implant bed will not be spread to aid in creating primary stability (Figures 13.25, 13.26).

At least 3–4 mm of intact bone should be left apical to the fracture to allow a proper recipient site preparation and to achieve primary stabilization of the implants. The buccal plate should remain no less than 1.5 mm wide.

If there is a gap of less than 3 mm, Jenson et al. (2009) recommends placement of a collagen sponge, thereby saying that there is no need for any bone graft placement. The flaps are sutured back using single interrupted sutures (Figures 13.27, 13.28).

The healing period for implants inserted with the ERE technique appears to be the same as regularly placed implants (Scipioni et al. 1999; Figures 13.29 and 13.30).

THE USE OF PIEZOSURGERY

The use of the piezoelectric ridge expansion technique permits implant placement in anatomic situations previously impossible to accomplish in a single-stage surgical operation. Piezoelectric scalpels separate the bone flaps without the risk of fracture caused by the excessive trauma that can result when using the chisel and osteotome technique. Vercelloti (2000) showed that the peri-implant healing is predictable because the piezoelectric inserts do not overheat the bone, which leads to a well-vascularized area.

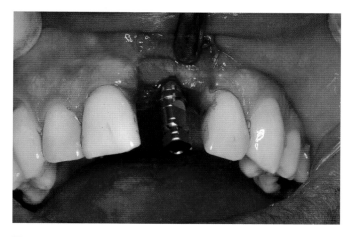

Figure 13.25 The implant is inserted.

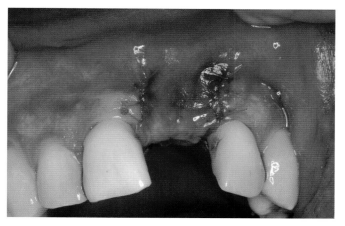

Figure 13.28 Flap is sutured with single interrupted sutures.

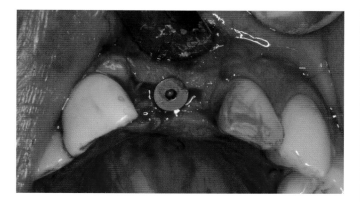

Figure 13.26 The implant mount had been removed and the healing screw inserted.

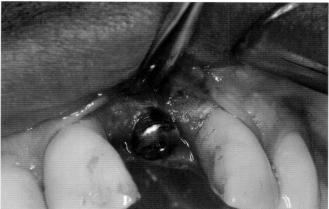

Figure 13.29 Uncovering surgery at 4 months; notice the amount of bone around the implant.

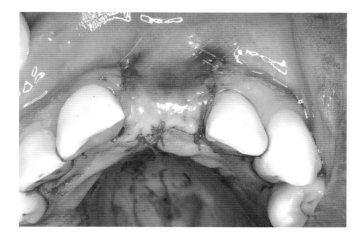

Figure 13.27 A periosteal release has been created for the buccal flap, allowing for primary closure.

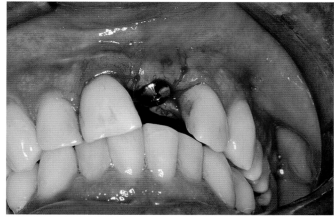

Figure 13.30 Healing abutment placed and flaps sutured.

Also the piezoelectric inserts have a smaller diameter compared to the surgical burs, thereby leading to preservation of the ridge. When the alveolar ridge is less than 3 mm and there is very little cancellous bone left, the use of piezoelectric inserts makes it possible to expand the ridge and place implants at the same time (Vercellotti 2000; Figures 13.31–13.33).

Piezoelectric inserts cut in a selective manner, thereby protecting the important structures such as nerves and the sinus membrane (Danza, Guidi, Carinci 2009). Also, the presence of a cooling irrigation fluid helps in visibility of the surgical site. A BS5 insert (Piezotome, Satelec, Acteon Group) is particularly useful (Figure 13.34). At the end of the crestal osteotomy, the bone loss due to the cuts is minimal (unlike the bur) (Figure 13.35). The buccal plate is displaced delicately to increase the buccal-lingual distance, and osteotomies using implant drills are carried out prior to implant placement (Figures 13.36, 13.37). Bone is grafted (Figure 13.38), and flaps are sutured back using single interrupted sutures. A postoperative radiograph illustrate the favorable outcome of the procedure (Figure 13.39).

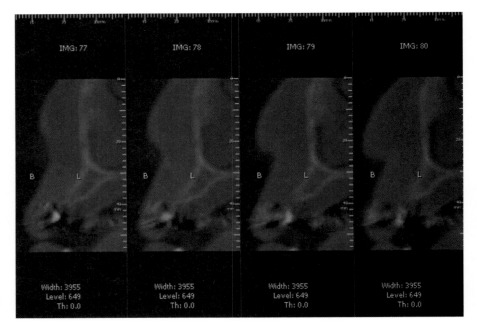

Figure 13.31 Preoperative CT scan prior to one-stage surgery.

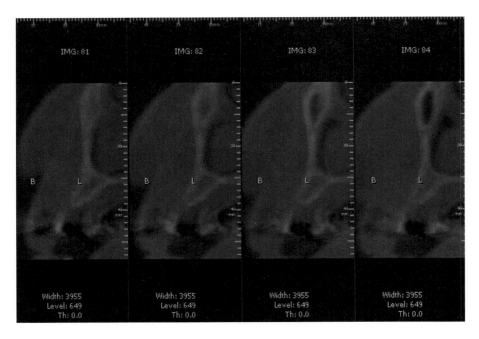

Figure 13.32 Preoperative CT scan prior to one stage-surgery (#11, #13).

Two-Stage Ridge Splitting of the Mandible

This two-stage technique is used mainly in the mandible because of the cortical nature of the bone and the higher chance for buccal plate fracture. After thorough radiographic evaluation (Figure 13.40) and local anesthesia, a midcrestal mucoperiosteal flap is elevated. One crestal groove is done using a #15 blade, then two vertical grooves are placed mesially and distally of the "bony flap" using a #2 round bur. A horizontal decortication is done at the base in order to weaken that buccal-cortical plate and allow for expansion (Figure 13.41). Then, the crestal groove is continued apically past the cortical bone into the cancellous bone. Relocation of the buccal plate of bone is done carefully and in a facial direction (Figure 13.42). Guiding pins should be wedged between the two cortices to hold the space (Figure 13.43) that was created

by splitting the ridge. The two screws are placed through the buccal plate and into the lingual plate to hold and stabilize the buccal plate (Figures 13.44, 13.45). The space created (Figure 13.46) is then filled with demineralized freeze dried bone (DFDBA) and Bio-Oss (Figure 13.47), and laminar bone can be used to cover the ridge (Figure 13.48). The flaps are sutured back with single interrupted sutures (Figure 13.49). A postoperative 6-month CT scan shows the successful outcome of the procedure (Figure 13.50).

One-Stage Ridge Splitting of the Mandible (with Implant Placement)

Using the Piezotome or the bur, a mucoperiosteal flap is elevated (Figure 13.51) and the ridge-splitting surgery performed as previously described (Figure 13.52). The buccal

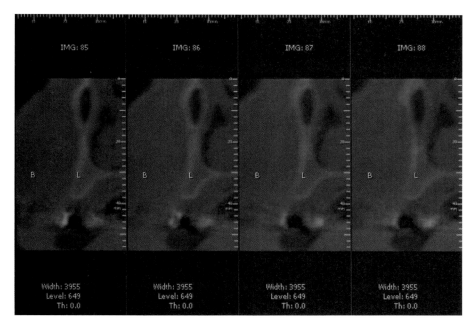

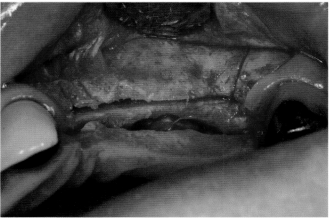

Figure 13.33 Preoperative CT scan prior to one stage surgery(#11, #13).

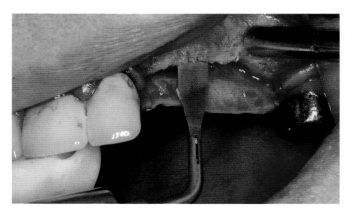

Figure 13.34 Insert BS5 from Satelec (Acteongroup, Merignac, France).

Figure 13.35 Bony crestal and "releasing" incisions. Notice how thin the osteotomy lines are when you use the piezotome

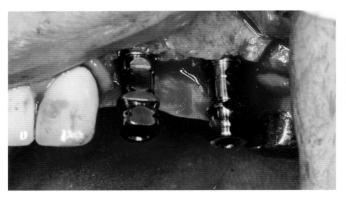

Figure 13.36 Implants placed in the position of teeth #11 and #13.

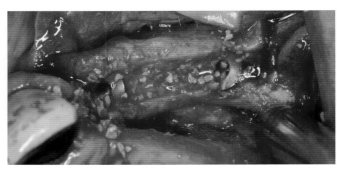

Figure 13.38 Bone graft placed in between the two corticals and around the implants.

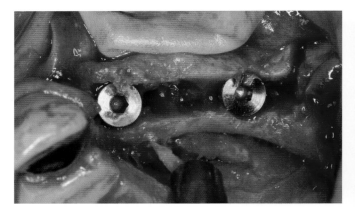

Figure 13.37 Occlusal view of the implants after placement of the healing screws.

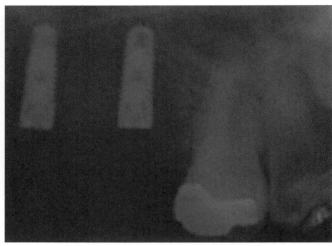

Figure 13.39 Postoperative radiograph showing proper position of the implants.

Figure 13.40 Preoperative CT scan of the lower posterior mandible that will require ridge splitting prior to implant placement. In this case, a two-stage procedure was chosen.

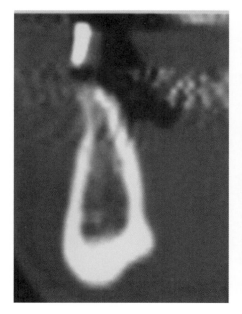

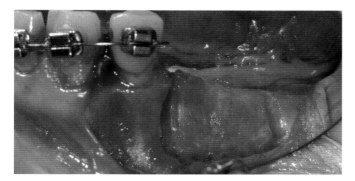

Figure 13.41 Mandible (area #19, #20) ERE with no implant placement.

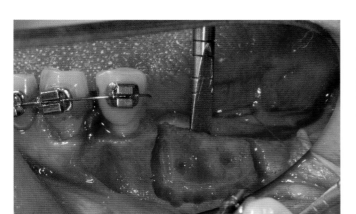

Figure 13.42 The buccal cortex is gently displaced using a bone chisel.

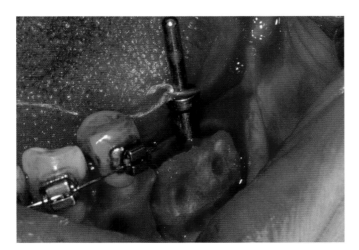

Figure 13.43 The buccal cortex, now displaced buccally, is kept in place with the help of a guiding pin inserted between the two cortices.

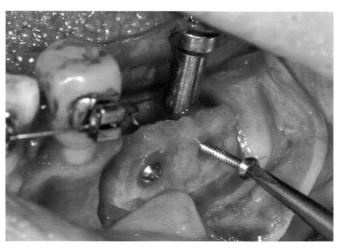

Figure 13.44 Two screws are placed to ensure the immobility of the cortical plate in its new position.

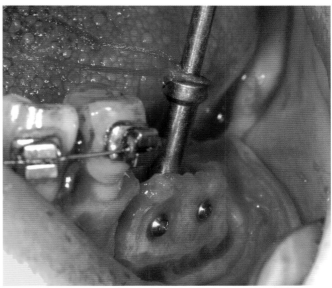

Figure 13.45 Buccal plate is now secured in its final position, and the internal space is ready for grafting.

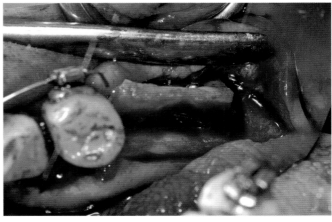

Figure 13.46 Occlusal view showing the extent of the ridge splitting and displacement of the buccal plate.

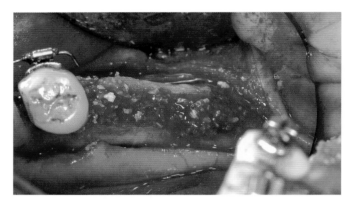

Figure 13.47 Area grafted with an allograft.

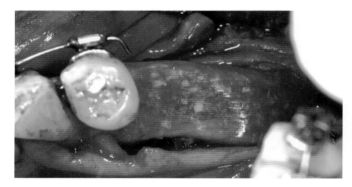

Figure 13.48 Membrane put on top of the graft.

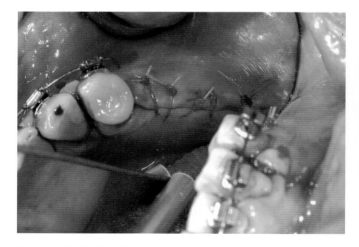

Figure 13.49 The flaps are sutured.

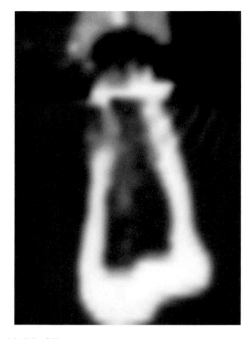

Figure 13.50 CT scan of that area 6 months later showing the new ridge width.

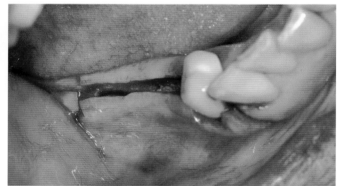

Figure 13.51 One-stage ridge splitting with implant placement site #29 and #30.

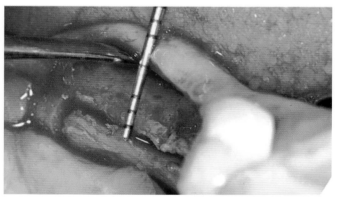

Figure 13.52 Crestal osteotomy.

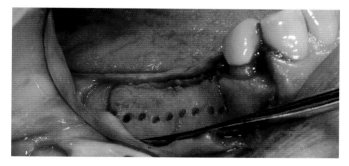

Figure 13.53 Weakening of the buccal plate with a round bur osteotomy.

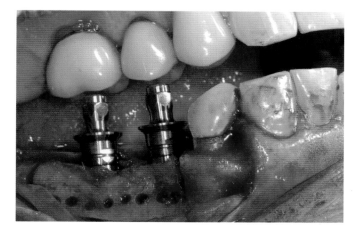

Figure 13.54 Placement of the two implants to replace teeth #29 and #30.

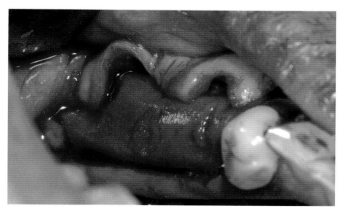

Figure 13.55 Guided bone regeneration (membrane and bone allograft).

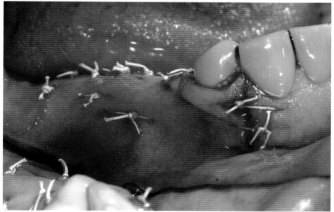

Figure 13.56 Flaps sutured with ePTFE sutures.

cortex is weakened with a "dotted line osteotomy" that goes from the external cortex to the midcrestal osteotomy's internal cut (Figure 13.53). This apical portion of the bony flap should not exceed 70% of the planned implant length. (For example, if the implant length is 10 mm, the distance between the crest of the bone and the apical dotted line osteotomy should not exceed 7 mm so that there is at least 3 mm of apical bone to ensure primary stability of the implant).

Once the buccal cortex has been displaced 3–4 mm, the implant drill sequence is used to create the implant osteotomy, and the fixtures are inserted (Figure 13.54). The implant mounts are removed, and a long-lasting collagen membrane is placed (Figure 13.55). The flap is sutured together with single interrupted and horizontal mattress sutures (Figure 13.56). A radiograph taken a year later shows the favorable outcome of the procedure (Figure 13.57), which is confirmed at the time of reentry for second-stage surgery (Figure 13.58). The case is restored with splinted prosthetic crowns shortly thereafter (Figure 13.59).

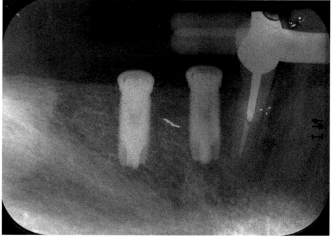

Figure 13.57 Radiograph of the area 1 year later.

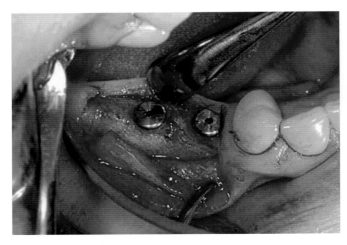

Figure 13.58 Uncovering of the area 1 year later; notice the bone fill.

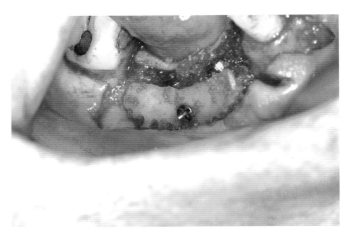

Figure 13.60 Fractured buccal plate that has been secured with a screw (the screw engages the lingual cortex and provides stabilization).

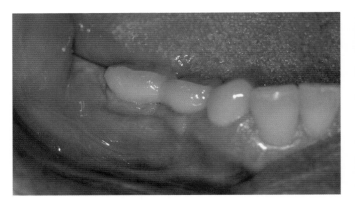

Figure 13.59 Prosthetic crown placement replacing teeth #29 and #30.

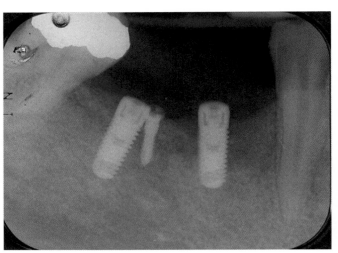

Figure 13.61 Radiograph of the area 6 months later.

Postoperative Treatment and Healing Period

After surgery, all patients received:

1. Oral antibiotics for 8 days

2. Nonsteroidal analgesics for 8 days

3. Detailed instructions about oral hygiene (mouth rinses with 0.2% chlorhexidine for 2 weeks).

Sutures were removed 8–15 days after surgery. For all implants inserted in the maxilla in conjunction with the split crest technique, the waiting time before the prosthetic phase was 3 months to allow an adequate amount of time for osseointegration.

COMPLICATIONS

The main complication is a fracture of the buccal plate (this will happen mainly in the mandible). When this occurs, the fractured segment is treated as a block graft and stabilized using screws (Figures 13.60–13.62) or a plate (Figures 13.63–13.67) with concomitant particulate grafting and membranes.

Another complication is membrane exposure in the mandible 1 week after the surgery. This could be minimized by proper buccal periosteal release as well as lingual release (blunt dissection of the lingual flap with a periosteal elevator at first and finger afterward). This slight release of the mylohyoide during the finger dissection will allow for a slight raising of the floor of the mouth and an easier suturing of the flaps. In the maxilla, when soft tissue closure is a problem, one can use a "pedicle" flap taken from the palate (Figures 13.68, 13.69).

Another complication is paroxysmal positional vertigo. According to Danza and colleagues (2009), "Benign parox-

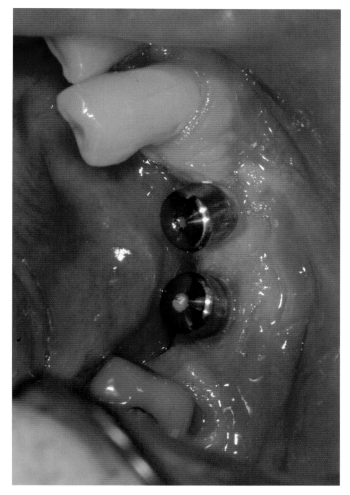

Figure 13.62 The area has been uncovered, and the healing abutments placed. It is ready for final restoration.

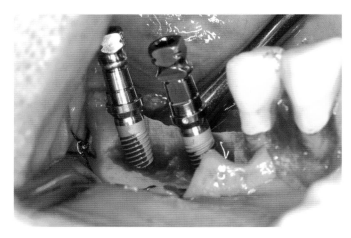

Figure 13.63 The buccal plate has fractured in two places and has been removed, the implants are inserted in the osteotomy.

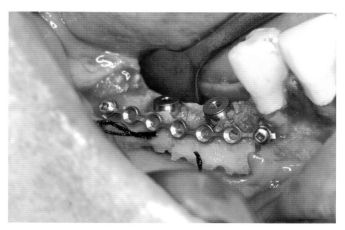

Figure 13.64 The pieces of the buccal plate are repositioned over the implants and secured with a metal plate.

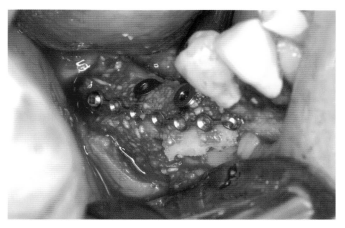

Figure 13.65 A bone allograft is placed prior to the use of a membrane for guided bone regeneration.

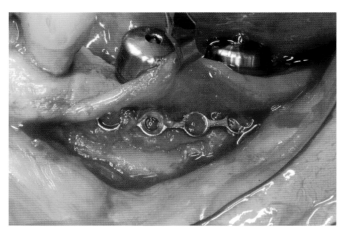

Figure 13.66 A year later, an incision is made in the muco-buccal fold to remove the metal plate.

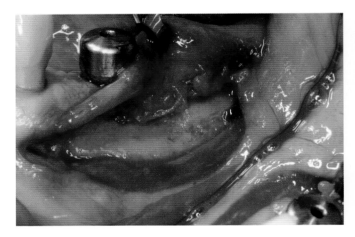

Figure 13.67 Once the plate has been removed, the healed buccal bone can be seen.

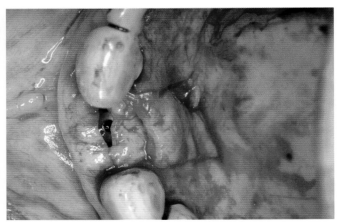

Figure 13.69 The flaps are ready to be sutured by primary intention with the help of that "extra" tissue taken from the inner palate.

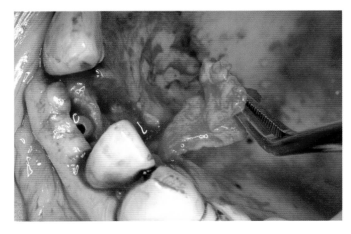

Figure 13.68 An inner palatal flap has been dissected from the palate. This will help achieve primary closure when the buccal soft tissue is scarce.

ysmal positional vertigo (BPPV) is a common vestibular end organ disorder characterized by short, often recurrent episodes of vertigo that are triggered by certain head movements in the plane of the posterior semicircular canals. BPPV may be idiopathic or secondary to a number of underlying conditions such as head injury, viral labyrinthitis, stapes surgery, and chronic suppurative otitis media."

The use of osteotomes and surgical hammers for implant bed preparation, especially in middle-aged patients, will lead to vertigo, which is an unpleasant and stressful situation for the patient. Although this condition resolves quickly with appropriate treatment, patients should be aware that this is a complication of the edentulous ridge expansion technique.

SURVIVAL RATE

Sciopioni showed that after 7 months of healing following surgical ridge expansion and implant installation, the amount of bone that was in intimate contact with the fixture surface was similar at test implants and at controls placed in normal alveolar bone.

In a 10-year multicenter retrospective clinical study of 1,715 implants placed with the edentulous ridge expansion technique (Bravi et al. 2007). The overall success rate over the 10-year follow-up period was 95.7%. Success rate in the mandible was higher than in the maxilla. The percentage of failures of cylindrical implants was about two times greater than that for root-form implants .The survival rate in the mandible was 100% and 94.7% in the maxilla, in line with the trend observed for classical implant placement. In contrast to normal implant placement procedures, the posterior region was more successful than the anterior one, 99.5% versus 82%, respectively.

This high survival rate was also shown by Sethi and Kraus (2000) and Ferrigno and Laureti (2005).

CONCLUSIONS

Ridge expansion is a fairly simple procedure that is well tolerated by patients. It could be a valid alternative to techniques that require extra bone augmentation. However, the limitation of this technique is the inability to create bone vertically. Use of the Piezotome gives good results with fewer complications.

REFERENCES

Basa S, Varol A, Turker N. 2004 Alternative bone expansion technique for immediate placement of implants in the edentulous posterior mandibular ridge: A clinical report. *Int J Oral Maxillofac Implants*. 19:554–58.

Blus C, Szmukler-Moncler S. 2006. Split-crest and immediate implant placement with ultra-sonic bone surgery: A 3-year life-table analysis with 230 treated sites. *Clin Oral Impl Res*. 17:700–707.

Bravi F, Bruschi GB, Ferrini F. 2007. A 10-year multicenter retrospect clinical study of 1,715 implants placed with the edentulous Ridge Expansion Technique. *Int J Periodontics Restorative Dent*. 27:557–65.

Bruschi GB, Scipioni A. 1990. Alveolar augmentation: New applications for implants. In Heimke G, ed. *Osseointegrated Implants*. Vol II. Implants in Oral and ENT Surgery. Bocca Raton, FL: CRC Press. p 35.

Chiapasco M, Ferrini F, Casentini P, et al. 2006. Dental implants placed in expanded narrow edentulous ridges with the Extension Crests device. A 1–3 year multicenter follow-up study. *Clin Oral Impl Res*. 17:265–72.

Coatoam G, Marioti A. 2003. The Segmental Ridge-Split Procedure. *J Periontol*. 74:757–70.

Danza M, Guidi R, Carinci F. 2009. Comparison between implants inserted into piezo split and unsplit alveolar crests. *J Oral Maxillofac Surg*. 67:2460–65.

Eggers G, Klein J, Blank J, et al. 2004. Piezosurgery: An ultrasound device for cutting bone and its use and limitations in maxillofacial surgery. *Br J Oral Maxillofac Surg*. 42:451–53.

Enisilidis G, Wittwer G, Ewers R. 2006. Preliminary report on a staged ridge splitting technique for implant placement in the mandible: A technical note. *Int J Oral Maxillofac Implants*. 21:445–49.

Ferrigno N, Laureti M. 2005. Surgical advantages with ITI TEs implants placement in conjunction with split crest technique: 18-month results of an ongoing prospective study. *Clin Oral Impl Res*. 16:147–55.

Jensen OT, Cullum DR, Baer D. 2009. Marginal bone stability using 3 different flap approaches for alveolar split expansion for dental implants: A 1-year clinical study. *J Oral Maxillofac Surg*. 67(9):1921–30.

Jensen OT, Ellis E III, Glick P. 2009. The book flap. In Jensen OT, ed. *The Osteoperiosteal Flap*. Chicago: Quintessence Publishing.

Koo, S, Serge D, Weber, H-P. 2008. Ridge-splitting technique with simultaneous implant placement. *Compend Contin Educ Dent*. 29:106–10.

Pace-Balzan A, Rutka JA. 1991. Non-ampullary plugging of the posterior semicircular canal for benign paroxysmal positional vertigo. *J Laryngol Otol*. 105:901.

Penarrocha M, Perez H., Garcia A, et al. 2001. Benign paroxysmal positional vertigo as a complication of osteotome expansion of the maxillary alveolar ridge. *J Oral Maxillofac Surg*. 59:106–107.

Scipioni A, Bruschi GB, Giargia M, et al. 1997. Healing at implants with and without primary bone contact. An experimental study in dogs. *Clin Oral Impl Res*. 8:39–47.

Scipioni A, Bruschi GB, Calesini M, et al. 1999. Bone regeneration in the edentulous ridge expansion technique: Histological and ultrastructural study of 20 clinical cases. *Int J Periodontics Restorative Dent*. 19:269–77.

Scipioni A, Bruschi GB, Calesini M, et al. 1994. The edentulous Ridge Expansion Technique: A five year study. *Int J Periodontics Reststorative Dent*. 14:451–59.

Sethi A, Kaus T. 2000. Maxillary ridge expansion with simultaneous implant placement: 5-year results of an ongoing clinical study. *Int J Oral Maxillofac Implants*. 15:491–99.

Summers RB. 1994. A new concept in maxillary implant surgery: The osteotome technique. *Compendium*. 15:152, 154–6, 158 passim; quiz 162.

Tatum H. 1986. Maxillary and sinus implant reconstructions. *Dent Clin North Am*. 30:207–29.

Vercellotti T. 2000. Piezoelectric surgery in implantology: A case report—a new piezoelectric ridge expansion technique. *Int J Periodontics Restorative Dent*. 20:358–65.

Zijderveld SA, ten Bruggenkate CM, van Den Bergh JP, et al. 2004. Fractures of the iliac crest after split-thickness bone grafting for pre-prosthetic surgery: Report of 3 cases and review of the literature. *J Oral Maxillofac Surg*. 62:781–86. Review.

Chapter 14 Autogenous Block Graft

Luigi Montesani, MD, DMD

Onlay grafting is a method in which the graft material is placed over the defective area to increase width and/or height of the alveolar jawbone when there is insufficient volume to accommodate endosseous implants, hence the need for bone reconstructive treatment (Collins 1991). This method can also be used to level deformities in the bone contour or to cover dehiscence. In minor graft procedures, small pieces of bone may be harvested from the chin or retro-molar area or tuberosity (intraoral source), and the host bed is usually perforated by means of a small round bur to stimulate the formation of a blood clot between graft and recipient bed. The graft is immobilized with screws and plates or with dental implants (Kahnberg, 1989; Kahnberg, Nystrom and Bartholdsson 2005). In major graft procedures, bone from the iliac crest or calvaria (extraoral source) is most commonly used to repair defects due to severe bone deficiency.

All these grafts are called "autogenous" (or "autografts"), because the missing bone is replaced with bone from the patient's own body, that is, by transplanting the bone tissue from one site to another (recipient site) within the same individual. The sources of autogenous bone grafts may be either intraoral or extraoral. The two main intraoral sources of block grafts are the mandibular symphysis and the mandibular ramus. As already mentioned, one extraoral source of block grafts include the iliac crest; but due to its endochondral origin, it has been shown to have increased resorptive properties (Zins 1983), whereas the resorption observed for mandibular sites seems to be lower. In addition, with the iliac crest harvesting procedure, an increase in morbidity is observed, associated with the need for hospitalization (Shwartz-Arad 2005). Implant reconstruction does not require the harvesting of as large a bone volume as that harvested from the iliac crest; therefore, this latter donor site is not indicated other than for large reconstructive surgeries. Moreover, recent advances in piezoelectric surgery (PS) have allowed easier harvesting from the mandibular ramus and symphysis, which in turn facilitates the procurement of even larger-size bone grafts because the piezoelectric cutting tip allows a more precise bone-saving cut (Vercellotti et al. 2005).

After a thorough exploration of the morphology of the bony defect to select a suitable bone-promoting technique, most commonly an autogenous bone graft is chosen. Indeed, autografts are considered the gold standard in bone grafting since they are essentially living tissues with their cells intact. Thus, no immune reaction is to be expected, and the outcome—especially in terms of healing and prognostic predictability—is very often successful as compared to other techniques using alloplastic and allogenic materials. Also, autogenous block grafts have superior biological and mechanical properties, and—being autogenous in nature (i.e., osteoconductive and osteoinductive)—represent an ideal choice for grafting large defects, ranging from Seibert class I to Seibert class III defects.

Importantly, all types of autografts have similar regenerative processes, but the success of the grafting procedure basically depends from the quality and intensity of revascularization(Burchardt 1983). In the absence of blood supply, the bone tissue dies and the bone collapses. However, besides the quality of the donor site, the graft revascularization also depends on the regenerative potential of the recipient site, which is generally unknown prior to surgery. Thus it is necessary to resolve the problem of improving graft regeneration and revascularization while maintaining bone density and osseointegration properties. In this regard, it is worth mentioning some theories addressing this issue, such as, for example, the so-called osteoblast theory by Wolff in 1863 (Glicenstein 2000), according to which grafted bone healing occurs by osteogenesis. In 1893, Barth introduced the "framework theory," stating that regeneration takes place through osteoconduction (colonization of the mineral part by osteoblasts from the recipient site). Today, studies mainly support the osteoinduction principle (osteoinduction implies the recruitment of immature cells and their stimulation to develop into preosteoblasts, thus inducing osteogenesis) for regeneration (Boyne, 1997), but all three confirm the graft of autogenous bone as the most advantageous in terms of regenerative capacity.

ADVANTAGES OF CHIN BONE HARVESTING

The chin, or menton, the lowest point of the mandibular symphysis, has been reported in the literature as an important donor site in preprosthetic reconstructions because the bone

Practical Osseous Surgery in Periodontics and Implant Dentistry, First Edition. Edited by Serge Dibart, Jean-Pierre Dibart.
© 2011 John Wiley & Sons, Inc. Published 2011 by John Wiley & Sons, Inc.

in this region is usually dense (mean volume obtained from a symphyseal harvest, about 4.71 mL). Multiple advantages of chin bone harvesting have been documented in the literature (Reddi 1987; Pikos 2005a, 2005b). As previously stated, onlay grafts are used especially when bone height or width are an issue, and chin block grafts (self-donated chin bone) are often successfully used to reconstruct the ridge defect before implant placement. The areas of the chin bone from which bone is extracted are known to regenerate very quickly and to provide what is considered to be the healthiest and best source of augmentation material, with only minimal complications and significantly less resorption. In addition, intra-membranous bone grafts maintain more volume than endochondral ones, possibly due to their faster revascularization. Indeed, the symphyseal region can provide higher quantities of bone compared with other intraoral sites. However, in order to avoid excessive resorption of the chin graft, it is recommended that fixture installation be performed within 4 months from the graft placement, except in particular cases (Sindet-Pedersen and Enemark 1990; Pikos 1995).

Moreover, another main advantage of chin bone harvesting is the ease of access to the harvest site, with enhanced proximity to the donor site. The bone harvested from the symphysis is an embryonic one, which means that it is vascularized quickly, and this leads to less resorption, making chin bone a good graft material for the preparation of the implant bed. It has been documented that the highest concentrations of promoter proteins, such as bone morphogenetic protein (BMP) or osteogenin, are found in the cortical structure (Urist, Mikulski and Lietze 1979; Urist and McLean 1952).

Furthermore, because harvesting of chin grafts is generally done under local anesthesia, after local infiltration and blocking of both mental nerves to reduce intraoperative bleeding, there is no need for hospitalization, which, taken together with minimal morbidity, a short healing period, and absence of cutaneous scars, represents an attractive option for the patient.

Chin grafts may be useful in managing both maxillary and mandibular reconstruction procedures, especially when small- to medium-size blocks are needed (Pikos 1996).

ADVANTAGES OF RAMUS BONE HARVESTING OVER SYMPHYSIS GRAFT (MISCH 2000; CAPELLI 2003; TOSCANO ET AL. 2010)

The mandibular ramus block graft can provide sufficient bone for medium- to long-span reconstructions, with augmentation of 3 to 4 mm being achieved both in the horizontal and vertical directions (Pikos 2005a, 2005b), In fact, ramus grafts are indicated in moderate to severe localized defects, for example,

in one- to four-tooth edentulous spans. If the third molars have been extracted or congenital missing of teeth is observed, or if there is not enough bone to harvest from the chin area, the ramus site can be used. In addition, a bilateral harvest from both rami gives the option to harvest a larger volume of bone when reconstructing a large edentulous area. Thanks to the thickness of the ramus cortical bone blocks, it is possible to obtain rectangular grafts of appreciable size, although some trouble exists in accessing this donor site. However, when harvesting bone from the mentum, there is a risk of altered facial contour, which is why the donor area should be grafted with particulate bone after harvest; this is not a concern when harvesting from the ramus. Moreover, the proximity of the ramus to the mandibular recipient sites makes it an excellent donor source. Mostly cortical bone is harvested from the ascending ramus of the mandible; with these grafts, a lower incidence of complications is observed than during chin graft procedures. The advantages of this donor site over the chin also include a decrease in complaints of postoperative sensory disturbances of the face and teeth by the patient and absence of aesthetic concerns (Pikos 1996; Misch and Misch 1995). Overall, fewer complications are reported with ramus bone harvesting than with the chin, and resorption rates are more than acceptable. Furthermore, long-term morbidity associated with mandibular ramus bone grafts is reported to be slightly lower than with symphyseal bone grafts. As already mentioned above, however, the surgical access is somewhat limited, and in a few cases there might be some damage to the mandibular neurovascular bundle. In any case, it appears that more ramus grafts are performed than chin blocks. Actually, the use of the mandibular ramus as a donor site is often preferable because of associated lower morbidity and postoperative pain. Symphyseal bone grafts offer bone quantity and quality, and chin ptosis is not a concern, as long as the inferior border is not exceeded and the mentalis muscle is managed well. Nevertheless, the ramus graft requires a short healing period (4 to 5 months) and shows minimal bone resorption while providing a high-density bone quality (Capelli, 2003).

More generally speaking, it is also important to note that classical studies, as well as several reviews conducted on both ramus and symphysis grafts, report a range of about 1- to 7-mm, with an average 4-mm, augmentation width increase. There are also advantages of blocks in terms of better bone quality for implants and faster integration (implants can be placed in 4 months vs. 6–9 months, compared with guided bone regneration). However, there is a lack of long-term studies on blocks. It is known that osteocytes in the block do not survive, and the block is turned over by gradual penetration of osteogenic tissue into the site to form new bone (creeping substitution). Resorption is known to be about 25% between the time of the block graft and the implant placement, but it would be important to know how much bone is resorbed and reconstructed over time. No such reports, however, are yet available in the literature (Toscano et al. 2010).

The rationale for using barrier membranes is the prevention of graft resorption, although the reviews of the efficacy of barrier membranes have been complicated by the inclusion of uncontrolled studies. Despite that, the current best evidence would suggest that it is reasonable to state that membranes show some preventative effects on graft resorption. (Rasmusson et al. 1999, Gielkins et al. 2007)

Ramus grafts are contraindicated in the following cases: the width of the ramus is less than 10 mm; the mandibular canal is positioned superiorly; the patient has limited jaw mobility or has previously undergone a sagittal split osteotomy; and the presence of third molar pathology may also potentially affect the harvested bone. Also, it is important to remember that thickness and morphology of the bone grafts harvested from the ascending ramus are not homogeneous and that, from a qualitative point of view, they are monocortical, with little or no cancellous bone.

Both the donor sites considered share a common embryological origin (first and second brachial arches) and, being membranous, have slow resorption rates.

SURGICAL TECHNIQUES

Chin Graft

The incision design is either intrasulcular or vestibular. The intrasulcular design is contraindicated in the presence of healthy periodontium, crown and bridge work, and thin biotype (Pikos 1996; Figure 14.1). Similar to any other flap procedure, some crestal bone loss can be expected with this procedure. In addition, dehiscences and fenestrations could be exposed by this technique, and if the remaining bone is

thin, surgical trauma and loss of periosteal blood supply to one-third of the facial plate could induce irreversible bone loss at the crest, followed by soft tissue recession. Repositioning of the tissue is difficult, especially when the mentalis muscle is stripped from its attachment. Usually, the intrasulcular incision is made on the facial aspect of the lower anteriors as far distal as the canines, with a full-thickness flap to expose the anterior surface of the mentum (Figure 14.2).

The vestibular incision is made as a shallow incision at the bottom of the vestibule, between the first premolars and in continuity with the bilateral crestal incisions to give access to the symphyseal region, thus allowing the design of the grafts needed. Mucosa, muscle, and periosteum are cut in a through-and-through fashion. After the first vestibular incision, the blade is turned perpendicular to the periosteum and the attachment of the mentalis muscle is incised to allow later suturing of the loose muscle to the part remaining attached to the bone. A full-thickness flap is reflected to expose the donor site (Figures 14.3, 14.4). The advantages with this

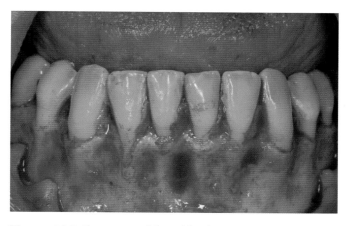

Figure 14.2 Exposure of the chin donor area after sulcular incision.

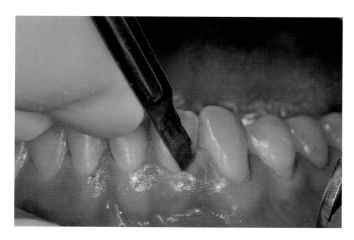

Figure 14.1 Sulcular incision.

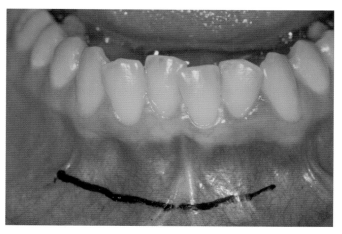

Figure 14.3 Vestibular design for incision.

Chapter 14: Autogenous Block Graft **181**

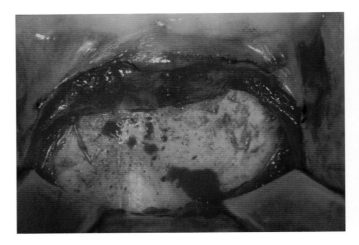

Figure 14.4 Chin donor area after exposure.

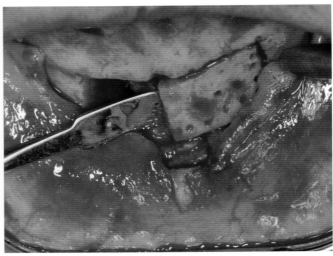

Figure 14.6 Removal of the block graft with the scalpel.

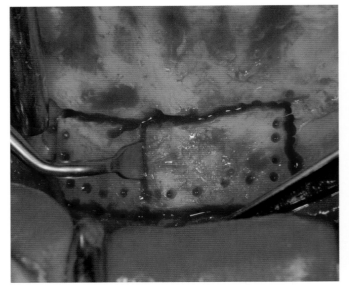

Figure 14.5 Outline of the incision with piezosurgery.

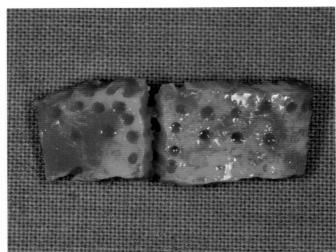

Figure 14.7 Block graft.

approach are that it does not interfere with the periodontium of the lower anterior teeth, that incisions are faster, and that the lateral access is greatly enlarged, although more morbidity and impaired postoperative recovery might be observed. After the initial incision and the reflection of the flap to expose the bone, the amount of bone needed is measured with a probe and an outline is drawn. To avoid morbidity, the most important rule to be followed is to use 5-mm safety margins— that is, 5 mm apical to the roots of the lower mandibular dentition, 5 mm anterior to the position of the mental foramen, and 5 mm coronal to the inferior border of the mandible. The bur or piezo insert used for the harvesting should be angled less than 90 degrees and undercuts avoided so that the resulting graft is easy to separate using a scalpel (Figures 14.5–14.7). A resorbable biomaterial is then placed to control bleeding and to enhance the formation of new bone to avoid altering the facial contour. Suturing is done in two steps: muscles are sutured first, and then the mucosa is sutured. Studies indicate that a block of $18 \times 6.5 \times 6$ mm can be expected as the minimal size (Montazem et al. 2000).

However, in both cases the dissection is made carefully, and the use of a sharp periosteal elevator is recommended to detach muscular insertions that appear at the inferior border from the bone. To preserve the mental nerve from injury, the dissection is not performed under the periosteal layer.

Usually, for safety purposes, the so-called 5s rule is applied to the harvesting procedure; that is, a mandatory distance of 5 mm is maintained from root apexes, mental foramen, and inferior border of the mandible. This is crucial for the vitality of the teeth and avoids contact with the anterior branch of the inferior alveolar nerve. The methods of graft procurement can differ based on the amount of bone required and the defect size.

A cheap but effective harvesting tool is the fissure bur, with which it is possible to perform sensitive control of the cut and to obtain suitable groove width for further positioning of the chisel. Trephines (of variable diameters) are indicated for harvesting small cores of corticocancellous bone, thus leaving the lingual cortex intact with neither violation of the mouth floor nor associated bleeding risks. Blades and oscillating saws are also used during this procedure so that thin cuts are made with minimal trauma. Discs, though very effective, are potentially dangerous instruments and must be used with extreme caution to avoid damage to the surrounding tissues. Furthermore, when total symphyseal harvesting is required, it is possible to reduce the risk of graft fracture by cutting the graft in the middle, which helps to achieve maximum harvesting from the mandibular symphysis safely.

When particulate bone is needed, it is necessary to grind the harvested block with a bone mill; in addition, it is advisable to mix the ground bone with platelet-rich plasma (PRP) as its cohesive and adhesive nature can help graft transportation (Anitua 2001).

Also, it is strongly recommended that the donor area be closed before taking any subsequent steps to avoid excessive bleeding and risk of infection. Persistent bleeding, if any, can be controlled by using local hemostatic agents. The donor site can be filled with bovine bone matrix and PRP to accelerate regeneration (Figures 14.8, 14.9).

Grafts must be trimmed to fit perfectly in the defects. Usually, two screws are sufficient to fix and avoid rotation of a block.

Once grafts are well integrated at the host site, the screws can be removed. If reconstruction is stable enough, graft placement and implant insertion can be done simultaneously.

RAMUS GRAFT

After careful evaluation and preparation of the recipient site to determine size and shape of the graft, it is important to extend the initial incision high enough to reach the ascending ramus to avoid possible challenges in accessing the donor site in some patients.

The incision should be made no higher than the level of the occlusal plane, as this minimizes the risk of cutting the buccal artery or exposing the buccal fat pad (Figures 14.10, 14.11). The incision also should be made distal to the second molar on the buccal aspect of the crest and then extended

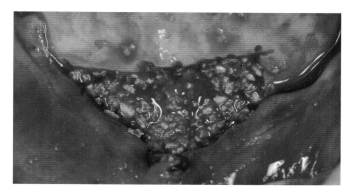

Figure 14.9 Filling the donor site with particulated bone chips to avoid loss of contour.

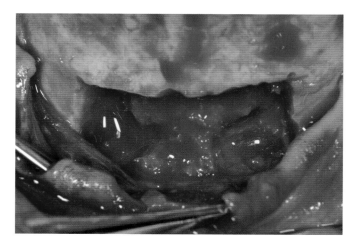

Figure 14.8 Donor site after harvesting.

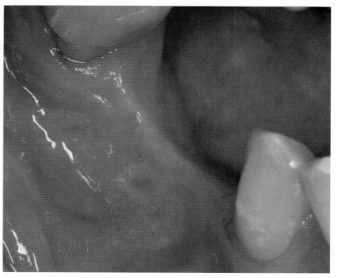

Figure 14.10 Preoperative picture.

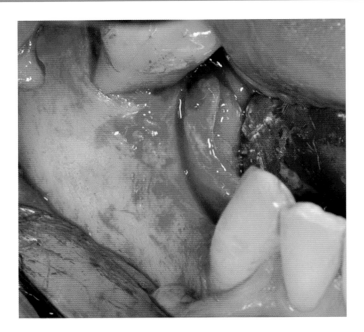

Figure 14.11 Preoperative picture showing loss of horizontal dimension.

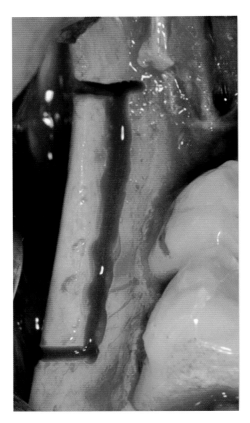

Figure 14.12 Exposure of the donor site after full thickness mucoperiosteal flap elevation.

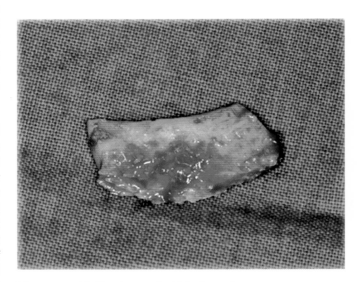

Figure 14.13 The harvested block graft.

anteriorly and laterally to expose the ramus (Figures 14.12–14.14). When making the incision, it is very important to proceed to palpation of the anterior border of the ascending ramus to avoid deviations to the lingual side that might cause trauma to the lingual or the inferior alveolar nerves. A full mucoperiosteal flap should be reflected. The size of the graft is then measured; at this point, an outline can be drawn to help in cutting. The length of the cuts obviously depends on the size of the graft required; moreover, the cut should be made only through the cortical bone.

A piezo insert can be used (BS2 tip) to make the vertical and horizontal cuts, and care should be taken to avoid injury to the inferior alveolar nerve. A preliminary CT scan analysis will show the exact dimension and location of the mandibular canal; moreover, the use of piezosurgery will limit the injury to the nerve. In this regard, it is also worth remembering that the medullary bone thickness has been found to be greatest at the distal half of the first molar; this is important to know in order to avoid possible damage, given that the position of the mandibular canal is variable and cannot be determined exactly. Also, the graft should be manipulated carefully by using a chisel parallel to the lateral surface of the ramus to avoid accidental injury or transposition of the nerve.

It is not mandatory to graft the area after harvest, but if it is done, then a decrease in bleeding and a shorter healing time will be observed. In general, the ramus yields a rectangular piece of bone approx 4 mm thick, 3 cm or more long, and up to 1 cm high (Misch 1997). After harvesting the bone graft, a bur or file is used to smooth possible sharp edges around the ramus. In addition, the cortex of the recipient site should be perforated before the placement of the bone harvested to improve revascularization (Figure 14.15).

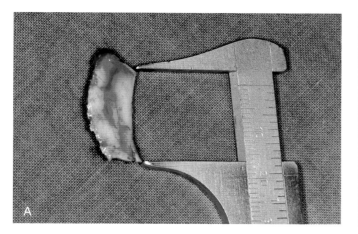

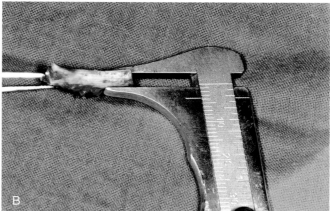

Figure 14.14 (A) Shows block graft length. (B) Shows block graft width.

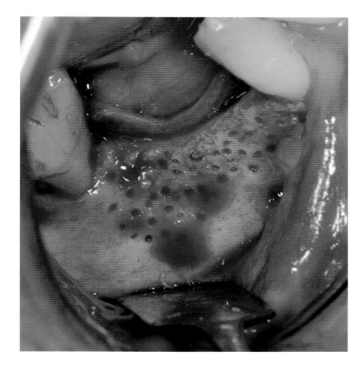

Figure 14.15 Recipient site after decortication and perforations with fissure bur 702L.

Duration of surgery and anesthesia, as well as associated morbidity, are considerably reduced thanks to the proximity of the donor and recipient sites. Also, because the procedure can be done on an outpatient basis and IV sedation and local anesthesia can be used, patient compliance and satisfaction are greatly increased.

RECIPIENT SITE

The exposure of the recipient site for the graft prior to bone harvest should be performed in all cases to ensure the minimal time between graft procurement and placement, as well as to allow measurement of the exact donor graft size required. Incisions slightly distant from the residual ridge crest—performed on the palatal side of the maxilla or on the lingual side of the mandible—and divergent releasing incisions far from the defect should be used both to facilitate closure and maintain blood supply (Figure 14.16). This is also obtained by using beveled or split-thickness incisions. Moreover, recipient sites and graft undersurfaces should be recontoured to improve bone-to-graft contact, when necessary. The underlying host bone should be decorticated and perforated with a bur (Figure 14.17). The procedure of decortication and perforation gives origin to the RAP, or regional acceleratory phenomenon (Frost 1983, Shin and Norrdin 1985).

RAP is a local response to a noxious stimulus, causing tissue forms faster than normal. It is more evident in cortical bone than in trabecular bone, with release of growth factors it is accompanied by a systemic response (systemic acceleratory phenomenon, or SAP).

The block grafts should be fixed with small-diameter titanium alloy screws (Figure 14.18) OsteoMed kit. Prior to fixation, the edges of the donor block graft should be rounded. The periosteum at the base of the flap should be incised to allow stretching of the mucosa and subsequent tension-free adaptation of the flap, which is the key to the success of all procedure (Figure 14.19).

Also, it is worth remembering that a successful bone union prognosis is usually enhanced by an intimate adaptation of the donor graft. In fact, empty spaces will remain between the graft and the recipient site if adaptation is defective, and ingrowth of fibrous tissue or infections might occur (Figure 14.20, 14.21). Establishing this intimate contact can be challenging at times as the bony block can be irregular in shape and size. The use of a proper bur kit to trim the block and

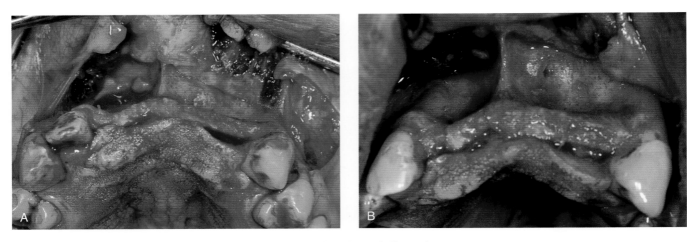

Figure 14.16 (A, B) Preoperative picture showing loss of horizontal dimension.

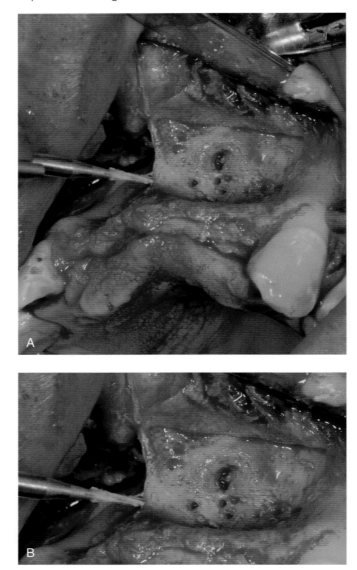

Figure 14.17 (A, B) Recipient site preparation decortication and perforation with 702L straight fissure bur (Brasseler USA, Savannah, GA).

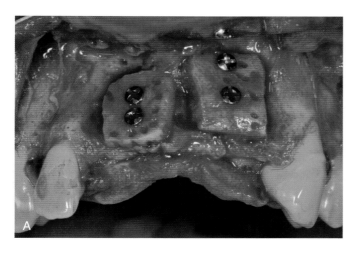
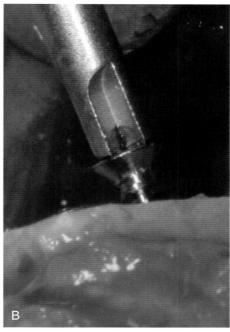

Figure 14.18 (A) Fixation of block graft with at least two screws to avoid rotation. (B) Fixation of the graft with screw.

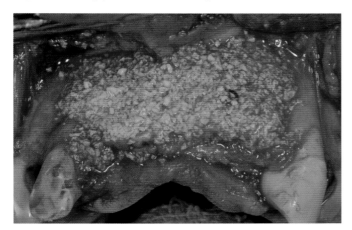

Figure 14.19 Passive adaptation of the flap of the surgical area.

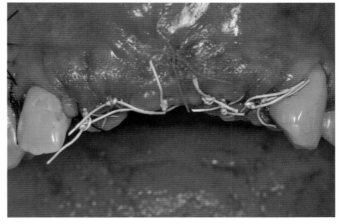

Figure 14.21 Resorbable membrane for graft protection.

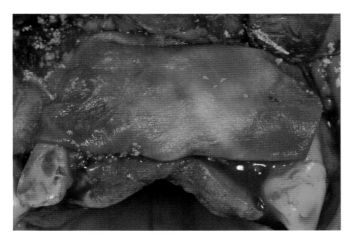

Figure 14.20 Bone particles to fill void spaces.

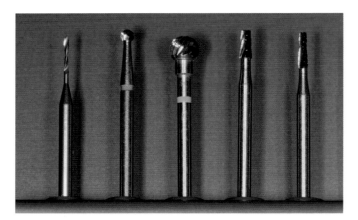

Figure 14.22 Pikos Bur Kit (Salvin Dental Specialties, Charlotte, NC) for preparation of the recipient site. The 702L straight fissure bur can also be used for donor site preparation.

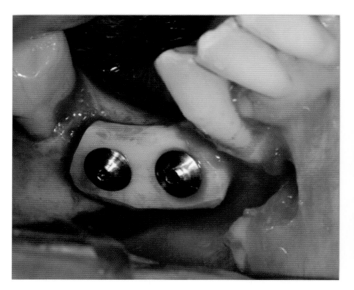

Figure 14.23 Fixation of the bone graft.

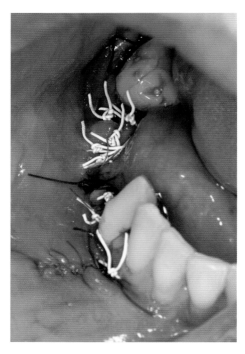

Figure 14.24 Wound passive closure.

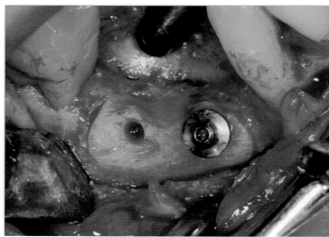

Figure 14.25 Four months later.

establish an intimate contact with the recipient site is essential (Figures 14.22–14.24). Four months after the graft the implants can be placed successfully in the newly grafted bone (Figures 14.25–14.27). The final prosthesis is completed after full osseointegration of the implants (in general 3–4 months after surgery) (Figures 14.28–14.30).

Prior to performing graft surgery, the recipient site must be completely healed. It is strongly recommended that complete removal of any foreign bodies, soft tissue surgery, and tooth extractions be done at least 8 week prior to grafting. In order to measure size and morphology of the bony defect, the reflection of the recipient site for the graft should be performed prior to graft harvest. Surgical trauma of the recipient site flap can be minimized by careful handling of soft tissues.

When the recipient site is the edentulous posterior mandible, a split-thickness incision lateral to the mucogingival junction and supraperiosteal dissection can be continued anteriorly to the most distal tooth to facilitate primary closure over the graft (Misch and Misch 1995).

MORBIDITIES (COMPLICATIONS): CHIN

Some intraoperative complications are possible with this type of procedure. Damage to the neuromuscular structure will lead to altered or loss of sensation in the chin and lip area. Damage to the roots or the pulp vascularity will cause loss of

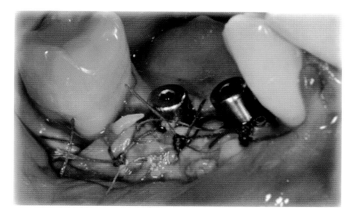

Figure 14.26 Placement of implants with healing abutment. Soft tissue grafting to improve the quality of tissue for better maintenance.

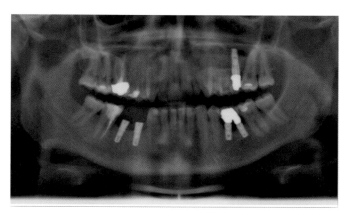

Figure 14.27. Radiographic image after implant insertion.

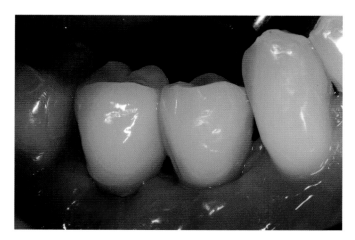

Figure 14.28 Prosthetic rehabilitation (technician M. DiPietro).

vitality of the anterior mandibular teeth, and this in turn will lead to root canal treatment. An improper incision will result in a ptosis. Injury to the mental or incisal nerve might occur; therefore, an appropriate knowledge of anatomy is important when attempting these procedures. Should a tension-free

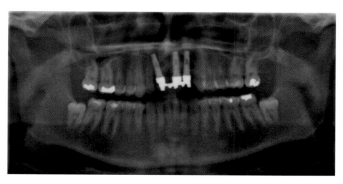

Figure 14.29 Radiographic image 6 months after implant insertion.

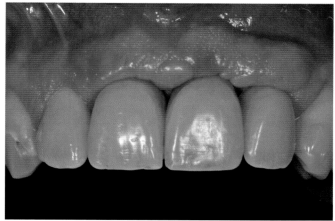

Figure 14.30 Prosthetic rehabilitation (technician M. DiPietro).

closure not be achieved, then an incision line opening might occur. Sometimes, indeed, the dental implant incision line opens—for a number of reasons. Usually, the underlying reason is that the area of bone exposed is very large, and the great amount of gum pulled up off of the jawbone cannot keep its blood supply. All human tissues, when they do not receive enough blood, have survival problems and can undergo necrosis. Infections in the dental surgery site can also decrease the blood supply and result in incision line opening.

Some long-term neurosensory disturbances have been described following symphyseal bone harvesting. Grafting of the area is important after harvest to avoid weakening of the symphysis, which might lead to fracture (Raghoebar et al. 2001; Nkene et al. 2001).

Postoperative sequelae include variable degrees of swelling and pain, but when the transection of muscle fibers from the chin region is avoided by using intrasulcular incisions and subperiosteal dissections, less swelling and pain can be expected.

MORBIDITIES (COMPLICATIONS): RAMUS

There are potential intraoperative complications to mention for the ramus, as well. Fracture, trismus, incision line opening, and damage of the inferior alveolar nerve/bundle are the most frequent complications that can be expected with the ramus bone harvesting procedure. These, however, can be avoided if proper surgical technique is followed. In addition, as already stated, the use of piezosurgery, the palpation of the anterior border of the ramus, and the careful retraction of the flaps can greatly reduce the risk of injury to nerves, and the ascending branches of the facial artery will be kept safe if the dissection of the lower border of the mandible is done at a subperiosteal plane (Nkene et al. 2001).

Postoperative complications include mild to moderate swelling, as well as pain, particularly due to disinsertion or cutting of muscles. Edema and hematoma are also frequently observed. Infections are possible, and in this regard a prophylactic antibiotic treatment—to be continued postoperatively for 5 days—is recommended. Sensory disturbances during the postoperative period can be expected when the inferior alveolar nerve has been exposed during surgery. Anti-inflammatory corticosteroids are administered in such cases. Using pressure dressings and topical ice packs may prevent early complications following this type of surgery.

POSTOPERATIVE INSTRUCTIONS

After surgery, all patients are treated as follows:

1. Oral antibiotics are given for 5 or 8 days.

2. Nonsteroidal analgesics are given for 3–5 days.

3. Detailed instructions are provided regarding oral hygiene. (mouth rinses with 0.2% chlorhexidine for 2 weeks).

4. Dexamethasone is given (to decrease the swelling).

5. Ice pack is applied on the surgical area for 5–7 hours (to decrease the swelling).

6. Chin area is bandaged to minimize hematoma.

REFERENCES

Anitua E. 2001. The use of plasma rich growth factors in oral surgery. *Pract Proced Aesthet Dent*. 13:487–93.

Boyne PJ, Marx RE, Nevins M, et al. A feasibility study evaluating rhBMP-2/absorbable collagen sponge for maxillary sinus floor augmentation. *Int J Periodontics Restorative Dent*. 17:11–25.

Burchardt H. 1983. The biology of bone graft repair. *Clin Orthop*. 174:28–42.

Capelli M. 2003. Autogenous bone graft from the mandibular ramus: A technique for bone augmentation. *Int J Periodontics Restorative Dent*. 23:277–85.

Collins TA. 1991. Onlay bone grafting in combination with Branemark implants. *Oral Maxillofac Surg Clin North Am*. 3:893–902.

Frost H. 1983. The regional acceleratory phenomenon, a review. *Henry Ford Hosp Med*. J 31:3–9.

Gielkins PF, Bos RR, Raghoebar GM, et al. 2007. Is there evidence that barrier membranes prevent bone resorption autologous bone graft during the healing period? A systematic review. *Int J Oral Max Facial Impl*. 22:390–98.

Glicenstein J. 2000. History of bone reconstruction [trans. from French]. *Ann Chir Plast Esthet*. 45:171–74.

Kahnberg KE. 2005. *Bone grafting techniques for maxillary implants*. Ames, Iowa: Blackwell Munksgaard.

Kahnberg KE, Nystrom E, Bartholdsson L. 1989.Combined use of bone grafts and Branemark fixtures in the treatment of severely resorbed maxillae. *Int J Oral Maxillofac Implants*. 4:297–304.

Misch CM. 1997. Comparison of intraoral donor sites for onlay grafting prior to implant placement. *Int J Oral Maxillofac Implants*. 12:767–76.

Misch CM. 2000. Use of the mandibular ramus as a donor site for onlay bone grafting. *J Oral Implantol*. 26:42–49.

Misch CM, Misch CE. 1995. The repair of localized severe ridge defects for implant placement using mandibular bone grafts. *Impl. Dent*. 4:261–67.

Montazem A, Valauri DV, St-Hilaire H, et al. 2000. The mandibular symphysis as a donor site in maxillofacial bone grafting: A quantitative anatomic study. *J Oral Maxillofac Surg*. 58:1368–71.

Nkenke E, Schultze-Mosgau S, Radespiel-Tröger M, et al. 2001. Morbidity of harvesting of chin grafts: A prospective study. *Clin Oral Implants Res*. 12:495–502.

Pikos MA. 1995. Facilitating implant placement with chin grafts as donor sites for maxillary bone augmentation, Part I. *Dent Impl*. (Update). 6(12):89–92.

Pikos MA. 1996. Chin grafts as donor sites for maxillary bone augmentation, Part II. *Dent Impl*. (Update). 7(1):1–4.

Pikos MA. 2005a. Atrophic posterior maxilla and mandible: Alveolar ridge reconstruction with mandibular block autografts. *Alpha Omegan*. 98(10):34–35.

Pikos MA. 2005b. Mandibular block autografts for Alveolar ridge augmentation. *Atlas Oral Maxillofac Surg Clin North Am*. 13(9):91–107.

Raghoebar GM, Louwerse C, Kalk WW, et al. 2001. Morbidity of chin bone harvesting. *Clin Oral Implants Res*. 12:503–07.

Rasmusson L, Meredith, N, Kahnberg, K. 1999. Effect of barrier membranes on bone resorption and implant stability in onlay bone grafts. *Clin Or Imp Res*. 10(8)267–77.

Reddi AH, Wientroub S, Muthukumaran N. 1987 Biologic principles of bone induction. *Orthop Clin North Am*. 18:207–12.

Schwartz-Arad D, Levin L. 2005. Intraoral autogenous block onlay bone grafting for extensive reconstruction of atrophic maxillary alveolar ridges. *J Periodontol*. 76:636–41.

Shin MS, Norrdin RW. 1985. Regional acceleration of remodeling during healing of bone defects in beagles of various ages. *Bone*. 6(5):377–79.

Sindet-Pedersen S, Enemark H. 1990. Reconstruction of alveolar clefts with mandibular or iliac crest bone grafts: A comparative study. *J Oral Maxillofac Surg*. 48:554–58; discussion 559–60.

Toscano N, Holtzclaw D, Mazor Z, et al. 2010. Horizontal ridge augmentation utilizing a composite graft of demineralized freeze-dried allograft, mineralized cortical cancellous chips, and a biologically degradable thermoplastic carrier combined with a resorbable membrane: a retrospective evaluation of 73 consecutively treated cases from private practices. *J Oral Implantol*. 36:467–74. Epub 2010, Jun 14.

Urist MR, Mc Lean F. 1952. Osteogenic potency and new bone formation by induction in transplants to the anterior chamber of the eye. *J Bone Joint Surg (Ann)*. 34:443–52.

Urist MR, Mikulski A, Lietze A. 1979. Solubilized bone morphogenetic protein. *Proc Natl Acad Sci USA*. 76:1828–32.

Vercellotti T, Nevins ML, Kim DM, et al. 2005. Osseous response following respective therapy with piezosurgery. *Int J Periodontics Restorative Dent*. 25:543–49.

Zins JE, Whitaker LA. 1983. Membranous versus endochondral bone: Implications for craniofacial reconstruction. *Plast Reconstr Surg*. 72:778–85.

Section 4
Osseous Surgery in Orthodontic Therapy

Chapter 15 Piezocision: Minimally Invasive Periodontally Accelerated Orthodontic Tooth Movement Procedure

Serge Dibart, DMD

INTRODUCTION

Surgical interventions on the alveolar ridges that are aimed at facilitating orthodontic treatment are not new. From the late 1800s to the late 1900s, we see the predominance of a mechanical concept that is prevalent in the surgical community: The orthodontic tooth movement is impaired by the physical presence of the alveolar cortex. Therefore, it becomes necessary to disrupt this cortical bone via surgery to allow for faster tooth movement. In 1892, Bryan (Guilford 1898) is credited with the first report in the literature in which alveolar corticotomy is used to correct a malocclusion. Several years later Kole (1959a, 1959b, 1959c), Generson (1979), and Suya (1991) use various types of corticotomies to achieve the same results. They cut through the alveolar cortex and created movable "blocks of bone" where the teeth are connected only by medullary bone. They believed that shorter treatment is due to removal of the cortical layer.

This concept was challenged by the Wilcko brothers in the late 20th century. They questioned the mechanical concept of bony block movement after reviewing radiographs and CT scans of their patients who had undergone corticotomy-facilitated orthodontic therapy. They noticed that following periodontally accelerated osteogenic orthodontics (PAOO), a demineralization of the jaw was taking place, followed by a remineralization. They hypothesized that rapid tooth movement resulted from marked but transient decalcification-recalcification process of the alveolus. This concept is known in the orthopedic literature as the regional accelerary phenomenon (RAP), as described by Frost in 1983. He reported localized increased osteoclastic and osteogenic activity at the site of osseous surgery. There was a decrease in regional bone density accompanied by increased bone turnover. He noticed that the RAP begins within a few days of the surgery and usually peaks in 1–2 months. The Wilckos had understood and witnessed this occurrence in their own patients. The elevation of buccal and lingual full-thickness flaps, with extensive decortications of the buccal and lingual alveolar

bone, resulted in a physical injury that was responsible for the initiation of a temporary demineralization process coupled with an increased regional bone turnover that characterizes the RAP. They surmised that this transient osteopenia (diminished bone density, same bone volume) is responsible for the rapid tooth movement, as the teeth move in a more "pliable" environment. Their pioneering work, combining alveolar decortication concomitant with bone grafting to expand alveolar volume and allow for rapid tooth movement into the newly expanded sites, stands out as seminal (Wilcko et al. 2001).

In 2007, Vercelotti and Podesta introduced the use of piezosurgery in conjunction with the conventional flap elevations to create an environment conducive to rapid tooth movement. Although quite effective, these techniques are also quite invasive in nature as they require extensive flap elevations and osseous surgery. They have the potential to generate postsurgical discomfort as well as postoperative complications. Because of these shortcomings, they have not been widely embraced by the patient or dental communities. Park et al. in 2006 and Kim et al. in 2009 introduced the corticision technique as a minimally invasive alternative to create surgical injury to the bone without flap reflection. In this technique, the authors use a reinforced scalpel and a mallet to go through the gingiva and cortical bone without raising a flap bucally and lingually. The surgical injury created is enough to induce the RAP effect and move the teeth rapidly during orthodontic treatment. This technique, although innovative, has two drawbacks: the inability to graft soft or hard tissues during the procedure to correct inadequacies and reinforce the periodontium and the repeated malleting, which may cause dizziness after surgery. We are describing here a new minimally invasive procedure that we called "piezocision." This technique combines microincisions limited to the buccal side that will allow for the use of the piezoelectic knife and selective tunneling that allows for hard or soft tissue grafting.

Practical Osseous Surgery in Periodontics and Implant Dentistry, First Edition. Edited by Serge Dibart, Jean-Pierre Dibart.
© 2011 John Wiley & Sons, Inc. Published 2011 by John Wiley & Sons, Inc.

INDICATIONS

Indications for using the piezocision technique include the following:

- Class I malocclusions with moderate to severe crowding (nonextraction)
- Correction of deep bite
- Selected class II malocclusions (end-on)
- Rapid adult orthodontic treatment
- Rapid intrusion and extrusion of teeth
- Simultaneous correction of osseous and mucogingival defects
- Prevention of mucogingival defects that may occur during or after orthodontic treatment.

ARMAMENTARIUM

The equipment needed to perform a piezocision include the following:

1. Topical and local anesthetic
2. Scalpel with blade #15C
3. Periosteal elevator (24G, Hu-Friedy, Chicago, IL)
4. Piezotome (Satelec, Acteon Group, Merignac, France), with insert BS1
5. Bone allograft or xenograft
6. 5-0 Chromic gut suture
7. Castroviejo needle holder
8. Surgical scissors
9. Peri-acryl, cyanoacrylate glue
10. Coe Pack if soft tissue grafting is needed

TECHNIQUE

Piezocision is performed 1 week after the placement of orthodontic appliances (Figure 15.1). The patient is anesthetized using Xylocaine 2% with 1:100.000 epinephrine in infiltration. Once complete anesthesia is achieved, a small vertical incision is performed buccally and interproximally in the attached gingiva or mucosa. The incision into the attached gingiva is preferable as it will give less visible postoperative scarring. A midlevel incision is made between the roots of the teeth involved, keeping in mind that the soft tissues and the periosteum need to be cut to create an opening that will allow the insertion of the piezoelectric knife.

At this point, it is important to emphasize the following concept: Piezocision has a localized and selective effect on the bone. Only the teeth or arch(es) to be moved need to be operated on. The areas not undergoing surgery have a higher anchorage value because they are not affected by the demineralization process and thus can be used as such in the global treatment plan. Once the vertical interproximal incisions are completed on the maxillary and mandibular arches or in localized segments, the tip of the Piezotome (BS1) is inserted in the openings previously made, and a 3-mm piezoelectrical corticotomy is done (Figures 15.2–15.4).

The first mark on the BS1 insert can be used as the landmark for the decortication depth as it is located 3 mm from the tip. One has to be very careful not to get too close to the interproximal papilla or to the roots, as irremediable damage may occur. In the areas with thin or little gingiva (recessions) or

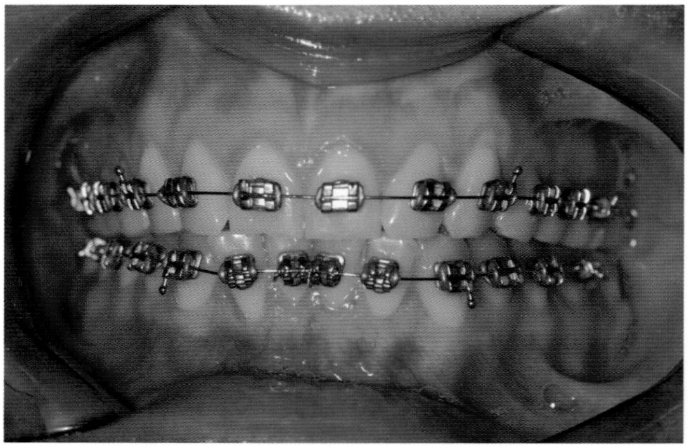

Figure 15.1 Class I malocclusion with moderate anterior crowding. Notice the mucogingival defect on tooth #11.

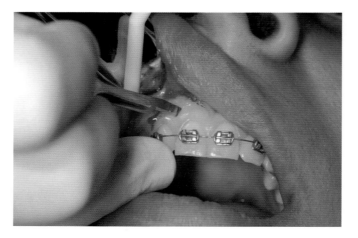

Figure 15.2 Interproximal incisions done with blade #15.

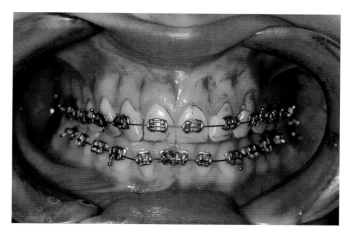

Figure 15.3 Interproximal incisions completed in the maxilla.

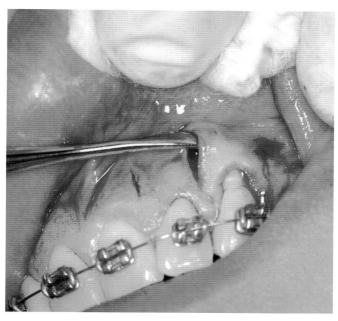

Figure 15.5 Tooth #11 presents with a gingival recession that will be corrected during piezocision. A thin periosteal elevator (24 G, Hu-Friedy) is used to create a tunnel from one vertical incision to another. This tunnel will host the connective tissue graft needed to correct the recession.

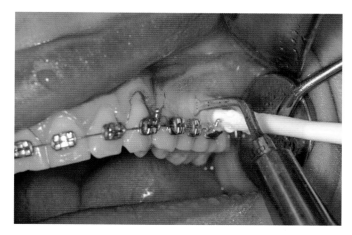

Figure 15.4 Piezoelectric corticotomy done with Piezotome (tip BS1; Satelec, Acteon).

with thin or no cortical buccal bone (dehiscence, fenestration), hard and soft tissue grafts can be added using a tunneling procedure (Figures 15.5, 15.6).

From one of the vertical openings, a periosteal elevator (24G, Hu-Friedy, Chicago, IL) is inserted between the periosteum and the bone, and a blunt dissection is carried forth. This will create a tunnel that will host soft tissue or a bone graft. Once the tunnel has been created, the piezoelectric corticotomy is done between the roots of the teeth, and a bone graft or soft tissue graft is then added (Figures 15.7, 15.8).

In the anterior mandible, this can be a little tricky, as only three vertical incisions in the soft tissue are made: between canines and laterals and between the two lower central incisors. This allows for a longer pouch, helping with the retention of the bone graft. Once the procedure is finished, only the areas that have been tunneled will require suturing with 5-0

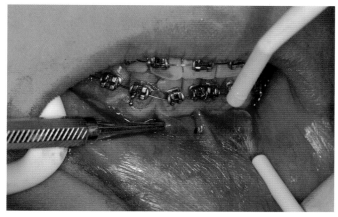

Figure 15.6 Tunneling is being done with the periosteal elevator from canine to canine to accommodate the bone graft needed to expand the mandibular alveolar bony envelope. This added bone will allow for the safe movement of the lower incisors forward.

chromic gut interrupted sutures. A few drops of cyanoacrylate glue (Periacryl) can also be useful to protect these sutures.

The remaining areas (verticals with corticotomy that have not been tunneled) do not need suturing or gluing.

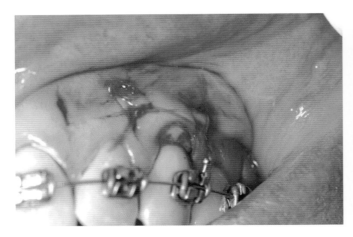

Figure 15.7 The subepithelial connective tissue graft has been harvested from the palate and placed into the tunnel and secured with 5-0 chromic gut sutures.

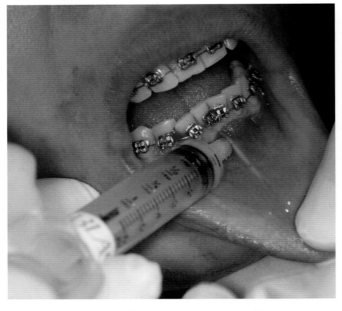

Figure 15.8 A bone allograft is being syringed into the prepared tunnel. This will enhance the bone volume and allow for anterior tooth movement with minimal risk.

POSTOPERATIVE CARE

The patient is seen a week after the surgery for a follow-up visit and 2 weeks after surgery to start the active phase of the orthodontic treatment. It is critical for the patient to be seen every 2 weeks thereafter by the orthodontist in order to benefit from the temporary demineralization phase created by piezocision and to allow for faster tooth movement and early completion of treatment (Figures 15.9, 15.10).

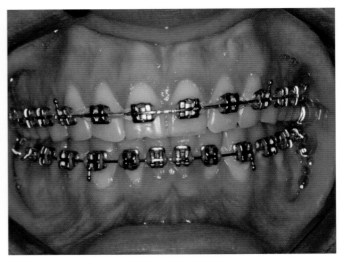

Figure 15.9 Three months into treatment, notice the correction of the recession on tooth #11 and the appearance of tooth #26.

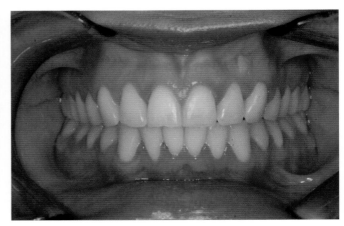

Figure 15.10 Case completed after 12 months.

POSSIBLE COMPLICATIONS

Complications could include loss of the interdental papilla (Figure 15.11). This may happen if the incision and the piezocision are done too close to the interdental papilla. It is of paramount importance to stay away from the papilla and do the incisions at mid-root level.

There may also be damage to the roots. This may happen due to not using the proper tip or not evaluating properly the underlying anatomy. In case of close root proximity, it is best, if unsure, to skip that site.

ADVANTAGES OF PIEZOCISION

There are several advantages to using the piezocision technique.

1. It is a minimally invasive, innovative procedure.

2. There is minimal postoperative discomfort.

3. There is short surgical time.

4. It allows concomitant soft and/or hard tissue augmentation.

5. It is very versatile and can be used in orthodontic therapy or included as part of a comprehensive interdisciplinary treatment approach (large perio-prosthetic-implant rehabilitations).

6. There is a high level of patient acceptance.

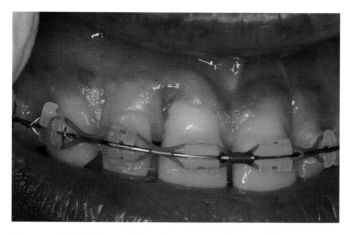

Figure 15.11 Piezocision done too close to interproximal papilla resulting in gingival recession on tooth #8. The defect has been present for 2 months.

CONCLUSION

It is important to remember that this is an orthodontically guided surgical procedure, designed by the orthodontist and performed by the periodontist/oral surgeon. After thorough data collection and analysis, the orthodontist and the surgeon will discuss the surgical treatment plan for the case. At this point, the orthodontist has made the diagnosis and created the treatment plan. The orthodontist will tell the surgeon which teeth or segments are going to move and where and will identify the areas that will need hard or soft tissue augmentation. The surgeon will then offer input regarding the feasibility of the procedure, the incision design, place of incision, type of graft. etc. The outcome of this meeting is the creation of a surgical "road map" that the surgeon will bring into the operating room and will follow (Figure 15.12).

This new treatment approach, which combines minimally invasive surgery and orthodontics, is a powerful tool in the armamentarium of the 21st-century dental team. The technique is extremely versatile as it allows for soft tissue as well as hard tissue grafting in the areas of need. These areas are

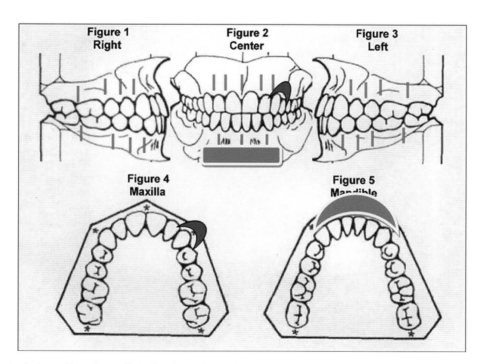

Figure 15.12 Surgical sheet ("road map") indicating where the cuts are going to take place (red), the bone graft (blue), and the soft tissue graft (dark red).

determined after thorough clinical and radiographic examination by the treatment team (Figures 15.13, 15.14).

I cannot emphasize enough the need for thorough presurgical data gathering and communication between the orthodontist and the surgeon. When a breakdown in communication or insufficient planning takes place, some unfortunate results may occur, as seen in Figures 15.15 and 15.16. These results could have been easily avoided through clear communication between the specialists.

The novelty of piezocision resides in the "one-sided" buccal approach, where there is no need to operate palatally or lingually. This combination of buccal interproximal microincisions and localized piezoelectric corticotomies is able to create a significant amount of demineralization all around the teeth in the areas of tooth movement, making this a very attractive alternative to the conventional and more aggressive techniques. Unlike conventional orthodontics, and during the course of treatment, a sharp increase in tooth mobility is observed, resulting from the transient osteopenia induced by the surgery. This is normal and expected. Also important is the fact that higher forces are applied to the teeth in order to maintain mechanical stimulation of the alveolar bone and the transient osteopenic state allowing for rapid treatment. Finally,

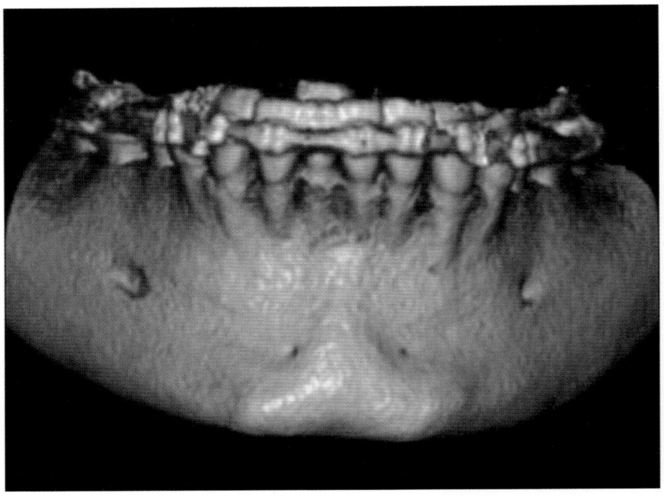

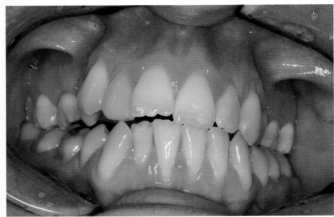

Figure 15.15 Initial picture prior to piezocision. No soft or hard tissue grafting was planned.

Figure 15.13 Three-dimensional view of the lower mandible, highlighting the need for a bone graft from canine to canine prior to labial orthodontic tooth movement.

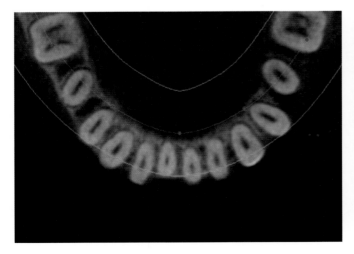

Figure 15.14 Horizontal cross-sections of mandible shown in Figure 15.13, confirming the need for bone graft in the lower anterior region prior to orthodontic tooth movement.

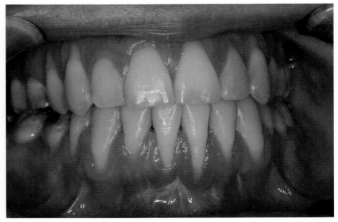

Figure 15.16 Orthodontic treatment completed. Notice the aggravated gingival recessions. These could have been avoided with hard and soft tissue grafting during piezocision.

it is of paramount importance for the orthodontist and surgeon to understand that the surgically induced high tissue turnover is restricted to the surgical areas, creating what might be referred to as a localized spatiotemporal window of opportunity. Attention must be given to performing the bony incisions only around the teeth where tooth movement is planned. As such, the relative anchorage value of the teeth away from the surgical site remains high, and anchorage value of teeth adjacent to the surgical site is low. RAP is transient, but the continuous mechanical stimulation of the teeth would prolong the osteopenic effect induced by the procedure, hence the need to see the patient and adjust the orthodontic appliance every 2 weeks during treatment.

Piezocision is an innovative, minimally invasive technique that allows rapid orthodontic tooth movement without the downside of the extensive and traumatic classical surgical approach. Piezocision proves to be efficient from the patient's and clinician's standpoint and offers advantages that should lead to greater acceptance in the dental and patient communities.

REFERENCES

Baloul SS, Gerstenfeld LC, Morgan EF, et al. 2011. mechanism of action and morphological changes in the alveolar bone in response to selective alveolar decortication facilitated tooth movement. *Am J Orthod*. 139(Suppl):S83–101.

Dibart S, Sebaoun JD, Surmenian J. 2009. Piezocision: A minimally invasive, periodontally accelerated orthodontic tooth movement procedure. *Compend Contin Educ Dent*. 30:342–44, 346, 348–50.

Frost HA. 1983. The regional acceleratory phenomena: A review. *Henry Ford Hosp Med J*. 31:3–9.

Frost HM. 1989a. The biology of fracture healing. An overview for clinicians. Part I. *Clin Orthop Relat Res*. 248:283–93.

Frost HM. 1989b. The biology of fracture healing. An overview for clinicians. Part II. *Clin Orthop Relat Res*. 248:294–309.

Generson RM, Porter JM, Zell A, et al. 1988. Combined surgical and orthodontic management of anterior open bite using corticotomy. *J Oral Surg*.36:216–19.

Guilford FH. 1898. *Orthodontia or Malpositions of the Human Teeth: Its Presentations and Remedy*. Philadelphia: T.C Davis and Sons.

Kim SJ, Park YG, Kang SG. 2009. Effects of corticision on paradental remodeling in orthodontic tooth movement. *Angle Ortho*. 79:284–91.

Kole H. 1959a. Surgical operations on the alveolar ridge to correct occlusal abnormalities. *Oral Surg Oral Med Oral Pathol*. 12:277–88.

Kole H. 1959b. Surgical operations on the alveolar ridge to correct occlusal abnormalities. *Oral Surg Oral Med Oral Pathol*. 12:413–20.

Kole H. 1959c. Surgical operations on the alveolar ridge to correct occlusal abnormalities. *Oral Surg Oral Med Oral Pathol*. 12:515–29.

Park YG, Kang SG, Kin SJ. 2006. Accelerated tooth movement by corticision as an osseous orthodontic paradigm. *Kinki Tokai Kyosei Shika Gakkai Gakujyutsu Taikai, Sokai*. 28:6.

Sebaoun JD, Kantarci A, Turner JW, et al. 2008. Modeling of trabecular bone and lamina dura following selective alveolar decortication in rats. *J Periodontol*. 79:1679–88.

Suya H. 1991. Corticotomy in orthodontics. In Hosl E, Baldauf A, eds., *Mechanical and Biological Basics in Orthodontics Therapy*. Heidelberg, Germany: Hütlig Buch, p. 207.

Vercellotti T, Podesta A. 2007. Orthodontic microsurgery: A new surgically guided technique for dental movement. *Int J Periodontics Restorative Dent*. 27:325–31.

Wilcko WM, Ferguson DJ, Bouguot JE, et al. 2003. Rapid orthodontic decrowding with alveolar augmentation: Case report. *World J Orthod*. 4:197–205.

Wilcko WM, Wilcko T, Bouquot JE, et al. 2001. Rapid orthodontics with alveolar reshaping: Two case reports of decrowding. *Int J Periodontics Restorative Dent*. 21:9–19.

Wilcko MT, Wilcko WM, Marquez MG, et al. 2007. The contribution of periodontics to orthodontic therapy. In Dibart S, ed., *Practical Advanced Periodontal Surgery*. Ames, Iowa: Wiley-Blackwell Publishing.

Section 5
Future Directions and Dilemmas

Chapter 16 Computer-Assisted Implant Dentistry: Possibilities and Limitations

Saynur Vardar-Sengul, DDS, PhD, CAGS

INTRODUCTION

Implant-supported restorations have become an increasingly common treatment option for edentulous and partially edentulous patients worldwide. The number of implants placed has been increasing every year in the United States. With developments in regenerative techniques and materials, implant placement has been made possible even in patients with bone deficiencies that were previously considered unsuitable for implants. In the early years of dental implantology, implants were placed based on available residual bone. Many studies have shown that implant placements disregarding prosthetic and biomechanical demands leads to compromised definitive prosthesis with jeopardized occlusal scheme, poor aesthetics, and unfavorable biomechanics, even though implants were osseointegrated (Stanford 1999, Kopp, Koslow and Abdo 2003; Duff and Razzoog 2006; Widmann and Bale 2006; Azari and Nikzad 2008a). Implants inclined to a buccal or lingual position are not working in their long axes and are exposed to detrimental lateral forces creating biomechanical problems and even breakages (Rangert et al. 1995; Stanford 1999; Azari and Nikzad 2008a).

To meet functional and aesthetic demands, a philosophy of prosthetic-driven implant dentistry had been adopted as a treatment modality, which combines functional and aesthetic concepts. In prosthetic-driven implant placement, diagnostic casts and diagnostic wax-up of the prosthetic restoration guide the position of implants (Garber 1996; Widmann and Bale 2006). With the concept of "prosthetic-driven implantology," both the available bone and teeth to be replaced were taken into consideration.

Developments in computer technology have changed diagnostic and surgical possibilities in dental implant dentistry. In modern dental implantology, the goal is not only to improve the precision and predictability of implant placement but also to change an invasive surgical protocol to a minimally invasive procedure and eventual immediate loading with less surgical time (Katsoulis, Pazera and Mericske-Stern. 2009). Pre-operative planning of the number of implants to be placed, their size, position, inclination, has been made possible with developments in imaging systems and software programs, and this allows the dental implant surgeon to concentrate on the patient and surgery itself while also shortening the surgical time (Vercruyssen et al. 2008).

In this chapter, we will discuss the current status of computer-assisted implant dentistry, with all its possibilities and limitations. We will first describe what prosthetic-driven implantology means and then will talk about radiographic methods, with an emphasis on computerized tomography (CT) and software planning. A review of surgical guides; a description of advanced computer-assisted design (CAD), computer-assisted manufacturing (CAM), and navigation techniques; and indications and limitations of flapless surgery will be discussed. We will end this chapter with a case report where we combined virtual implant planning with conventional implant surgery.

PROSTHETIC-DRIVEN IMPLANTOLOGY

Prosthetic-driven implantology (PDI) is a modality that combines functional and aesthetic concepts of implant dentistry. In this concept, dental implants are placed according to prosthetic demands. To achieve this goal, the planned prosthesis is brought into the CT images. This way, implant planning takes into account both the jaw bone anatomy and the planned superstructure, which improves the biomechanics and the aesthetics. It is important that the implant axes coincide with the teeth of the fixed denture and fall within the circumference of the occlusal plane of the tooth (Sethi and Sochor 1995; Becker and Kaiser 2000, Vercruyssen et al. 2008, Azari and Nikzad 2008a).

In the early days of implant dentistry, clinicians who believed in the prosthetic-driven implantology concept used wax-up prostheses and/or surgical templates made on hard gypsum surfaces of master casts. To overcome the problem

Practical Osseous Surgery in Periodontics and Implant Dentistry, First Edition. Edited by Serge Dibart, Jean-Pierre Dibart.
© 2011 John Wiley & Sons, Inc. Published 2011 by John Wiley & Sons, Inc.

of transferring the prosthetic plan to the operative site, customized radiographic and surgical templates have become a routine part of treatment (Pesun and Gardner 1995; Garber 1996; Becker and Kaiser 2000). However, after a while, the hard surface of casts was found not to equal the soft tissue surface of the oral cavity. Templates fabricated on the diagnostic casts without knowledge of the exact anatomy below the surface was also found to be unreliable (Lal et al. 2006; Widmann and Bale 2006; Azari and Nikzad 2008a). It was soon understood that this type of template cannot be used during radiographic pre-evaluation of bony structures, and this precludes "show-through" of the proposed teeth in the radiographs (Basten 1995; Wat et al. 2002). Working on the subject instead of casts led to double-purpose templates, which can be used not only for radiographic examination and evaluation of the patient but also during surgery and placement of the implants (Cehreli, Aslan and Sahin 2000). Before three-dimensional imaging came into play, conventional dental panoramic tomography and plain film tomography were usually performed with the patient wearing a radiographic template with integrated metal spheres at the position of the wax-up. Based on the magnification factor and the known dimensions of the metal sphere, the depth and dimensions of the implants could be estimated. In fact, double-purpose templates may somewhat relieve the problem of directing the implant to a good position. However, it was soon well established that all x-ray transmission–based radiographs suffer the limitation of being two-dimensional projections of complex, intrinsically three-dimensional anatomy. Conventional radiography has important diagnostic limitations such as expansion and distortion, setting errors and position artifacts (Azari and Nikzad 2008a). Soon after, three-dimensional imaging was introduced, and the prosthetic-driven implantology concept was adapted to three-dimensional imaging.

IMAGING METHODS IN DENTISTRY

Two-Dimensional Radiography

The most commonly used radiographs available to dentists are periapicals, bitewings, and panoramic radiographs. They are useful in providing diagnostic information regarding identifiable landmarks, pathology, and initial estimates of bone availability. They are also readily accessible, simple, and emit acceptable amounts of radiation. Even though in the early days of dental implantology dental surgeons relied on two-dimensional radiography, the use of these radiographs are limited in advanced implant treatment planning. Because of a lack of three-dimensional viewing, radiographs provide limited information regarding anatomical limitations, such as maxillary sinus, bone height estimate, bucco-lingual dimensions, concavities, and inferior alveolar nerve proximity (Jabero and Sarment 2006). Linear tomography can be used in planning of dental implants for a bucco-lingual estimate of

bone, but it does not provide accurate imaging; nor does it produce volume images of adjacent structures for precise planning and placement in advanced cases.

Introduction of Three-Dimensional Imaging to Implant Dentistry

One of the most important technological advancements that dramatically enhanced the clinician's ability to diagnose and plan dental implants has been the computed tomography (CT) scan. Although computerized axial tomography (CAT) scans have been available for medical use since 1973 (Hounsfield 1973), it was not until 1987 that this innovative technology became available for dental applications (Schwarz et al. 1987a, b). One of the major features that draw the dentist's attention to CT technology is the ability to avoid the superimposition of structures, which makes CT scans more desirable than conventional radiography as a morphometric tool (Azari and Nikzad 2008a).

CT is the most advanced radiographic methodology for dental implant diagnosis (Todd et al. 1993; Gher and Richardson 1995; Jacobs et al. 1999). This technology is different from previous methods in that it includes a radiographic source with circular movements, a digital receptor, and advanced software reformatting processes. The result is a series of axial images that the computer can reformat to provide images in cross-sectional, panoramic, and three-dimensional views. Contrary to other radiographs, there is no exposure onto a radiographic film. Instead, computer files can be seen using software (Jabero and Sarment 2006). CTs are used for the following purposes (Iplikcioglu, Akca and Cehreli 2002):

1. To determine the quality and the quantity of bone

2. To evaluate the potential sites for implant placement

3. To evaluate intra-osseous pathologies

4. To follow up regions where extensive surgery is performed.

CT is now a very common imaging technique. For maxillofacial applications, dedicated software was developed capable of reformatting the data of the axial slices into panoramic images and multiplanar cross-sectional images (Schwarz et al. 1989). Today, the availability of three-dimensional planning software, which, furthermore, allows a reliable transfer of the virtual implant planning into the surgical field through drilling templates, helps the surgeon to achieve an adequate oral implant placement (Van Steenberghe et al. 2002).

Advantages of CT

One of the most promising advantages of CT is its high level of accuracy in comparison to other modalities. There is almost no magnification error caused by geometric distortions, whereas such errors are common in conventional dental radiographs. Some researchers have compared the degree of accuracy and distortion of conventional radiographs and CT (Jemt 1993; Bahat 1993). According to these studies, the least accurate methods were panoramic views (17%), conventional tomography (39%), and peri-apical views (53%), whereas the CT has accuracy as high as 95% (Bassi et al. 1999). Sonick et al. (1994) also compared accuracy of two-dimensional and three-dimensional imaging. The differences between the actual caliper and radiograph were as follows:

- Periapical: 0.5–5.5 mm/average 1.9 mm
- Panoramic: 0.5–7.5 mm/average 3.0 mm
- CT: 0–0.5 mm/average 0.mm

The radiographic distortion differences are:

- Periapical: 8–24%/average 14%
- Panoramic: 5–39%/average 23.5%
- CT: 0–8%/average 1.8%

CT also has ability to measure bone density. Also in CT, multiplanner reformatting allows one to reformat a volumetric dataset in axial, coronal, and sagittal cuts and to build multiple cross-sectional and panoramic views (Schwarz et al. 1987a, b). For the time being, these advantages make CT the most precise and comprehensive radiological technique for dental implant planning.

From the introduction of modern implantology, it was proposed that the success rate of dental implant therapy is influenced by both the quality and the quantity of bone (Ulm et al. 1999; Azari and Nikzad 2008a), and clinical reports have indicated that implant prognosis is significantly affected by bone quality (Jaffin and Berman 1991; Jemt et al. 1992). Conventional dental radiographs, including periapical, panoramic, lateral cephalometric, or even conventional tomography are less useful for diagnosing the bone density.

Concerns Regarding High-Dose Radiation with CT

Studies have demonstrated that the use of CT is associated with significantly higher doses of radiation compared to conventional radiography (Ekestubbe et al. 1993; Frederiksen, Benson and Sokolowski 1994, 1995). The American Academy of Oral and Maxillofacial Radiology (AAOMR) and the European Association for Osseointegration (EAO) recommend the cross-sectional imaging modality for patients receiving implants (Tyndall and Brooks 2000; White et al. 2001; Harris et al. 2002). On the other hand, CT scanner systems have been developed to such an extent that dramatic advances

have been. As scanners improved in the speed of image acquisition, so did their versatility. Multiphase scanning with well-defined phases can now be achieved where larger body volumes may be scanned with little relevant time penalty, at a very low possible dose of radiation, and with rapid screening in a variety of guises (Dawson 2004; Azari and Nikzad 2008a).

Cone-Beam Computed Tomography

Continued advancements in CT scanning technology have led to the development of cone-beam CT (CBCT). The cone-beam technique requires only a single rotation to capture the entire object. Scanning time is reduced to 10–40 seconds. While the rotation takes place, a high number of projections are rapidly captured. Later, a reconstruction algorithm renders cross sections. CBCT has become the most advanced type of radiographic technique when compared to traditional spiral and helical CT, based on the following advantages: reduced cost; decreased radiation; decreased scanning time, resulting in less patient movement; smaller and more convenient machinery; and more precise imaging (CBCT: 0.2–0.4 mm slices; CT: 0.5–1 mm) (Jabero and Sarment 2006). CBCT requires 30–90 times less radiation than the conventional CT scanner (Van der Zel 2008). Therefore, the introduction of CBCT, offering imaging at low dose and relatively lower costs, has increased the applicability and feasibility of three-dimensional–based presurgical planning. The surgeon can properly position implants in a virtual reality (Vercruyssen et al. 2008). Data acquisition, slice thickness, and interval of the reconstruction can determine the imaging resolution. One of the characteristics of these CBCT systems is being able to select the region of interest in accordance with the clinical demands (Guerrero et al. 2006).

CT Scanning Appliances

To address the requirements of the concept of prosthetic-driven implantology, some type of radio-opaque CT scan template incorporating information about the position, occlusion, form, and contour of missing teeth gives the data that can be viewed in relationship to the underlying structures (Israelson et al. 1992; Klein, Cranin and Sirakian. 1993; Verde and Morgano 1993; Basten 1995; Borrow and Smith 1996; Amet and Ganz 1997; Azari and Nikzad 2008a). In this way it will be possible for a restorative dentist to visualize the location of planned implants from an aesthetic and biomechanical standpoint. There are three generations of scanning appliance designs described (Rosenfeld, Mandelaris and Tardieu 2006, Azari and Nikzad 2008a).

1. A barium-coated silhouette of the proposed prosthesis
2. A radiopaque tooth from the vacuum-formed template filled with acrylic resin/barium
3. The Tardieu Scannoguide, which is a differential barium gradient–scanning appliance.

The Tardieu Scannoguides allow the clinician to transfer the prosthetic outcome and define the soft tissue on the CT. This offers the potential for fabrication of specialized surgical drilling guides for flapless implant surgery (Rosenfeld, Mandelaris and Tardieu 2006).

It is necessary to have some degree of expertise to correctly interpret the CT's printed images, and this is not easy in routine dental practice. The images obtained from CT are really two-dimensional, which requires a process of mental integration of multiple sections by the observer to derive three-dimensional information (Gillespie and Isherwood 1986). These two-dimensional views are easier to show on the computer, but they are basically a digitized version of printed images. To overcome these obstacles, we need systems that allow simultaneous visualization of two-dimensional reformatted images as well as three-dimensional–derived bone surface representations. In this way we have the opportunity for interactive placement of implant-like CAD models on the images obtained from CT data (Azari and Nikzad 2008a).

FROM IMAGES TO PRACTICE

Virtual Implant Planning

By using software programs, clinicians have the ability to view and interact with the CT scan data to place the implant presurgically and visualize the restorative implications virtually. It is possible to reformat the CT scan data to provide an accurate three-dimensional view of the anatomy of the bone in which the clinician can interactively introduce implant planning into the CT images (Jabero and Sarment 2006; Azari and Nikzad 2008a). Today, many specific software programs have been developed for planning dental implant surgery in the maxilla and mandible. Specific software applications have been developed that can directly import Digital Imaging and Communication in Medicine (DICOM) data into a diagnostic and interactive treatment planning tool (Vercruyssen et al. 2008). All reconstructed images, as well as three-dimensional virtual reconstructions, are visible, and measurements of bone height, width, and density are always available. Tracing of anatomical landmarks such as the mandibular nerve is possible, and placement of virtual implants to select an appropriate size and position is simple (Jabero and Sarment 2006). These software programs allow the clinician to plan the best position, angulation and size of the implant relative to the designed prosthesis and proximity of vital structures (Figure 16.1). After implants are virtually placed in the best position, it is possible to see the bone density around the implants. This allows the implant surgeon to have an idea of what the primary stability would be; therefore, the surgeon can plan final drill sizes to get best primary stability since surgical guides make it difficult to feel bone density during drilling. Most of the surgical guides are designed for medium bone density, which could be hard to have in posterior maxilla.

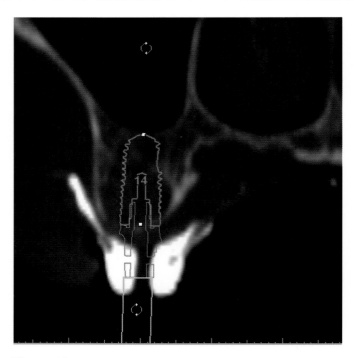

Figure 16.1 Virtual implant planning using software to verify implant size and relationship to prosthesis and vital structures.

Transferring Computer Plan into Surgical Site

Transferring the computer plan into actual patient treatment has been made possible first by the revolutionary CAD/CAM techniques.

There are mainly two guided-surgery systems: (1) static guides and (2) dynamic systems.

Static Surgical Guides

Traditional surgical guides are acrylic appliances used during surgery to place implants properly by conveying the decisions for implant positions made during the diagnostic and treatment planning stages. These templates are made by duplicating the diagnostic teeth or reproducing the long axis of future restorations using. However, providing a surgical guide does not guarantee the recommended location of implants because bone may not be available to accommodate the desired positions or anatomical limitations. Use of traditional surgical guides designed from stone models with the assistance of periapical, bitewing, and panoramic x-rays can lead to multiple limitations for advanced implant guidance that may compromise the overall execution of treatment (Jabero and Sarment 2006). Therefore, radiographic surgical guides and CAD/CAM technology came into play.

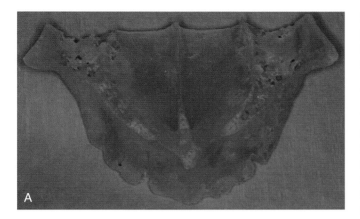

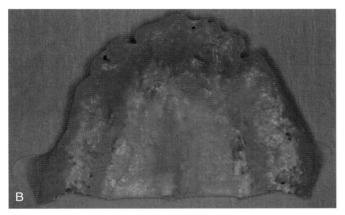

Figure 16.2 (A and B) Physical models of maxilla.

CAD/CAM Surgical Guide

To address concerns inherent in traditional surgical guides, further computer software programs have been developed using sophisticated modalities of CAD as well as fabrication of surgical guidance models with CAM. CAD/CAM technique was the first attempt to bring virtual planning into reality. Early data regarding the incorporation of CAD/CAM techniques into implant dentistry were for eliminating the surgical bone impression phase of the subperiosteal implant modality (Truitt et al. 1988). With CAD/CAM technology, for the first time it was possible to physically feel the area of interest, such as maxilla or mandible. Physical models are very helpful because they offer the opportunity to hold the model in the hand, which provides the clinician with a direct understanding of complex anatomical details that otherwise cannot be obtained from imaging on a screen (Figure 16.2).

CAM methods for implant applications include three-dimensional printing techniques or computer-driven model drilling. These guides are used during surgery to improve accuracy, confidence, and rapidity. CAD/CAM surgical guides require CT scanning and computer software programs that assist in diagnosis and planning. Once the CT data and

implant planning procedures have been determined, surgical guide fabrication can be manufactured in a variety of three-dimensional printing or computer-driven drilling systems (Jabero and Sarment 2006).

Three-Dimensional Printing Guides—Rapid Prototyping

The layer data format of CT scanners quickly prompted the realization that it may be possible to convert the data to be compatible with rapid prototyping (RP) machine requirements. By definition, RP refers to the fabrication of three-dimensional physical models directly from a CAD model. Currently, the most developed CAD/CAM surgical guide methods use three-dimensional printing. The model is built layer by layer according to three-dimensional data (Jacobs 1992; Cooper 2001). This type of mechanical prototyping is capable of quickly fabricating complex shaped, three-dimensional parts directly from CAD models. This may differ from just milling, which has been a routine procedure in normal CAD technology (Azari and Nikzad 2008a).

One of the three-dimensional printing methods called *stereolithography* uses a laser-cured resin model (SurgiGuide, CSI Materialise, Glen Burine, MD) (Ganz 2003). The process begins with the patient receiving a CT scan. It is preferable to provide a scanographic template. Implant planning is performed with final prosthetic planning being visible. After acquisition, the CT files are submitted to the company, and reformatting is performed. The implant planning team then receives a small proprietary file via e-mail that contains all images. Planning takes place using software (Sim-Plant, CSI Materialise, Belgium), and alterations can be made until a satisfactory treatment plan is agreed upon. The planning files can then be submitted by e-mail for processing. For tooth-supported CAD/CAM guides, a stone model must also be mailed together with the file because a separate optical scanning of the model is necessary. The rapid modeling process can then begin, using a computer-driven laser that cures a thin layer of liquid polymer, followed by additional stacked layers, resulting in a three-dimensional model. Once the process is complete, metal sleeves are inserted into the guide, providing guidance for implant placement. This method also produces a three-dimensional template of the anatomical model. A series of guides are produced to accommodate drill size (Jabero and Sarment 2006).

There are many software programs in the marketplace for CT-based modeling and RP-made surgical templates, such as Simplant, Implant 3D, Vimplant, NobelGuide, Implant Master, CADImplant, Galileos, 10DR, and DDent/DDent plus I.

Computer-Driven Drilling

Another method of CAD/CAM surgical guide fabrication uses computer-driven drilling without producing three-dimensional models. One of these systems (CADImplant, CADImplant Inc.,

Medfield, MA) uses such drilling. The process begins with the fabrication of a surgical template from prosthetic study models. A registration cube is then attached to the template, producing a scanographic guide specific for CADImplant technology. The patient is then referred for CT scanning with the scanographic guide. After completion of the examination, files are sent back to the clinician who imports them into CADImplant computer software. Following virtual implant placement, the scanographic guide, model, and planning data are sent back to a CADImplant drilling center. Planning data and models are matched using the cube attached to the scanographic guide. The computer-driven drilling is performed followed by insertion of metal sleeves. The scanographic guide perforated with guiding tubes has become the surgical guide (Jabero and Sarment 2006).

Advantages of rapid prototyping (three-dimensional modeling) and computer drilling systems include the use of software for virtual implant placement, which allows the dentist to view the field three-dimensionally and to transfer implant planning to the surgical site. These procedures enhance surgical execution that is prosthetically acceptable.

Dynamic Surgical Guides—Navigation Systems

Navigation systems started as an attempt to incorporate robotics principles into implant planning. Development of image-guided surgery in the medical field has opened new avenues for implant treatment planning and placement. Navigation is another option for transferring a surgical plan to the operative field. This technology requires a CT scan, during which a specialized acrylic splint is required to assist in the registration (three-dimensional matching) of the patient's position. During implant surgery, the patient must wear this acrylic template. The splint and dental hand-piece are equipped with strategically positioned infrared emitters enabling camera detectors located in the room to track movement during surgery. Therefore, the matching of jaw position and hand-piece with the patient's CT scan and planning are performed instantaneously (Casap et al. 2004, 2005; Jabero and Sarment 2006). This setup allows real-time updates and feedback to the surgeon who is continuously informed of the osteotomy location and its relationship to the desired implant location.

Navigation systems were principally designed to relieve the common drawbacks of RP technology. If the jaw is severely atrophied, it is difficult to handle the templates without dislodgement. Moreover, it is always a matter of concern to control the distance of the drill tip from critical structures, such as inferior alveolar nerve, floor of the nasal cavity, or maxillary sinus during surgery (Azari and Nikzad 2008a). Navigation systems allow the dental surgeon to follow preestablished drill sequences and make modifications during surgery.

How Does the Navigation System Work?

Navigation systems provide sensors as well as software programs to transfer the presurgical plan to the patient. They also provide automated monitoring of the surgical procedure. Basically, the system produced by this concept uses marker-based referencing methods (registration points, fiducial markers, etc.) to establish the transference of the tool's coordinate system to the patient. By incorporating the light or sound generator markers, the clinician is able to be guided audially and/or visually to set the implant by simply moving the drill in the appropriate position with the support of the navigation system. The system assists the surgeon during the preoperative planning and also during the intraoperative procedure (Azari and Nikzad 2008a).

Accuracy of Navigation Systems

The accuracy of a computer-aided intraoperative navigation system (IGS) during implant surgery depends on the precision of the surgical navigation system and the skill of the surgeon to interpret positional data displayed on the computer screen during the drilling of the implant socket (Wanschitz et al. 2002). Similar to the RP–CT method, intraoperative computerized navigation also mandates that an interfacing template be firmly attached to the operated jaw (usually by bone screws) throughout the surgery (Azari and Nikzad 2008a).

There are also difficulties in using navigation with patients under local anesthesia due to jaw movements and the need for regular recalibration toward a fixed reference point. The greatest problem is the large deviations reported between the position and orientation of implants at planning and the result obtained at surgery (Wagner et al. 2003).

There are currently many systems available in the marketplace providing surgical guides and navigation systems (Table 16.1).

ACCURACY OF COMPUTER-ASSISTED IMPLANT SURGERY

The accuracy of an image-guided procedure is defined as the deviation in location and angle of the plan compared to the outcome. It includes all possible errors from image acquisition to surgical implant positioning (Widmann and Bale 2006). Deviations from the plan can vary according to the system used. The errors are accumulative and interactive and can occur at any stage, such as CT scan data collection, proper positioning of the radiological template, segmentation, stereolithographic or CAD/CAM modeling, fixation of the surgical guide to the jaw bone, and whether high-precision sleeves are used or not. Theoretically, all errors can add up, even if they compensate each other. Therefore, it is of utmost importance when using a system to be aware of the largest deviation reported (Vercruyssen et al. 2008).

Table 16.1. Currently available static and dynamic systems in computer-assisted implant dentistry.

Application	Website	Company	Drill Guide Production
Surgical Guides			
Biodental Models	www.biodental.com	BioMedical Modeling, USA	RP
Implant3D	www.implant3d.com	Media Lab, Italy	RP
3D-Doctor	www.ablesw.com	Able Software, USA	CDD
Cyrtina guide	www.cyrtina.nl	Oratio, Netherlands	RP
DentalSlice	www.bioparts.com.br	BioParts, Brazil	RP
EasyGuide	www.keystonedental.com	Keystone Dental, USA	CDD
GPI S	www.gpitechnology.net	GPI Technology, Germany	CDD
ILS	www.tactile-tech.com	Tactile Technologies, Israel	Custom tubes
ILUMA DigiGuide	www.imtec.com	IMTEC, USA	RP
InVivoDental	www.anatomage.com	Anatomage, USA	CDD
AnatoModel	www.anatomage.com	Anatomage, USA	CDD
implant3D	www.med3d.de	med3D GmbH, Germany	CDD
Implant Master	www.ident-surgical.com	I-Dent Imaging, USA	RP
Scan2Guide	www.ident-surgical.com	I-Dent Imaging, USA	RP
OnDemand3D	www.cybermed.co.kr	Cybermed, Korea	RP
Oralim Oral Implant Planning System	www.medicim.com	Medicim, Belgium	RP
NobelGuide	www.nobelguide.com	Nobel Biocare, USA	CDD
Simplant Master	www.materialise.com	Materialise, Belgium	RP
Simplant Planner	www.materialise.com	Materialise, Belgium	RP
Simplant Pro	www.materialise.com	Materialise, Belgium	RP
VIP	www.implantlogic.com	Implant Logic Systems, USA	CDD
Navigation Systems			
coNavix	www.codiagnostix.de	IVS Solutions, Germany	None
MONA-DENT	www.drheuermann.de	MSc Implantologie, Germany	None
NaviBase, NaviDoc, NaviPad	www.robodent.com	Robodent, Germany	None
Treon	www.medtronicnavigation.com	Medtronic, USA	None
IGI	www.image-navigation.com	Image Navigation, Israel	None
VISIT		University of Vienna, Austria	None

RP, rapid prototyping; CDD, computer-driven drilling.

Accuracy of Image Acquisition

Accurate assessment of bony architecture and measurements of anatomic structures are prerequisites for appropriate implant planning (Benjamin 2002; Widmann and Bale 2006). In general, accuracy of CT data depends on the slice thickness and the influence of possible artifacts. The thinner the slice thickness and the smaller the voxel size, the higher the resolution and accuracy of measurements (Vannier et al. 1997; Odlum 2001; Widmann and Bale 2006). Movement and metallic artifacts of dental restorations may lead to geometric distortions and invalid data acquisition.

Accuracy of Registration

The precise transfer of virtual planning to the surgical site depends on the accuracy of the registration procedure. This is known as the image-to-physical transformation. Dental implant surgery requires the most accurate registration. It was reported that mean accuracies of surgical templates obtained by a drilling machine was 0.6 mm for maxilla and 0.3 mm for mandible, with a maximum deviation of 1.5 mm (Besimo,

Lambrecht and Guindy 2000). Van Steenberghe et al. (2002) found mean accuracies of rapid prototyping templates of 0.8 mm at the base and 0.9 mm at the tip of the implant. Wanschitz et al. (2002) reported mean accuracy of 0.5–0.6 mm at the base (maximum deviation 1.5 mm) and about 1.4 mm at the tip (maximum 3.5 mm) with the image-guided bur tracking-navigation systems. The accuracy at the base and accuracy at the tip of implant needs to be distinguished as the tip is situated in the vicinity of vital anatomical structures. In image-guided template production, errors may be the result of unstable fixation of the surgical template. Precise mechanical fitting of the template into the patient's mouth is of major importance. Also, if the bur tube diameter is too large, imprecise drilling results in the angular deviation (Widmann and Bale 2006).

Human Error

Flapless implant surgery has been promoted to general practice dentists to make implant placement an easier procedure. However, clinical success is dependent upon the skill of the surgeon to interpret and execute data during drilling. Human error is attributed to all the steps of image-guided surgery, including imaging, planning, and transfer errors. Therefore, every step needs to be carefully controlled and meticulously done. Positioning of registration devices, motionless CT data acquisition, precise planning, verification of registration accuracy, and constant attention to stable and precise fit of the registration template is required to get the most precise outcome.

Accuracy Studies

Computer-assisted systems offer clear benefits, although precision of the systems, investment, and cost–benefit ratio of such treatment strategies are still controversial. Katsoulis et al. (2009) analyzed 40 patients for virtual implant planning in the maxilla and observed that four implants for over-denture support could be located in sufficient bone and adequate position in 70% of the patients and 79% of the implants. Reduced implant diameter and the need for guided bone regeneration (GBR) were regarded as necessary for another 21% of the implants. This demonstrates that often a thin bone wall in the anterior region is present. Increasing numbers of implants are necessary for fixed prosthesis, and their placement in a more posterior zone becomes critical and is conflicted with reduced bone height and deep sinus floor. The need for transcrestal or lateral sinus membrane elevation is needed in most of the cases. In this study, the prerequisite for the installation of all six implants by means of a guided flapless procedure worked for only 30% of the patients (Katsoulis et al. 2009). Therefore, case selection and interpretation of CT data are crucial in choosing computer-assisted implant surgery, and it is only 30% of the time that it is possible to do using the flapless approach.

In a recent systematic review by Jung et al. (2009), nine systems were tested, and a meta-analysis was done. The majority of the systems were dynamic systems (navigation), and two out of nine systems used drill guides based on computer-assisted implant planning. Overall mean deviation error in the horizontal direction at the entry point of the drill was 0.74 mm (95% CI: 0.58–0.9 mm) with a maximum of 4.5 mm, whereas mean error at the apex was 0.85 mm (95% CI: 0.72–0.99 mm) with a maximum of 7.1 mm (Jung et al. 2009). With systems using surgical guides, the mean error was 1.12 mm (95% CI: 0.82–1.42 mm; max 4.5 mm) at the entry point and 1.2 mm (95% CI: 0.87–1.52 mm; max 7.1 mm) at the apex. For dynamic intraoperative navigation, the mean error was 0.62 mm (95% CI: 0.43–0.81 mm; max 3.4 mm) at the entry point and 0.68 mm (95% CI: 0.55–0.80 mm; max 3.5 mm) at the apex. Dynamic systems showed a statistically significantly higher mean precision by 0.5 mm ($P = 0.0058$) at the entry point and by 0.52 mm ($P = 0.0354$) at the apex. Implants positioned in humans showed a higher mean deviation at the entry point and apex compared to implants or drills in cadaver studies and studies on models (Jung et al. 2009). Overall mean error in angulations was 4.0 degrees, with a maximum of 20.43 degrees. The mean annual implant failure rate for all clinical studies (13 human studies) was 3.36%, ranging from 0% to 8.45% after an observation period of at least 12 months, with a 96.6% success rate. However, there are no long-term data. Ten out of 13 clinical human studies reported on intraoperative complications including interocclusal distances that were too limited to perform guided implant placement, limited primary stability, or the need for additional grafting. Intraoperative complications or unexpected events were observed 4.6% (95% CI: 1.2%–16.5%) in the implant placements. Dynamic systems showed a 2.2 times higher incidence of complications, although this was not significant ($P = 0.5282$) (Jung et al. 2009).

CONCERNS AND DISADVANTAGES OF COMPUTER-ASSISTED SURGERY

The major concern for the transfer of the planning to the operative field is the maximum deviation between the planned position of the implants and the postoperative outcome. Even if such deviation occurs only once, it should be taken into account for both the patient's safety and because of its legal implications. The maximal deviation ever recognized should be taken into account to determine which safety zone should be respected at surgery. The best data available at the clinical level still report a 1 mm–1.5 mm maximum deviation (Vercruyssen et al. 2008).

When prosthetic-driven implant positioning is taken into consideration and when safe positioning of implants at optimal length and accurate estimation of bone density is desired, the clinician and patient can benefit from the advantages of computer-assisted implantology (Azari and Nikzad 2008a). However, this sophisticated technology requires substantially more cost, meticulous effort (CT imaging, fabrication of a registration template, etc.), and a high level of training. Furthermore, the potential for thermal injury secondary to reduced access for external irrigation during osteotomy preparation must be considered. The implant surgeon also must be familiar with the clinical goals and guidelines for surgical management of peri-implant soft tissues. It was shown that the clinical goal of flapless surgical management is to establish an adequate zone, approximately 3 mm in the apicocoronal dimension (width) of attached nonmobile, preferably keratinized, soft tissue that is circumferentially adapted to the transmucosal implant structures (Schwarz et al. 1987a). Long-term clinical observations indicate that ideal tissue thickness is somewhere between 2.5 and 3 mm and that the presence of adequate soft tissue thickness greatly contributes to the maintenance of a stable peri-implant soft tissue environment (Schwarz et al. 1987b; Azari and Nikzad 2008b). Although long-term success is possible with less than the recommended 3 mm of keratinized tissue surrounding an implant restoration, predictability is far greater with the recommended amount because the tissues are better able to withstand the trauma of prosthetic procedures, abutment connection, and reconnection; the forces of mastication and oral hygiene maintenance; and the mechanical challenges presented by removable implant prosthesis secured by resilient prosthetic attachments (Sclar 2007). In addition, the combination of adequate soft tissue thickness and apico-coronal dimension of keratinized tissue surrounding an implant restoration helps resist recession, protects peri-implant crestal bone levels, and provides aesthetic masking of underlying metal components. Furthermore, at the ideal tissue thickness, a reduction in the apicocoronal width of keratinized tissue may become acceptable (Berglundh and Lindhe 1996, Sclar 2007).

The implant surgeon should be familiar with criteria for optimal flap designs used in dental implant surgery when deciding whether to use flapless or flap surgery. These criteria include preserving circulation and alveolar ridge topography; providing access for required implant instrumentation; allowing identification of vital structures; providing access for modifying osseous contours and/or local bone harvest when indicated; providing closure away from submerged fixture installation or augmentation sites; minimizing postsurgical bacterial contamination; facilitating flap elevation, retraction, and wound closure; and achieving circumferential adaptation of good-quality tissues around emerging implant structures (Sclar 2007). Considering the knowledge and skills needed for computer-assisted implant surgery, it seems more for experienced and trained surgeons. Computer-assisted surgery does not make implant surgery easier for beginners; however, it is promising for better prosthetic outcome in implant dentistry.

FLAPLESS VERSUS FLAP SURGERY

Today the implant-supported oral restorations are among the most validated treatment options for treating edentulous and partially edentulous patients. With the introduction of in-office cone beam computed tomography, improved access to conventional CT scanning, and new dental implant treatment planning software allowing three-dimensional evaluation of potential implant sites, the use of flapless surgery as a minimally invasive surgical approach for implant placement has been gaining popularity among implant surgeons. To fulfill this goal, flapless surgery has been advocated by many clinicians (Azari and Nikzad 2008b). Flapless surgery involves using a tissue punch device to gain access to the alveolar ridge for implant placement or abutment connection. Although the flapless approach was initially suggested for general practitioners, the successful use of this approach often requires advanced clinical experience and surgical judgment.

Indications of Flapless Surgery

The flapless (tissue punch) surgery is indicated when the surgeon has confidence that the underlying osseous anatomy is ideal relative to the planned implant diameter and three-dimensional placement in the alveolus. In cases where site preservation is performed at the time of tooth removal, the surgeon should closely observe and document the dimensions of the remaining alveolar housing and the morphology of any socket wall defects. This information will allow the surgeon to decide whether a flapless approach will be feasible for subsequent implant placement in most cases when delayed implant placement is planned after the tooth extraction (Sclar 2007).

The surgeon also must be able to determine whether an adequate volume of good-quality soft tissues will remain surrounding the emerging implant structures for optimal function and aesthetics. The quantity, quality, and position of the existing keratinized tissues relative to the planned implant emergence should be evaluated before surgery to decide which approach should be used, flapless versus flap, to minimize soft tissue complications that can jeopardize the long-term success of an implant restoration. Also, the implant surgeon must be prepared and competent when unexpected intraoperative complications necessitate additional access or visualization (Sclar 2007). Therefore, flapless surgery is not for everyone, but it's a viable option when all criteria are met, which could be judged by an experienced implant surgeon.

It has been shown that a flapless surgical approach has advantages, including preservation of circulation, soft tissue architecture, and hard tissue volume at the site; less postoperative bleeding and decreased surgical time; improved patient comfort; minor or no swelling; and accelerated recuperation, allowing the patient to resume normal oral hygiene procedures immediately after surgery (Azari and Nikzad 2008b; Sclar 2007).

According to Dr. Sclar (2007), "There are certain prerequisites for surgeons wishing to use the flapless approach for implant placement and uncovering procedures." These include in-depth knowledge of the criteria for optimal flap designs used in dental implant surgery, as well as the clinical goals for surgical management of peri-implant soft tissues. The surgeon should also be knowledgeable regarding the indications and techniques required for successful management of peri-implant soft tissues during conventional open-flap surgery. There are other minimally invasive techniques such as U-shaped peninsula flaps, abbreviated trapezoidal flaps, and pouch or tunnel dissections. If the implant surgeon is familiar with these techniques, these approaches may be more beneficial than the flapless tissue punch approach in many clinical situations. Flapless surgery is not the only minimally invasive approach in soft tissue management of dental implants.

Therefore, flapless approach has limited but viable indications, and its application needs experience and knowledge in implant dentistry and soft tissue management.

Despite many benefits, flapless implant surgery has generally been perceived as a blind procedure, and this approach does have some drawbacks. Some of these include the following:

- the surgeon's inability to visualize anatomic landmarks and vital structures
- the potential for thermal damage secondary to reduced access for external irrigation during osteotomy preparation
- the increased risk of malposed angle or depth of implant placement
- a decreased ability to contour osseous topography when needed to facilitate restorative procedures and to optimize soft tissue contours
- an inability to manipulate soft tissues to ensure circumferential adaptation of adequate dimensions of keratinized gingival tissues around implant structures.

CONCLUSION AND FUTURE DIRECTIONS

There have been objections against computer-assisted implant surgery among implant surgeons for various reasons. Surgeons often doubt that the technology provides sufficient precision, and they prefer to raise a flap and to use standard procedures with conventional surgical guides. Many surgeons think that computer technology with flapless surgery can be applied only in few patients—in those with sufficient bone and without the need for adjunctive surgical procedures such as guided bone regeneration or sinus floor elevation. Therefore, three-dimensional computer-guided planning would be advantageous even in cases when flapless procedures cannot be practiced.

Once the doctor is familiar with the software, three-dimensional analysis of computer tomograms and virtual implant placement are fast. A compensation of costs results from reduced chairside time when doing surgery and a reduction of follow-up visits for the patients. An efficient planning tool based on new computer technology facilitates final decision making in implant prosthodontic treatment (Katsoulis et al. 2009).

Accuracy in computer-assisted implant surgery is very important issue and should be assessed in clinical situations. Maximum deviation should be reported rather than the mean deviation to prevent damage to vital structures. The accuracy of these systems depends on all cumulative and interactive errors involved, from data set acquisition to the surgical pro-

cedure. The positioning, fixation, and stability of the surgical guide, and also a parallel and central positioning of the drill in the drill guide, is crucial to prevent the deviations. A discrepancy between the drill and the sleeve is needed to prevent heating and cutting of metal, but it unfortunately creates a deviation. Other materials can be used for the drill and guides that prevent heating so that the deviation can be further reduced (Jung et al. 2009; Van Assche and Quirynen 2010).

Although there is some evidence that higher accuracy can be achieved with computer-assisted implant surgery, it is unclear if surgical outcomes and long-term prosthetic success are improved because there are no long-term data in the literature. However, technology has been improving every day and it looks promising. Future long-term clinical studies are necessary to understand clinical indications and to justify efforts and costs associated with computer-assisted implant surgery. There is not yet enough evidence to suggest that computer-assisted implant surgery is superior to conventional procedures in terms of safety, outcomes, morbidity, and efficiency.

The three-dimensional view of the jaws allows the determination of the best implant position, the optimization of the implant axis, and the definition of the best surgical and prosthetic solution for the patient. Available data confirmed that a full flapless surgery is not available for many patients (Katsoulis et al. 2009). However, a protocol that combines a computer-guided technique with conventional surgical procedures becomes a promising option. An implant surgeon has to be aware that a combination of image-guided techniques with virtual implant planning and conventional surgery is feasible and may be advantageous. In this kind of scenario, the surgical guide can be used for the pilot drilling of all implants, allowing proper angulations and spacing; and after placing direction indicators, all areas can be evaluated to determine if it is feasible to proceed with further drilling in a flapless approach. Eventually, the implants are placed in a flapless way where sufficient bone is present. Then, the surgical guide can be removed and surgery is completed by raising a flap, followed by selective additional procedures such as sinus lift, guided bone regeneration, or bone splitting for the remaining implants. An example of this scenario is presented at the end of this chapter as a case presentation. The end result was quite pleasing from the surgeon's, restorative dentist's, and most importantly, from the patient's point of view. Virtual implant planning helped us to determine the best implant position, implant axis, and best surgical and prosthetic solution.

CASE REPORT

A 33-year-old African American male presented to Boston University, Goldman School of Dental Medicine, Post-

Graduate Periodontology Clinic. Clinical and radiographic evaluation and the family history of the patient led to diagnosis of generalized aggressive periodontitis (Armitage 1999). Upon periodontal examination, the marginal gingiva was inflamed, and bleeding on probing was ubiquitous throughout the mouth. Probing depths ranged from 2 to 11 mm with clinical attachment loss of ≥7 mm. Radiographic evidence of generalized moderate to advanced bone loss was observed (Figures 16.3–16.5).

Because of advanced generalized aggressive periodontitis with poor prognosis, extraction of all teeth was planned. Before extractions, oral hygiene instructions were given and full-mouth mechanical debridement was done. All teeth were extracted atraumatically with no socket grafting, and complete dentures were delivered right after extractions (Figure 16.6).

CT scans were taken 3 months after extraction and showed inadequate bone height for placing implants in posterior

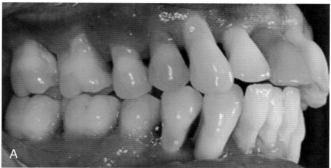
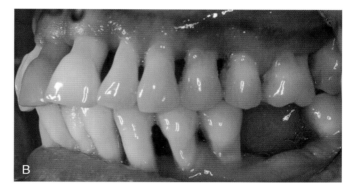

Figure 16.4 (A, B) Intraoral picture of the patient diagnosed with generalized aggressive periodontitis.

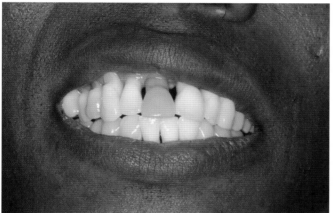

Figure 16.3 Extraoral view of the patient diagnosed with generalized aggressive periodontitis.

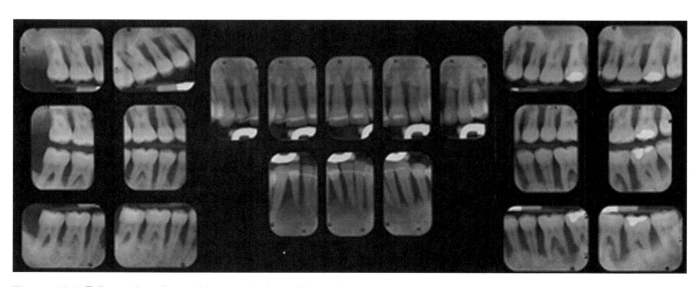

Figure 16.5 Full-mouth radiographic examination of the patient.

maxilla. Lateral wall sinus lift procedures were done by using piezosurgical instruments and were grafted with rhBMP-2 (Infuse) on one side and demineralized freeze-dried bone allograft (DFDBA) on the other. Seven months after sinus grafting, a second set of CT scans were taken (Figures 16.7, 16.8).

A CT scan was taken of the patient with the denture-like template in situ. Prior to the CT, records, aesthetics, fit of the denture base, functional aspects, occlusion, and vertical dimension of the complete dentures were checked clinically. The original denture was then converted into a denture-like surgical template, which was used for the CT. This denture template exhibited radio-opaque markers from gutta-percha (Figure 16.9).

In this case, the CT analysis and virtual implant planning was performed with the InVivo Dental software program (Anatomage, San Jose, CA). Accordingly, the best implant position was determined in relation to the bone structure and prospective tooth position (Figures 16.10, 16.11).

CT scan analysis and virtual implant planning showed the need for an internal sinus lift procedure since we had about 8 to 9 mm height in posterior maxilla. Lower anterior area also showed about 5 mm bone width. Therefore, we planned to reflect the flap and proceed with conventional surgery. Virtual implant planning helped us to determine the best implant position, implant axis, and best surgical and prosthetic solution.

Six implants were placed in the maxilla with simultaneous internal sinus lifts and seven implants in the mandible (bone level; SLActive surface, Straumann, Andover, MA). See Figures 6.12 through 6.16.

In a case report, Emrani et al. (2009) showed that periodontal pathogens can be retained for a prolonged period of time in non-dental sites, from where they can later colonize and compromise the health of dental implants. Therefore, during the uncovering procedure (Figure 16.16), we prescribed amoxicillin and metronidazole combination therapy to eradicate possible periodontopathogens from the oral environment to prevent recolonization around the implants. Six weeks after implant placement surgeries, the provisional prosthesis was inserted (Figure 16.17). The patient was motivated and instructed in good home care. The patient is in a maintenance program with 3-month recalls.

ACKNOWLEDGMENTS

I would like to thank Dhurata Shosho, Implant and CBCT Coordinator at Department of General Dentistry, Goldman

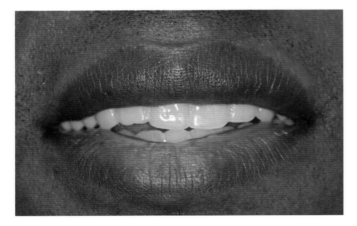

Figure 16.6 Patient's smile after complete denture delivery.

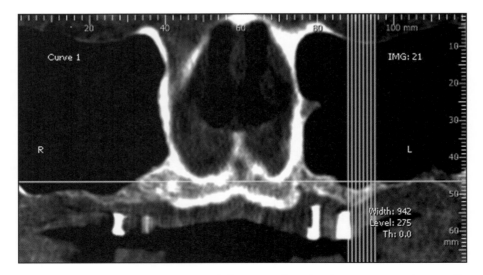

Figure 16.7 CT scan after extractions reveals not enough bone to place implants on posterior maxilla.

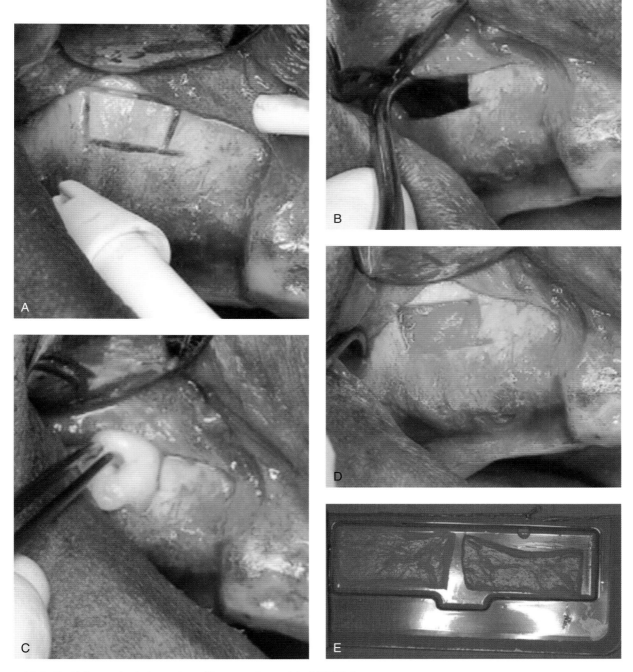

Figure 16.8 (A–E) Lateral window sinus lift procedure with rhBMP-2.

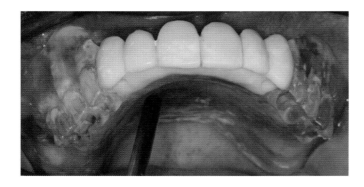

Figure 16.9 Denture-like templates with gutta-percha markers.

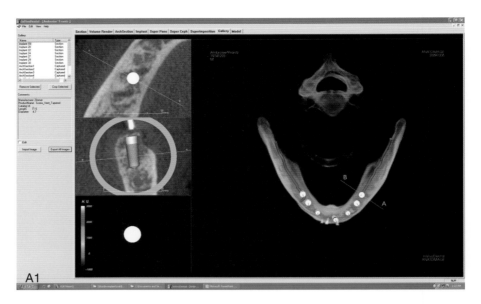

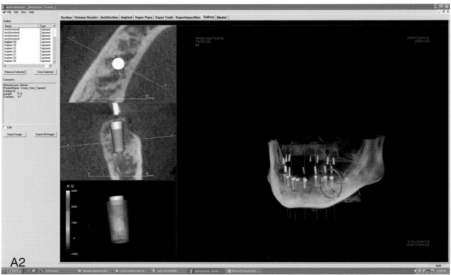

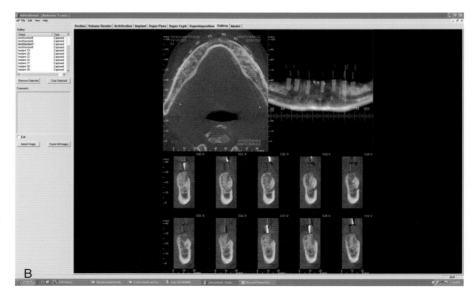

Figure 16.10 (A, B) CT scan analysis and virtual implant planning in mandible. Software program shows three-dimensional images of mandible and implants in place.

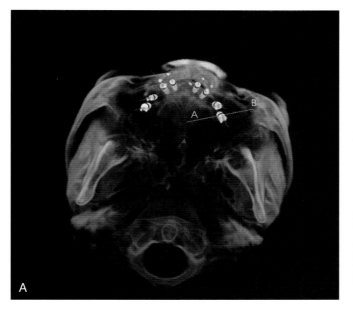 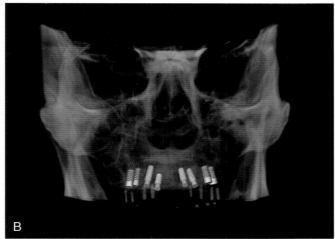

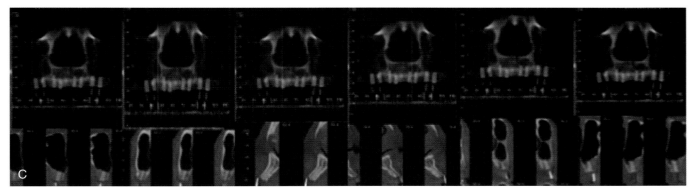

Figure 16.11 (A, B, C) CT scan analysis and virtual implant planning in maxilla. Software program shows three-dimensional images of maxilla and implants in place.

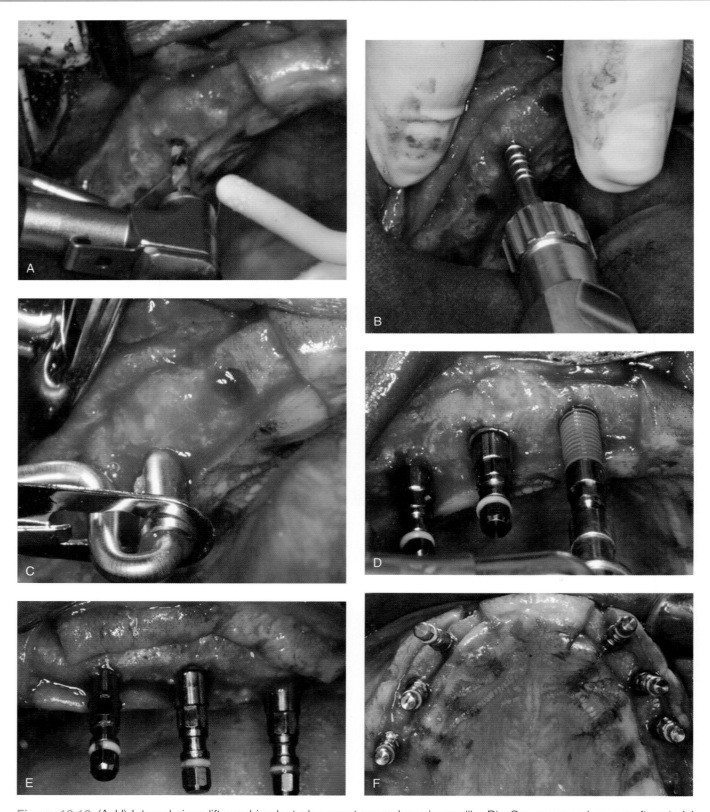

Figure 16.12 (A–H) Internal sinus lifts and implant placement procedures in maxilla. Bio-Oss was used as a graft material in sinus lift procedure.

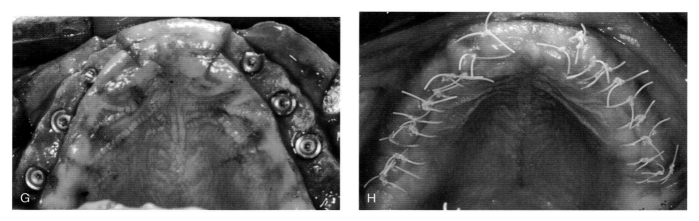

Figure 16.12 *Continued*

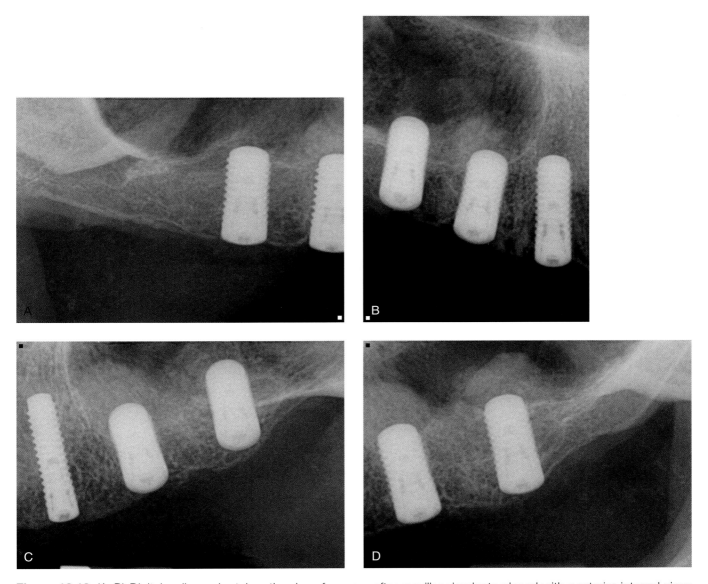

Figure 16.13 (A–D) Digital radiographs taken the day of surgery after maxillary implants placed with posterior internal sinus lift procedures.

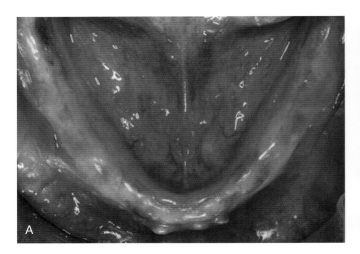

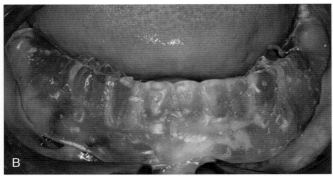

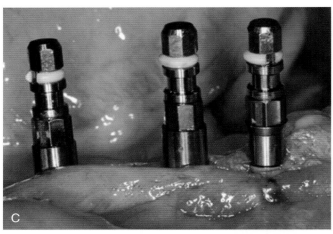

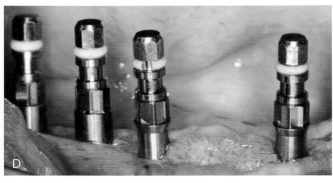

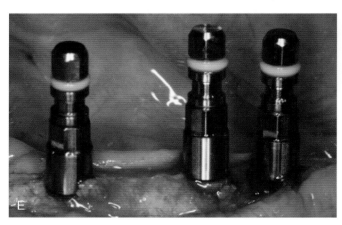

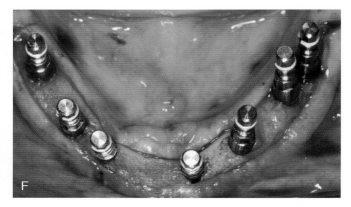

Figure 16.14 (A–H) Mandibular implant placement procedures.

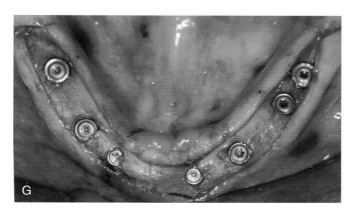

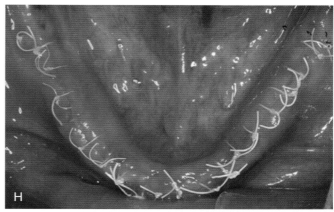

Figure 16.14 *Continued*

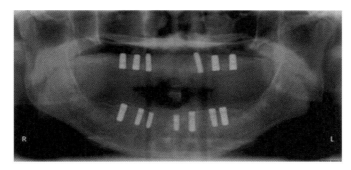

Figure 16.15 Panoramic radiograph of the patient after maxillary and mandibular implant placements.

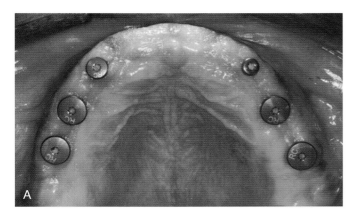

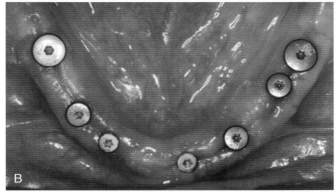

Figure 16.16 (A, B) Uncovering procedure was done 4 weeks after implant placements. Combination of amoxicillin 250 mg and metronidazole 250 mg three times a day for 10 days was prescribed on the day of the uncovering procedure.

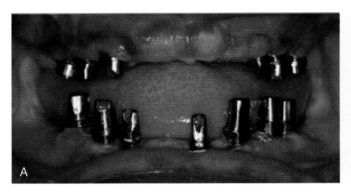
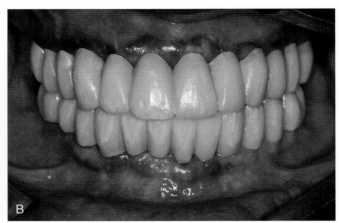

Figure 16.17 (A and B) Patient with provisional prosthesis.

School of Dental Medicine, Boston University, who helped me take CT scans and worked with me on software programs for virtual implant planning. I appreciate her effort and time. Also I would like to thank Dr. Serge Dibart with whom I worked on the case for giving me this opportunity. I would like to thank Dr. Arthur O'Connor and Dr. Gurkan Goktug from the Prosthetic Department. They did an amazing job with the treatment planning and prosthesis of the patient.

REFERENCES

Amet EM, Ganz SD. 1997. Implant treatment planning using a patient acceptance prosthesis, radiographic record base, and surgical template. Part 1: Presurgical phase. *Implant Dent*. 6:193–97.

Armitage GC. 1999. Development of a classification system for periodontal diseases and conditions. *Ann Periodontol*. 4:1–6.

Azari A, Nikzad S. 2008a. Computer-assisted implantology: Historical background and potential outcomes—a review. *Int J Med Robotics Computer Assist Surg*. 4:95–104.

Azari A, Nikzad S. 2008b. Flapless implant surgery: Review of the literature and report of 2 cases with computer-guided surgical approach. *J Oral Maxillofac Surg*. 66:1015–21.

Bahat O. 1993. Treatment planning, placement of implants in the posterior maxillae: Report of 732 consecutive nobelpharma implants. *Int J Oral Maxillofac Impl*. 8:151–61.

Bassi F, Procchio M, Fava C, et al. 1999. Bone density in human dentate and edentulous mandibles using computed tomography. *Clin Oral Impl Res*. 10:356–61.

Basten CH, Kois JC. 1996. The use of barium sulfate for implant templates. *J Prosthet Dent*. 76:451–14.

Basten CH. 1995. The use of radiopaque templates for predictable implant placement. *Quintessence Int*. 26:609–12.

Becker CM, Kaiser DA. 2000. Surgical guide for dental implant placement. *J Prosthet Dent*. 83:248–51.

Benjamin LS. 2002. The evolution of multiplanar diagnostic imaging: Predictable transfer of preoperative analysis to the surgical site. *J Oral Implantol*. 28:135–44.

Berglundh T, Lindhe J. 1996. Dimension of the periimplant mucosa. Biological width revisited. *J Clin Periodontol*. 23:971–73.

Besimo CE, Lambrecht JT, Guindy JS. 2000. Accuracy of implant treatment planning utilizing template-guided reformatted computed tomography. *Dentomaxillofac Radiol*. 29:46–51.

Borrow JW, Smith JP. 1996. Stent marker materials for computerized tomograph-assisted implant planning. *Int J Periodontics Restorative Dent*. 16:60–67.

Casap N, Tarazi E, Wexler A, et al. 2005. Intraoperative computerized navigation for flapless implant surgery and immediate loading in the edentulous mandible. *Int J Oral Maxillofac Implants*. 20:92–98.

Casap N, Wexler A, Persky N, et al. 2004. Navigation surgery for dental implants: Assessment of accuracy of the image guided implantology system. *J Oral Maxillofac Surg*. 62:116–19.

Cehreli MC, Aslan Y, Sahin S. 2000. Bilaminar dual-purpose stent for placement of dental implants. *J Prosthet Dent*. 84:55–58.

Cooper KG. 2001. *Rapid Prototyping Technology: Selection and Application*, Marcel Dekker, Inc., New York, USA.

Dawson P. 2004. Patient dose in multislice CT: Why is it increasing and does it matter? *Br J Radiol*. 77 (Special issue):S10–S13.

Duff RE, Razzoog ME. 2006. Management of a partially edentulous patient with malpositioned implants, using all-ceramic abutments and all-ceramic restorations: A clinical report. *J Prosthet Dent*. 96: 309–12.

Ekestubbe A, Thilander A, Gröndahl K, et al. 1993. Absorbed doses from computed tomography for dental implant surgery: Comparison with conventional tomography. *Dentomaxillofac Radiol*. 22:13–17.

Emrani J, Chee W, Slots J. 2009. Bacterial colonization of oral implants from nondental sources. *Clin Implant Dent Relat Res*. 11:106–12.

Frederiksen NL, Benson BW, Sokolowski TW. 1994. Effective dose and risk assessment from film tomography used for dental implant diagnostics. *Dentomaxillofac Radiol*. 23:123–27.

Frederiksen NL, Benson BW, Sokolowski TW. 1995. Effective dose and risk assessment from computed tomography of the maxillofacial complex. *Dentomaxillofac Radiol*. 24:55–58.

Ganz SD. 2003. Use of stereolithographic models as diagnostic and restorative aids for predictable immediate loading of implants. *Pract Proced Aesthet Dent*. 15:763–71.

Garber DA. 1996. The esthetic dental implant: Letting restoration be the guide. *J Oral Implantol*. 22:45–50.

Gher ME, Richardson AC. 1995. The accuracy of dental radiographic techniques used for evaluation of implant fixture placement. *Int J Periodontics Restorative Dent*. 15:268–83.

Gillespie JE, Isherwood I. 1986. Three-dimensional anatomical images from computed tomographic scans. *Br J Radiol*. 59:289–92.

Guerrero ME, Jacobs R, Loubele M, et al. 2006 State-of-the-art on cone beam CT imaging for preoperative planning of implant placement. *Clin Oral Invest*. 10:1–7.

Harris D, Buser D, Dula K, et al. 2002. E.A.O. guidelines for the use of diagnostic imaging in implant dentistry. A consensus workshop organized by the European Association for Osseointegration in Trinity College Dublin. *Clin Oral Implants Res*. 13:566–70.

Hounsfield, GN. 1973. Computerized transverse axial scanning (tomography). 1. Description of system. *Br J Radiol*. 46:1016–22.

Israelson H, Plemon JM, Watkins P, et al. 1992. Barium-coated surgical stents and computer-assisted tomography in the preoperative assessment of dental implant patients. *Int J Periodontics Restorative Dent*. 12:52–61.

Jabero M, Sarment DP. 2006. Advanced surgical guidance technology: A review. *Implant Dentistry*. 15:135–42.

Jacobs R, Adriansens A, Verstreken K, et al. 1999. Predictability of a three-dimensional planning system for oral implant surgery. *Dentomaxillofac Radiol*. 28:105–11.

Jacobs PF, ed. 1992. *Rapid Prototyping & Manufacturing: Fundamentals of Stereolithography*, Society of Manufacturing Engineers, Dearborn, Michigan, USA.

Jaffin RA, Berman CL. 1991. The excessive loss of Branemark fixtures in type IV bone: A 5-year analysis. *J Periodontol*. 62:2–4.

Jemt T, Book K, Lindén B, et al. 1992. Failures and complications in 92 consecutively inserted overdentures supported by Brånemark implants in severely resorbed edentulous maxillae: A study from prosthetic treatment to first annual check-up. *Int J Oral Maxillofac Implants*. 7:162–67.

Jemt T. 1993. Implant treatment in resorbed edentulous upper jaws. A 3-year follow-up study in 70 patients. *Clin Oral Implants Res*. 4: 187–94.

Jung RE, Schneider D, Ganeles J, et al. 2009. Computer technology applications in surgical implant dentistry: A systematic review. *Int J Oral Maxollofac Implants*. 24:92–109.

Iplikcioglu H, Akca K, Cehreli MC. 2002. The use of computerized tomography for diagnosis and treatment planning in implant dentistry. *J Oral Implantol*. XXVIII:29–36.

Katsoulis J, Pazera P, Mericske-Stern R. 2009. Prosthetically driven, computer-guided implant planning for the edentulous maxialla: A model study. *Clin Implant Dent Relat Res*. 11:238–45.

Klein M, Cranin AN, Sirakian A. 1993. A computerized tomography (CT) scan appliance for optimal presurgical and preprosthetic planning of the implant patient. *Pract Periodontics Aesthet Dent*. 5:33–39.

Kopp KC, Koslow AH, Abdo OS. 2003. Predictable implant placement with a diagnostic/surgical template and advanced radiographic imaging. *J Prosthet Dent*. 89:611–15.

Lal K, White GS, Morea DN, et al. 2006. Use of stereolithographic templates for surgical and prosthodontic implant planning and placement. Part I. The concept. *J Prosthodont*. 15:51–58.

Odlum O. 2001. A method of eliminating streak artifacts from metallic dental restorations in CTs of head and neck cancer patients. *Spec Care Dentist*. 21:72–74.

Pesun IJ, Gardner FM. 1995. Fabrication of a guide for radiographic evaluation and surgical placement of implants. *J Prosthet Dent*. 73:548–52.

Rangert B, Krogh PH, Langer B, et al. 1995. Bending overload and implant fracture: A retrospective clinical analysis. *Int J Oral Maxillofac Implants*. 10:326–34.

Rosenfeld AL, Mandelaris GA, Tardieu, PB. 2006. Prosthetically directed implant placement using computer software to ensure precise placement and predictable prosthetic outcomes. Part 1: Diagnostics, imaging, and collaborative accountability. *Int J Periodontics Restorative Dent*. 26:215–21.

Schwarz MS, Rothman SL, Rhodes ML, et al. 1987. Computed tomography: Part I. Preoperative assessment of the mandible for endosseous implant surgery. *Int J Oral Maxillofac Implants*. 2:137–41.

Schwarz MS, Rothman SL, Rhodes ML, et al. 1987. Computed tomography: Part II. Preoperative assessment of the maxilla for endosseous implant surgery. *Int J Oral Maxillofac Implants*. 2:143–48.

Schwarz MS, Rothman SL, Chafetz N, et al. 1989. Computed tomography in dental implantation surgery. *Dent Clin North Am*. 33: 555–97.

Sclar AG. 2007. Guidelines for flapless surgery. *J Oral Maxillofac Surg*. 65:20–32.

Sclar AG. 1999. Preserving alveolar ridge anatomy following tooth removal in conjunction with immediate implant placement. The Bio-Col technique. *Atlas Oral Maxillofac Surg Clin North Am*. 7:39–59.

Sethi A, Sochor P. 1995. Predicting esthetics in implant dentistry using multiplanar angulation: A technical note. *Int J Oral Maxillofac Implants*. 10:485–90.

Stanford CM. 1999. Biomechanical and functional behavior of implants. *Adv Dent Res*. 13:88–92.

Sonick M, Abrahams J, Faeilla R. 1994. A comparison of the accuracy of periapical, panoramic, and computerized tomographic radiographs in locating mandibular canal. *Int J Oral Maxillofac Impls*. 9:455–60.

Todd AD, Gher ME, Quintero G, et al. 1993. Interpretation of linear and computed tomograms in the assessment of implant recipient sites. *J Periodontol*. 64:1243–49.

Truitt HP, James RA, Lindley PE, et al. 1988. Morphologic replication of the mandible using computerized tomography for the fabrication of a subperiosteal implant. *Oral Surg Oral Med Oral Pathol*. 65: 499–504.

Tyndall DA, Brooks SL. 2000. Selection criteria for dental implant site imaging: A position paper of the American Academy of Oral and Maxillofacial radiology. *Oral Surg Oral Med Oral Pathol Oral Radiol Endod*. 89:630–37.

Ulm C, Kneissel M, Schedl A, et al. 1999. Characteristic features of trabecular bone in edentulous maxillae. *Clin Oral Implants Res*. 10:459–67.

Van Assche N, Quirynen M. 2010. Tolerance within a surgical guide. *Clin Oral Impl Res*. 21:455–58.

Van der Zel JM. 2008. Implant planning and placement using optical scanning and cone beam CT technology. *J Prosthodon*. 17: 476–81.

Vannier MW, Hildebolt CF, Conover G, et al. 1997. Three-dimensional dental imaging by spiral CT. A progress report. *Oral Surg Oral Med Oral Pathol Oral Radiol Endod*. 84:561–70.

Van Steenberghe D, Naert I, Andersson M, et al. 2002. A custom template and definitive prosthesis allowing immediate implant loading in the maxilla: A clinical report. *Int J Oral Maxillofac Implants*. 17: 663–70.

Vercruyssen M, Jacobs R, Van Assche N, et al. 2008. The use of CT scan based planning for oral rehabilitation by means of implants and its transfer to the surgical fields: A critical review on accuracy. *J Oral Rehab*. 35:454–74.

Verde MA, Morgano SM. 1993. A dual-purpose stent for the implant-supported prosthesis. *J Prosthet Dent*. 69:276–80.

Wagner A, Wanschitz F, Birkfellner W, et al. 2003. Computer-aided placement of endosseous oral implants in patients after ablative tumour surgery: Assessment of accuracy. *Clin Oral Implants Res*. 14:340–48.

Wanschitz F, Birkfellner W, Watzinger F, et al. 2002. Evaluation of accuracy of computer-aided intraoperative positioning of endosseous oral implants in the edentulous mandible. *Clin Oral Implants Res*. 13:59–64.

Wat PY, Chow TW, Luk HW, et al. 2002. Precision surgical template for implant placement: A new systematic approach. *Clin Implant Dent Relat Res*. 4:88–92.

Widmann G, Bale RJ. 2006. Accuracy in computer-aided implant surgery—a review. *Int J Oral Maxillofac Implants*. 21:305–13.

White SC, Heslop EW, Hollender LG, et al. 2001. Parameters of radiologic care: An official report of the American Academy of Oral and Maxillofacial Radiology. *Oral Surg Oral Med Oral Pathol Oral Radiol Endod*. 91:498–511.

Chapter 17 Endodontic Microsurgery or Dental Implants?

Obadah Attar, BDS, Cert. Endodontics, Fellowship Implantology

INTRODUCTION

Nonsurgical root canal treatment has advanced over the past two decades in both materials and technique. This improvement has allowed practitioners to approach teeth with a complex root canal system efficiently and provide patients with much more predictable treatment. In year 2000, approximately 30,000,000 endodontic treatments were provided compared to 910,000 dental implants (Millennium Research Group and ADA; Figure 17.1). In the United States, evaluation of 1.4 million teeth with initial endodontic treatment resulted in a 97% survival rate over a period of 8 years. Only 0.7% of treated teeth required surgical root canal treatment. This is in part due to the high survival rate of nonsurgical root canal treatments (Salehrabi and Rotstein 2004; Figure 17.2). On the other hand, dental implants have also advanced surgically and prosthetically, promising highly aesthetic and functional results. Unfortunately, dental implants have been over-commercialized at the expense of other, highly advanced, predictable treatment modalities, namely, endodontic microsurgery. This has resulted in the overall trend of extracting teeth with failed root canal treatments and replacing them with implants instead of referring them to specialists for surgical management. The past experience with the traditional endodontic surgery and the lack of knowledge about the recent advances in the microsurgical approach reinforced this trend.

ENDODONTIC MICROSURGERY

Historically, surgical root canal treatment was approached with less enthusiasm by practitioners and educators due to lack of specialized surgical instruments, poor magnification, biologically incompatible materials, and low success rates. The introduction of the surgical operating microscope in endodontics in the 1990s allowed for the manufacturing of smaller, more convenient instruments, such as micro-mirrors, micro-condensers, and ultrasonics tips, which made the instrumentation and filling of the apical portion of the root

canal system more precise and convenient to operators. The introduction of biocompatible materials resulted in superior, more predictable healing outcomes. The overall advancements in microsurgery resulted in better operators confidence, greater treatment success rate, and better patient experience.

Definition, Objectives, Indications, and Considerations of Endodontic Microsurgery

Definition and Objectives

Endodontic microsurgery can be best defined as a clinical procedure intended to remove the root tips, place a biocompatible material, and remove the associated diseased soft tissue. The optimal objectives—just like any endodontic procedure—are to prevent adverse signs and symptoms, to achieve complete removal of the contents of the root canal system(s), to create radiographically well-obturated root canal system(s), to promote healing and repair of the periradicular tissues, and to prevent further breakdown (AAE Quality Assurance Guidelines).

Indications

The indications for surgical root canal treatment include the following (Ingle, Craig, and Baumgartner 2007):

- *Failure of nonsurgical root canal treatment or retreatment:* If endodontic treatment or retreatment was provided within the standard of care and the patient had persistent signs and symptoms for longer than 4 years, this indicates failure of either procedure. Clinical symptoms of failure may require earlier intervention. While radiographic signs of failure can be followed up and diagnosed objectively, practitioners should look for other causes of failure such as missed canals, inadequate instrumentation and/or obturation, coronal leakage, and fractures. Often, retreatment of a contaminated, well-treated root canal system will result in resolution of signs or symptoms or is necessary before any surgical intervention.

Practical Osseous Surgery in Periodontics and Implant Dentistry, First Edition. Edited by Serge Dibart, Jean-Pierre Dibart.
© 2011 John Wiley & Sons, Inc. Published 2011 by John Wiley & Sons, Inc.

- *Failure of nonsurgical "initial" treatment and retreatment is not possible or practical or would not achieve a better result:* The presence of a recent, serviceable crown or obstruction of the main root canal system by endogenous (e.g., calcification) or exogenous (e.g., post) reasons may render orthograde endodontic treatment impossible or impractical (Figure 17.3). It should be noted that if the initial endodontic treatment was done within the standard of care with no obvious reason for failure, practitioners should not attempt to retreat the tooth.

- *A biopsy is necessary:* If vertical root fracture is suspected, resecting the root apex followed by staining will often provide an accurate diagnosis of vertical root fracture (Figure 17.4). A biopsy for persistent infection (e.g., actinomycosis) can be done simultaneously with microsurgical root canal treatment.

Considerations

Almost any patient who is fit for oral surgical procedure is a good candidate for endodontic microsurgery, with few considerations:

- Patient medical status, including uncontrolled high blood pressure, recent myocardial infarction, subacute bacterial endocarditis, uncontrolled hematological problems, osteoradionecrosis, and uncontrolled diabetes

- Practitioner's skills and experience and lack of equipment.

- Anatomical considerations, such as sulcus height, buccal thickness of bone, and proximity of mental foramen and inferior alveolar canal (Figure 17.5).

Other Considerations in Endodonitic Microsurgery

Before the decision for surgical root canal treatment to is made, several tooth-related factors should be evaluated. The restorability and the current crown/root ratio should be considered. It is generally accepted that 1:1 crown/root ratio is required for favorable radicular support for the prosthetic superstructure. Teeth with compromised crown/root ratio should be carefully evaluated since root-end resection will

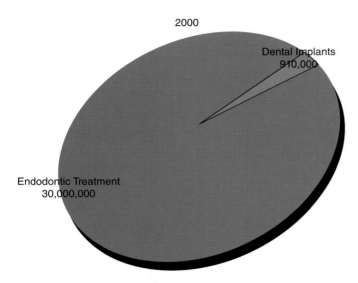

Figure 17.1 Pie chart illustrating number of endodontic treatment procedures done compared with dental implants in year 2000. (Data from Millennium Research Group and ADA).

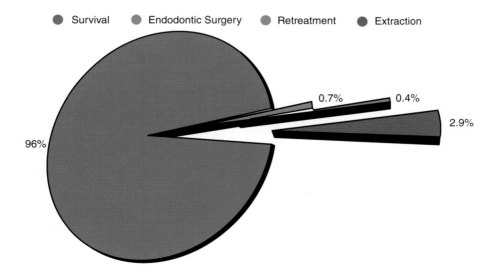

Figure 17.2 Pie chart illustrating the outcomes of 1,463,936 root canal–treated teeth with an 8-year follow-up. Data are from Delta Dental insurance database and represent patients from all 50 states of the United States. (Data from Salehrabi and Rotstein 2004).

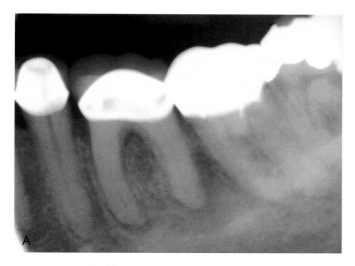

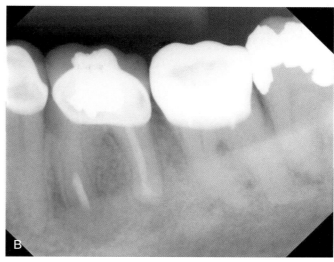

Figure 17.3 (A, B) Indications for endodontic microsurgery: Mesial root canals obstructed at the coronal two-thirds due to extensive calcification; non-surgical treatment was impossible. Apical root resection was performed. Six-month follow-up radiograph.

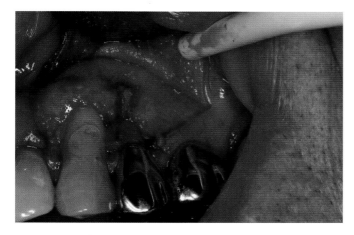

Figure 17.4 Tooth #12 had persistent periapical lesion determined radiographically after root canal treatment. Clinical examination during surgical root canal treatment showed vertical root fracture extending 6 mm from the root apex coronally.

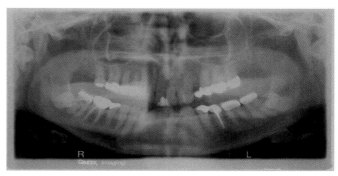

Figure 17.5 Anatomical considerations in endodontic microsurgery: Note the proximity of the mental foramen to the radiographic apex of tooth #20.

further compromise the root length. This is less important in multirooted teeth unless all roots will be resected (e.g., birooted premolars). It should be noted that surgical root canal treatment should be performed only if all other causes of endodontic failure are excluded. The current nonsurgical root canal treatment quality should be evaluated. Root canal–treated teeth should be assessed for radiographic obturation length, homogeneity, density, size, taper, and the presence of missed canals (Figure 17.6). Surgical treatment on a poorly done orthograde treatment does not satisfy the objective of endodontic treatment of complete removal of root canal content; retreatment should be chosen whenever possible as the first treatment approach over surgical treatment, provided

that the benefits of this retreatment outweigh the surgical treatment (Moiseiwitsch and Trope 1998). Studies showed that success of surgical root canal treatment combined with orthograde treatment is higher than surgical root canal treatment alone (Dorn and Gartner 1990; Grung, Molven et al. 1990). Cases where coronal access is impossible due to recent crown restoration, presence of post(s), or other intra-canal obstructions might render the retreatment difficult or impossible and should be assessed carefully since surgical treatment might be compromised by the previously done poor orthograde treatment. Adequate coronal restoration should be present since both a coronal and apical seal is required for successful endodontic treatment. Lack of adequate coronal seal results in coronal micro-leakage, which is an important cause of endodontic failure (Saunders and Saunders 1994). A retrospective study of 1,010 nonsurgical root canal treatments evaluating periradicular radiographic

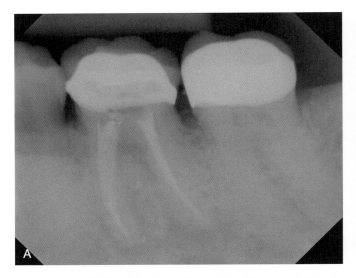

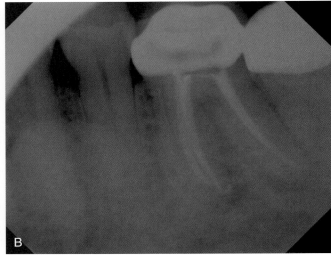

Figure 17.6 (A) Straight shot of a tooth with apparently adequate root canal obturation. Patient failed to have the temporary restoration replaced by permanent for a long period. (B) Shift shot radiograph revealed additional cause for failure at distal root. Note the eccentric position of the distal root canal filling and dual lamina dura at distal root that suggests the presence of additional root canal systems. Retreatment of this case is the ideal treatment plan.

status found that failure was attributed more to technical quality of coronal restoration than to quality of root canal treatment itself (Ray and Trope 1995). If coronal leakage is suspected, the tooth first should be retreated nonsurgically and properly restored to ensure adequate coronal seal and followed up for evidence of healing.

Surgical Procedure

Endodontic microsurgery follows the same basic steps as any other surgical procedure that requires the elevation of full-thickness mucoperiosteal flap (Figure 17.7). The basic steps are as follows:

1. Obtain patient's preoperative vital signs.
2. Review patient's health history.
3. Deliver appropriate anesthesia.
4. Reflect full-thickness mucoperiosteal flap.
5. Perform osteotomy.
6. Perform curettage of lesion (if present) to obtain tissue for biopsy.
7. Complete root-end resection (apicectomy or apicoectomy) and root-end inspection.
8. Perform root-end preparation (retropreparation).
9. Complete root-end filling (retrofilling).
10. Perform flap reapposition and suture.
12. Give postoperative instructions and prescriptions and take vital signs.
13. Recall.

Differences between Traditional and Modern Techniques in Endodontic Surgery

To be able to achieve the objectives of surgical root canal treatment, operators should be able to diagnose, access, and visualize the complex apical ramifications to ensure adequate cleaning and shaping and to be able to seal the remaining root canal system. Recent advances in endodontic microsurgery facilitated the diagnosis and management of failed initial endodontic treatments. Digital radiography introduced many potential benefits to endodontic practice with instant generation of high-quality images that allowed manipulation or processing of the captured image for enhanced diagnostic performance. Because patients needn't be reexposed due to retakes and because there is lower dose exposure compared with D-speed film, there is a safer environment for patients. The associated ease of archiving and use for long-distance consultation, shorter turnaround times, reduction in time between exposure and image interpretation, and digital documentation of patient records made digital radiography a convenient alternative for practitioners and patients (Wenzel and Grondahl 1995; Naoum et al. 2003). Anesthetic techniques have improved, offering better patient comfort and hemostasis. Before the introduction of surgical operating microscope in 1990s, operators had to establish larger osteotomy sizes to be able to visualize root apices and to accommodate the

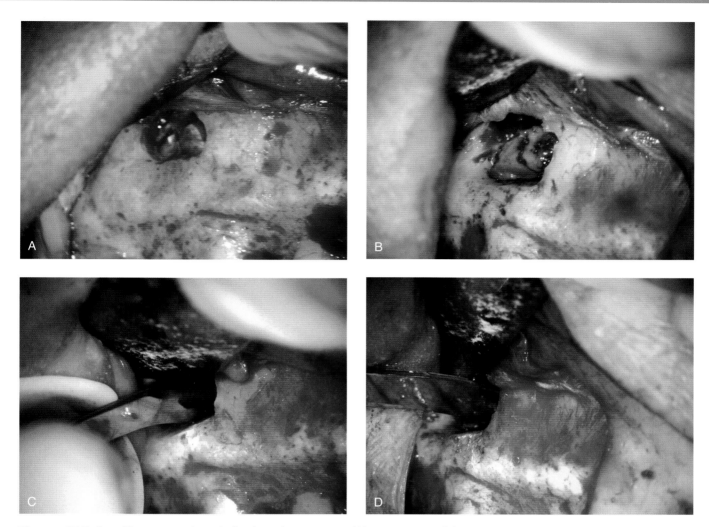

Figure 17.7 Specific steps of endodontic microsurgery: (A) osteotomy, (B) root-end resection, (C) retropreparation, (D) retrofilling.

larger instruments. Currently, osteotomy size is almost half the size and often dictated by the amount of root-end resection required. The introduction of micro-mirrors allowed better visualization of the resected root surface within the osteotomy. A steep bevel to allow better visualization and root-end preparation is no longer necessary, and operators are able to resect the root apex within 0–10 degrees. This conserves bone and root structure and reduces the amount of leakage due to exposure of dentinal tubules that result from steep bevels (Gilheany et al. 1994). The introduction of the surgical microscope allowed better inspection of the resected root surface to detect vertical root fractures, cracks, isthmuses, fins, and lateral canals. Commercially available ultrasonic instruments for microsurgeries became available in 1990s, and along with it came the introduction of superior handling and precise retropreparation within the root canal system compared to micro-hand-pieces that required bigger oste-

otomies and steep bevels. The use of amalgam is now considered below standard of care by most endodontists due to inferior biocompatability compared to the widely used mineral trioxide aggregate introduced in the 1990s. The introduction of finer monofilament suture materials resulted in superior soft tissue healing that allowed for early suture removal and superior patient experience. All those advancements resulted in bringing the overall success rate of endodontic microsurgery to a predictable range of 85%–96.8% compared to the wide-range success of 40%–90% before the microscope era.

Modern Advances in Microsurgical Instruments

The introduction of the surgical operating microscope in endodontics allowed the development of smaller, more precise instruments (Figure 17.8). With higher magnification power up

Table 17.1. Differences between traditional and microsurgical endodontics.

	Traditional	Microsurgery
Time period	Before 1990s	Beginning of 1990s
Radiographs	Plain film	Digital
Anesthesia	Nerve block and infiltration	Nerve block, infiltration, intraosseous and intraligamentary
Microscope use	Never	Always
Osteotomy size	Approx. 8–10 mm	3–4 mm
Bevel angle degree	45–65 degrees	0–10 degrees
Inspection of resected root surface	None	Always
Isthmus identification and treatment	Impossible	Always
Root-end preparation	Seldom inside canal	Always within canal
Root-end preparation instrument	Bur	Ultrasonic tips
Root-end filling material	Less biocompatible	More biocompatible
Sutures	4–0 silk	5–0, 6–0 monofilament
Suture removal	7 days post-op	2–3 days post-op
Healing success (over 1 year)	40%–90%	85%–96.8%

Adapted from Kim and Kratchman (2006).

to 30× and better illumination, the need for bigger instruments and the removal of critical bone and tooth structure is greatly minimized. The osteotomy size is dictated by the size of the removed root apex instead of the instrument itself. The micro-mirrors, ultrasonic tips, micro-condensers, and micro-pluggers are almost the size of the osteotomy, if not smaller. Many instruments come with different angulations to accommodate difficult access in posterior teeth.

The Use of Ultrasonics in Endodontics

The use of burs in a micro-hand-piece for retropreparation had many drawbacks. The difficulty in access resulted in cavities that were never parallel to the main root canal system, do not confer to the overall shape of the canal, and often resulted in lingual perforation of the root. The difficulty in creating retropreparation of enough depth to retain the retro-filling was a common problem, and a steep bevel of resected root surface to improve visibility and extra means of retention in the retropreparation removed critical root structure. The introduction of ultrasonics in endodontics revolutionized surgical endodontics. Historically, the use of ultrasonics or ultrasonic instrumentation was first introduced to dentistry for cavity preparations using an abrasive slurry (Catuna 1953). The concept of using ultrasonics in endodontics was first introduced by Richman in 1957. However, it was not until Martin et al. (Martin 1976; Martin et al. 1980a, 1980b) demonstrated the ability of ultrasonically activated K-type files to cut dentin that this application found common use in the preparation of root canals before filling and obturation. The term "endosonics" was coined by Martin and Cunningham

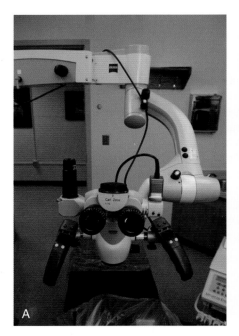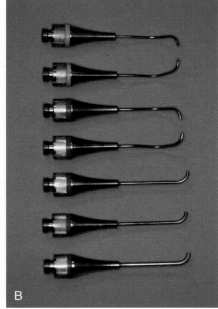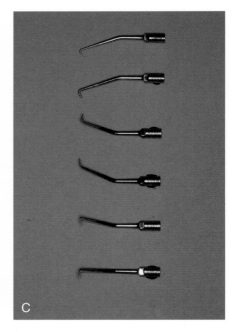

Figure 17.8 (A) Surgical operating microscope, (B) MAP system tips, (C) ultrasonic tips.

(1984, 1985) and was defined as the ultrasonic and synergistic system of root canal instrumentation and disinfection. The following is the most common use of ultrasonics in endodontics (Plotino et al. 2007):

- Access refinement, finding calcified canals, and removal of attached pulp stones.

- Removal of intracanal obstructions (separated instruments, root canal posts, silver points, and fractured metallic posts).

- Increased action of irrigating solutions.

- Ultrasonic condensation of gutta-percha.

- Placement of mineral trioxide aggregate (MTA).

- Surgical endodontics, including root-end cavity preparation and refinement and placement of root-end obturation material.

- Root canal preparation.

In the mid1980s, standardized instruments and aluminum oxide ceramic pins were introduced for retrograde filling. This system could not be used in cases with limited working space or in teeth with large oval canals (Keller 1990). Since sonically or ultrasonically driven microsurgical retro-tips became commercially available in the early 1990s (Pannkuk 1991), this new technique of retrograde root canal instrumentation has been established as an essential adjunct in periradicular surgery (Carr 1992). The use of ultrasonics in surgical endodontics overcomes many of the drawbacks that practitioners used to face when using burs. The small tips allow for better access and does not require large osteotomies to accommodate their size. Many tips come with different angulations for better access (Figure 17.9). The preparation is confined and parallel to the main root canal system and is of enough depth to retain the retrofilling material (Wuchenich

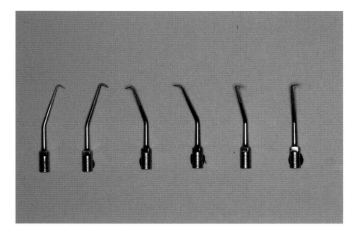

Figure 17.9 Ultrasonics come in various angulations to facilitate access to the resected root surface.

et al. 1994). The reduced bevel results in conservative root resection, reduces the number of exposed dentinal tubules that result from steep bevels, and minimizes leakage (Tidmarsh and Arrowsmith 1989). Ultrasonics produced less smear layer in a retro-end cavity compared to a slow-speed hand-piece (Gorman et al. 1995). Several studies focused on crack formation as a result of root-end preparation. Gutmann and Saunders (1994) were first to report that ultrasonics may produce cracks during instrumentation. Abedi and Torabinejad reported that crack formation at the root end is a dependent on power setting, time, initial cracks, and thickness or remaining dentin (Abedi et al. 1995). Frank and Bakland found that the use of ultrasonics on medium power with water spray reduces incidence of root infractions (Ingle 2007). Other studies did not detect any crack formation associated with ultrasonic preparation (Beling et al. 1997; Waplington et al. 1997). The effect of microfractures on success has been studied by several authors. It should be noted that apical resorption after healing may eliminate the surface defects and contribute to the overall success of treatment (Holland et al. 1998). In conclusion, the superior results obtained with ultrasonics over burs resulted in higher overall success rates in surgical root canal treatment (Refer to surgical outcome studies Table 17.4).

The Advancements in Retrofilling Materials

The indications for the retrofilling procedure are to create a good seal and to prevent leakage of irritants from the root canal system (RCS) to the periradicular tissues (Bondra et al. 1989). This will improve the fill of complex root canal anatomy that would be missed or impossible to fill by orthograde obturation. A higher chance of failure is seen in teeth without an adequate apical seal (Frank et al. 1992). Placement of a retrofilling material is considered standard in endodontic microsurgery except in very few cases. The current evidence shows that today we have materials with better biologic and physical properties than those used in orthograde fillings. For example, mineral trioxide aggregate (MTA) has proven to provide better biologic and sealing ability and favors healing (Koh et al. 1997; Torabinejad et al. 1997). Significant numbers of practitioners use cold burnishing of the gutta-percha after root-end resection. Cold burnishing of gutta-percha exposed after apical root resection of a well-obturated canal resulted in a poorer apical seal than did no burnishing. Likewise, cold burnishing the gutta-percha exposed after apical root resection of a poorly obturated canal resulted in an improved apical seal compared with no burnishing (Minnich et al. 1989). The importance of root-end filling has been studied in literature. Table 17.2 shows the result of selected studies of the root apex management after root-end resection. Note that most of those studies have smaller sample size, used older techniques and materials as root-end fillings that do not reflect the current understanding, and resected root apexes to a level that would eliminate complex root-end anatomy, yet

Table 17.2. Selected studies comparing root-end filled vs. nonfilled resected roots.

Author (year)	Sample Size	Follow-up Period	Results	Notes
Altonen and Mattila (1976)	93 Roots in 46 molars	1–6 Years	Orthograde better than retrograde filling	Resected 1/2 the root in selected cases
Lustmann et al. (1991)	136 Premolars and molars	6 Months to 8 Years	Better results with amalgam and Super EBA compared to nonfilled	Higher success in well-obturated cases
Rahbaran et al. (2001)	176 Teeth	+4 Years	Placement of root-end filling had significant effect on outcome	Presence of adequate coronal restoration had positive impact on outcome
Rapp et al. (1991)	424 Patients	6 Months	No significant difference in healing between root-end filled vs. nonfilled	Presence of adequate coronal restoration had positive impact on outcome
August (1996)	23 Teeth with root-end resection only 16 Root-end resection + amalgam retrofilling	+10 Years	Fewer healing with filled compared to resected only	

Note the small sample size, old materials and technique used, and extensive root resection.

compromise the root structure. Although conclusive information is absent in the literature, retrofilling the conservatively resected root apex to provide an adequate seal should be done routinely, except in certain cases such as difficult access in second molars where visualization and instrumentation of the resected root apex is difficult.

Several materials have been used as to fill the retropreparations. The ideal root-end filling material should have the following characteristics (Hargreaves 2006):

- Seal the contents of the root canal system within the canal
- Prevent egress of any bacteria, bacterial products, or toxic materials into the surrounding tissue
- Be Nnnresorbable
- Be biocompatible
- Be dimensionally stable over time
- Induce generation of the periodontal ligament (PDL)
- Exhibit good handling properties
- Provide reasonable working time.

It should be noted that no material has fulfilled those requirements as yet. Until a material does so, practitioners should seek the material that meets most of the requirements for better results. Many literature reviews have covered the retrofilling materials in detail (Torabinejad 1996). In recent years, MTA and zinc-oxide eugenol–based (ZOE-based) materials have shown higher success rate when compared to other materials, such as amalgam. In the next few paragraphs, MTA will be covered briefly.

Mineral Trioxide Aggregate (MTA)

MTA has been reviewed in depth in literature. It has been considered the most biocompatible root-end filling material and can be used with predictable outcomes in endodontic surgery (Kim and Kratchman 2006; Figure 17.10). MTA has been used for apexification, apexogenesis, noncommunicating perforation repair, direct pulp capping, and root-end filling (Torabinejad and Chivian 1999). MTA major ingredients are:

- Dicalcium silicate
- Tricalcium aluminate
- Tricalcium silicate
- Tetra calcium aluminoferrite
- Calcium sulfate hydrate
- Gypsum
- Bismuth oxide

The apparent advantages of MTA are: it is radio-opaque; it is the least toxic of retrofilling materials; it has the best biocompatibility of retrofilling material; it is hydrophilic (Torabinejad et al. 1995; Koh et al. 1997); it is noninflammatory; and it has a high pH that creates a poor living environment for most bacteria in the presence of moisture/blood (Pitt Ford and Roberts 1990).

The disadvantages include discoloration potential, presence of toxic elements in the material composition, difficult handling characteristics, long setting time, high material cost, an absence of a known solvent, and the difficulty of its removal after curing (Naik and Hegde 2005; Duggal and Al Ansary

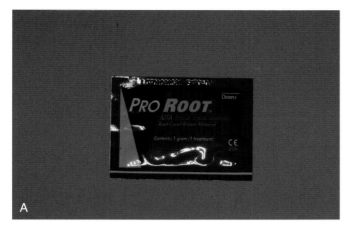

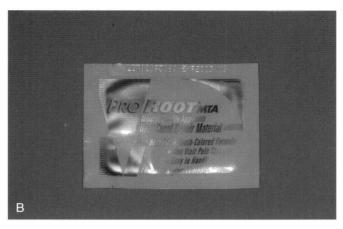

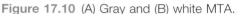

Figure 17.10 (A) Gray and (B) white MTA.

2006; Maroto et al. 2006; Percinoto et al. 2006; Watts et al. 2007; Boutsioukis et al. 2008; Ling et al. 2008; Park and Lee 2008; Silveira, Sanchez-Ayala et al. 2008; Bogen and Kuttler 2009).

MTA is considered biocompatible due to the histological findings of cementum formation adjacent to MTA and the non-inflammatory reaction of the surrounding tissue (Torabinejad et al. 1997). In vitro studies found osteoblasts to grow adjacent to MTA with elevated levels of cytokines (Koh et al. 1997). MTA provides superior sealing ability and demonstrated less bacterial leakage to *Staphylococcus* epidermis than did amalgam, Super EBA, or IRM at 90 days (Wuchenich et al. 1994). In vitro studies showed that MTA leaked less than Super EBA, amalgam, or IRM with or without blood contamination of the root-end cavities (Torabinejad et al. 1995).

The "Power" of Magnification

One of the most significant developments in the past decade in endodontics has been the use of the operating microscope for surgical endodontics (Kim 1997). The medical disciplines (e.g., neurosurgery, ENT, and ophthalmology) incorporated the microscope into practice 20 to 30 year previously (Kim and Kratchman 2006). The advantages of using the surgical operating microscope include the following:

- Better magnification so important anatomical structures are not missed
- Better illumination
- Improved documentation of cases
- Better ergonomics, increasing the operators' comfort during various endodontic procedures

The disadvantages of using the surgical operating microscope are its initial expense, the long-learning curve that

Table 17.3. Recommended magnification for different procedures.

Magnification	Procedure
Low (4× to 8×)	Orientation, inspection of the surgical site, osteotomy, alignment of surgical tips, root-end preparation, and suturing
Midrange (8× to 14×)	Most surgical procedures, including hemostasis. Removal of granulation tissue, detection of root tips, apicoectomy, root-end preparation, root-end filling
High (14× to 26×)	Inspection of resected root surface and root-end filling, observation of fine anatomical details, documentation

From Kim and Kratchman (2006).

would prevent many practitioners from using it, and its size. Companies provide several suspension systems (ceiling, wall, and floor mounting) for convenient incorporation in dental practice. Since 1998, all postgraduate endodontic programs must teach the use of magnification in accordance with the American Dental Association Accreditation Standard for Endodontic Graduate Programs (Commission on Dental Accreditation of the American Dental Association 2004).

Modern microscopes are capable of high magnification up to 30×. This does not directly relate to "usable power." Usable power is the maximum object magnification that can be used in a given clinical situation relative to depth and size of the field. With increasing magnification, the depth of field decreases and becomes narrower. At higher magnification, slight movement by the patient moves the field of view and changes the focus (Kim and Kratchman 2006). High magnification requires frequent adjustment that might become inconvenient when compared with lower magnification with a stable field and focus. Table 7.3 shows the recommended magnification level for different intraoral procedures.

Studies comparing the traditional surgical approach with no magnification to the modern surgical approach showed a better success rate when the surgical operating microscope is used (Refer to surgical outcome studies Table 17.4).

Outcomes Assessment Criteria for Microsurgical Root Canal Treatment

Unlike for dental implants, the evaluation of success and failure in endodontics has not changed much over years. Complete resolution of signs and symptoms has always been the ultimate goal of any endodontic procedure. In 1956, Strindberg proposed a system of criteria based on the absence or presence of radiographic rarification around the evaluated root apex. Periapical radiolucencies diagnosed at the end of a predetermined healing period should be considered a sign of biologic treatment failure. Although Strindberg found that sometimes complete healing did not occur until 10 years after healing, he proposed 4 years as a cut-off for success to be determined. Biopsies of periapical area of teeth with persistent periapical radiolucencies proved that healing with no inflammation (scar) might occur (Penick 1961), and it is difficult to determine if a large periapical radiolucencies PARL is scar tissue or inflammation in the healing periapical surgery area (Andreasen and Rud 1972). The diagnosis of healing/nonhealing cases is difficult to accomplish radiographically, and practitioners should evaluate the overall benefit/risk when evaluating asymptomatic teeth with residual periapical radiolucency because longer evaluation periods might be necessary. Criteria for clinical success of endodontically treated teeth are based on the following (Gutmann 1991):

- No tenderness to percussion or palpation.
- Normal mobility.
- No evidence of sinusitis
- No sinus tracts or periodontal pocketing.
- Tooth functional for at least 2 years
- No signs of infection or swelling
- Adjacent teeth respond normally to stimuli.
- No soft tissue scarring or discoloration.
- No evidence of subjective discomfort.

Criteria for clinical failure are:

- Persistent subjective symptoms
- Recurrent sinus tract or swelling
- Discomfort to percussion and/or palpation
- Evidence of irreparable fractured tooth

- Excessive mobility or progressive periodontal breakdown
- Inability to function with the tooth

Criteria for radiographic evidence of complete healing are:

- Normal periodontal ligament width or slight increase
- Rarefaction eliminated
- Normal lamina dura
- Normal osseous trabeculae
- No resorption evident

Criterion for radiographic evidence of healing is:

- Decrease in size of radiolucency after follow-up period shorter than 4 years

Criteria for diseased teeth (lack of healing) are:

- Increased width of periodontal ligament and lamina dura
- Circular rarefaction
- Symmetrical rarefaction with funnel-shaped borders
- Limited osseous trabeculae within rarefaction
- Evidence of resorption

Scoring indices for periapical radiographic assessment have been proposed for better accuracy and reproducibility. The periapical index (PAI) proposed by Orstavik (1988) is a simplified version of the radiographic method of interpretation used by Brynolf in 1967. The PAI is an ordinal scale index ranging from 1 (healthy) to 5 (severe periodontitis with exacerbating features). The validity is based on the use of reference radiographs of teeth with verified histological diagnosis. The following method is used in assigning a score:

- Find the reference radiograph where the periapical area most closely resembles the periapical area you are studying and assign the corresponding score to the observed tooth.
- When in doubt, assign a higher score.
- For multirooted teeth, use the highest of the scores given to the individual roots.
- All teeth must be given a score.

The use of indices in endodontic literature provides a strict, unbiased approach to evaluating the radiographic evidence of healing and disease. Newer indices keep emerging in endodontic literature to overcome the limitations of older indices. A recently proposed index based on cone beam computed tomography adds the expansion and destruction

Table 17.4. Summary of selected literature in surgical endodonitcs.

Author/Year	Category	Teeth (#)	Recall Period	Study Design	Inclusion/ Exclusion Criterial	Magnification	Retroprep	Retrofill Material	Success Rate
Tsesis et al. (2006)	Traditional vs. modern treatment techniques	88 teeth in 71 patients	2 years	Prospective RCT	Yes	Microscope vs. non	Bur vs. ultrasonics	IRM	91% success for the modern technique and 44.2% for the traditional
Wang, et al. (2004)	Healing > for teeth with small PAR	155 teeth in 138 patients	4–8 years	Prospective	No	No	Ultrasonics	Amalgam Composite Super EBA IRM or MTA	74%
Wesson and Gale (2003)	Complete healing at 1 year maintained in 75% of cases at 5 years	790 molars	5 years	Prospective	No	No	Bur	Amalgam	57%
Chong et al. (2003)	IRM vs. MTA 1 vs. 2 years	122/108	1 vs. 2 years	Prospective	Yes	Microscope	Ultrasonics	IRM vs. MTA	76%/87% IRM 84%/92% MTA
Maddalone and Gagliani (2003)		120 teeth	3 years	Prospective	No	Loupes	Ultrasonics	Super EBA	92.5
Schwartz-Arad (2003)	Did not advocate SRCT	122 from 101 patients	11.2 months mean	Retrospective	No	No	Bur	Amalgam and IRM	44.3%
von Arx et al. (2001)		39 roots in 25 molars	1 Year	Prospective	Yes	No	Ultrasonics	Super EBA	88%
von Arx and Bornstein (2003)	Endoscopy VS Micromirrors	129 Teeth	1 year	Prospective RCT	No	Endoscope	Ultrasonics	Super EBA	88.9% endoscopy 75.4 mirrors
Rubinstein and Kim (2002)		59 roots	5–7 years	Prospective	Yes	Microscope	Ultrasonics	Super EBA	91.5%
Rahbaran et al. (2001)	Endodontic VS OS clinic	167 Teeth	4 years	Retrospective	No	No	Ultrasonics VS Bur	Super EBA and amalgam	37.4% endo 19.4 OS
Rud et al. (2001)		834 roots in 520 Molars	1 year	Retrospective	No	Microscope	N/A	Dentin bonded resin	92%
Zuolo et al. (2000)	Periapical surgery	114	1–4 years	Prospective	Yes	No	Ultrasonics	IRM	91.2%
Testori et al. (1999)		302 roots in 181 teeth	4.6 years	Retrospective	No	No	Ultrasonics VS Bur	Super EBA and amalgam	68% Bur 85% ultrasonic

Continued

Table 17.4. *Continued*

Author/Year	Category	Teeth (#)	Recall Period	Study Design	Inclusion/ Exclusion Criterial	Magnification	Retroprep	Retrofill Material	Success Rate
Rubinstein (1999)		91 roots	1 year	Prospective	Yes	Microscope	Ultrasonics	Super EBA	96.8%
Rud et al. (1997)	Effect of root canal content on healing	551 teeth	2–4 years	Prospective	Yes	Microscope	Bur	Composite	92% healing with root filling to the apex
Danin et al. (1996)	Retreatment vs. surgical treatment	38 teeth	1 year	Prospective root canal treatment	No				Higher success for surgery than for conventional
Jesslen et al. (1995)	materials (amalgam vs. GI)	67 teeth in 64 Patients	1–5 years	Prospective RCT	No			Amalgam vs. glass ionomer	Overall 90% in one year and 85% in 5 years.
Molven et al. (1991)	Surgery	224 teeth	1–8 years	Prospective	No	Microscope	Bur	Amalgam	76.6% success
Molveneet al. (1991)	Surgery	474 teeth	1 year	Prospective	No	Microscope	Bur	Amalgam	250 teeth success
Rapp et al. (1991)	Apicectomy	424 teeth	6 months	Retrospective	No	No	Bur	Amalgam, IRM, Super EBA	65% Overall 68% IRM 70.8% Amalgam 65.4% EBA
Dorn and Gartner (1990)	Materials	488 teeth	6 months– 10 years	Retrospective	No	Unstated	Unstated	Amalgam, IRM, Super EBA	75% success for amalgam, 91% for IRM, 95% for Super EBA.

GI, glass ionomer; OS, oral surgery.

of the periapical cortical bone to the scoring system (Estrela et al. 2008).

Endodontic Literature on Surgery—Outcomes Assessment Studies

The problem in making treatment decisions based on outcome assessment studies is that in endodontic literature, many of the studies fall in the lower level of evidence-based research (cohort and case series). Most of the endodontic systematic reviews were conducted on literature that used materials and methods relevant to the era in which the text was written and does not reflect the advances in endodontics. It would be ideal to perform randomized clinical trials, where half the patients receive traditional endodontic surgery and the other half receives modern endodontic microsurgery. A study such as this would provide strong evidence of how the changes in technique and materials affected the success rate, but it would be unethical. The treatment decision should be based on the best available evidence with careful understanding of the limitations of the current literature. Table 17.4 summarizes selected outcome assessment studies.

In surgical endodontics literature, it is shown that as the endodontic technique and materials improved, the success rate improved as well. As mentioned earlier, studies in which no magnification was used, burs were used to prepare the retropreparations, and materials of lower biocompatability were used (such as amalgam) for retrofilling showed a lower success rate compared to those in which surgical operating microscope, ultrasonics, and biocompatible materials such as MTA were used.

Endodontic Literature on Resurgery—Outcomes Assessment Studies

Teeth with persistent radiographic evidence of failure should be assessed carefully because complete resolution of periapical radiolucencies can take up to 10 years (Strindberg 1956). Reit et al. recommended recalls annually for a minimum of 4 years, especially in questionable cases (Reit 1987). Studies showed that healing with scar formation can be the end result even after nonsurgical root canal treatment (Penick 1961). Andreasen and Rud concluded that it is difficult to determine if a large periapical radiolucency is scar tissue or inflammation in the healing periapical surgery area (Andreasen and Rud 1972). Failure of surgical root canal treatment can be attributed to many factors, such as materials used, technique, and coronal leakage. Amalgam retrofills have high leakage when compared to other materials such as MTA and Super EBA (Testori et al. 1999; Chong et al. 2009). Cases with steep bevels and bur retropreparations can be improved with contemporary microsurgery (Figure 17.11). Several studies focused on the prognosis or resurgery. Peterson et al. found 62.4% success rate at resurgery and that uncertain cases diminish over time (Peterson and Gutmann 2001). Gagliani

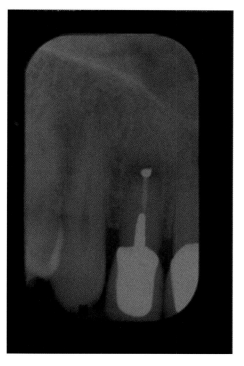

Figure 17.11 Traditional surgical root canal treatment case. Note the steep bevel, amalgam retrofill of inadequate length, and remaining root tip at the apical area. This tooth can be improved with modern microsurgery technique and materials, but extraction was done due to poor crown/root ratio.

et al. compared resurgery versus surgery and found the success rates to be 59% vs. 78% at 5 years, respectively (Gagliani et al. 2005). Taschieri et al. found 77% success rate when microscope and micro-instruments are used in resurgery (Taschieri et al. 2007). Saunders et al. compared surgery to resurgery and found 88.8% success compared to 74.5% with resurgery.

REVIEW OF ENDODONTIC AND IMPLANT LITERATURE:

Overview

Most of the current systematic reviews comparing endodontic treatment and dental implants focused on nonsurgical root canal treatment and implant-supported single crowns. Comparison between nonsurgical retreatment, surgical treatment, and retreatment, and implant-supported single crowns are largely missing in literature. On the other hand, implant-supported fixed partial dentures, implant-supported overdentures, and other complex implant restorations are not systematically reviewed. Systematic review of literature comparing the outcomes of all treatment modalities is required, yet it is missing. A review of literature on implant and nonsurgical root canal treatment revealed interesting findings. Comparing the cost of either one of the treatments, implants were found to be 70%–400% more expensive than root canal–treated restored teeth (Moiseiwitsch and Caplan 2001). This study did not take into consideration other adjunctive procedures such as sinus left and bone grafting. Dental implants required five times the posttreatment intervention compared to root canal–treated restored teeth (Doyle et al. 2007). In terms of posttreatment satisfaction, only 80% of patients were satisfied or extremely satisfied with dental implants (Gibbard and Zarb 2002). Surveys report a high (97%) level of patient satisfaction with a positive impact on quality of life after endodontic treatment. It should be noted that patients' previous experiences with either treatment are likely to greatly influence their decision (Dugas, et al. 2002). Recent implant success criteria adds aesthetic results into consideration. Aesthetic failures of dental implants outnumber the mechanical failures, especially in anterior restorations (Goodacre et al. 2003). Aesthetically, prevalence of papillary contracture after implant placement ranges from 5%–20% when compared with contralateral natural teeth (Chang, et al. 1999).

Problems When Comparing Dental Implants to Endodontic Treatment

Unlike dental implants, endodontic treatment aims to cure existing disease. Endodontic studies measure both healing of existing disease and the occurrence of new diseases. In dental implant studies, a single factor of disease presence/progression is measured. This adds and uncomparable environment for both treatments, with endodontic treatment being in a much more challenging disease state.

To answer the question of which treatment has better outcome, the Academy of Osseointegration's 2006 workshop on the state of the science of implant dentistry entrusted Iqbal and Kim to systematically review clinical studies of the survival of single-tooth implants and endodontically treated and restored teeth and to compare the results. Their conclusions are discussed next.

Success versus Survival

In implant literature, stringent success criteria are not routinely applied in much of the studies. Many studies use their own success criteria, and oftentimes survival rates are referred to as success. In endodontic literature, stringent criteria based on clinical and radiographic findings are employed in root canal prognostic studies. Unlike success, survival is defined as the retention of tooth or implant, depending on the studied intervention (Iqbal and Kim 2008). This will lead to exaggeration of the overall success of dental implants compared to the strictly evaluated and reported endodontic success. To establish comparable comparisons, it is critical that the same outcome measure be used to assess both procedures. Due to these differences in meanings of success, survival rates will permit less biased, but less informative comparisons. Life table analysis used in implant literature expresses retention during a length of time and gives a measure of expected outcome. However, life-table analyses can be misleading since patients who withdraw from the recall periods are both excluded or included in the analysis. Either method risks distortion of the clinically meaningful treatment effects (Iqbal and Kim 2008).

Who Is Doing the Treating?

Historically, dental implants were placed by specialists, and many endodontic studies were conducted on patients treated by dental students. Of 13,047 studies reviewed, 147 articles from the endodontic, prosthesis, and implant literature were systematically reviewed. None of these articles had implants placed by general dentists or students compared with 63% of the endodontic treatment provided by general dentists and students (Torabinejad et al. 2007). This should be considered when reviewing the outcome of modern endodontic treatment since endodontic microsurgery is almost exclusively done by endodontists. The use of a surgical operating microscope among endodontists increased from 52% in 1999 to 90% in 2007 (Kersten et al. 2008). This should have a positive effect on the outcome of surgical root canal treatment. None of the literature reviewed stated the trend of using the surgical operating microscope among oral surgeons, periodontists, general dentists, and students performing surgical root canal treatment. In contrast, dental implants are usually placed by specialists, and students are permitted to restore them. With the recent advances in dental implants, surgical protocols became easier to follow, and general dentists are beginning to place and restore dental implants (Figure 17.12). This should have an effect on the success of dental implants because recent studies suggest that the most significant factor in implant success is the operators' experience.

Case Selection

Appropriate case selection plays an important role in the success of any dental procedure. Cases selected in implant studies are usually subjected to strict inclusion/exclusion criteria. Most cases are selected based on favorable conditions such as patient's general health status, whether the patient smokes or has other habits, bone type, and so on. In endodontic literature, inclusion/exclusion criteria are usually absent. If the patient is fit for dental treatment, endodontic procedure is performed. Exclusion criteria in endodontics are usually followed to eliminate treatment variables rather than improve the treatment outcome. Most of endodontic procedures are done to treat existing disease conditions, and those performed for prosthetic purposes (e.g., overeruption) or trauma are excluded from the systematic review of literature.

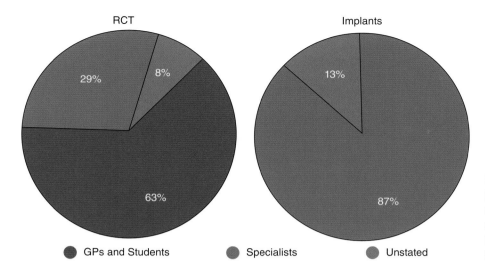

RCT

29% 8%

63%

Implants

13%

87%

● GPs and Students   ● Specialists   ● Unstated

Figure 17.12 Percentage of general practitioners and students, specialists, and unstated providers for (left) root canal treatment (RCT) and (right) dental implants. (Data from Torabinejad et al. 2007.)

Publication Bias

In implant literature, only 13% of studies had an evaluator different from the operator compared to 88% in endodontic literature (Torabinejad et al. 2007). Systematic investigation of dental implant literature confirmed the presence of publication bias and investigators recommended not basing treatment decisions on a limited number of studies (Moradi et al. 2006). Publication bias is more likely to exist when a particular brand of implant is studied, whereas endodontics is mostly generic (Brocard et al. 2000; Iqbal and Kim 2007).

Advancements

As mentioned earlier, both Iqbal and Kim's, as well as Torabinejad and colleagues', systemic reviews were conducted using material from previous decades and reflect the treatment approaches prevalent at that time.

Follow-Up Period

A systematic review of 23,000 root canal–treated teeth in 13 studies and 12,000 dental implants in 56 studies showed that the average follow-up period for root canal–treated teeth is 7.8 years compared to a 5-year follow-up period for dental implants (Torabinejad et al. 2007). Long-term studies on dental implants are often few in number, involve small numbers of patients, and suffer from attrition biases. Several studies involving large number of cases suggested that dental implant outcomes are excellent in the short term, but long-term outcome is still undefined. In contrast, endodontic treatment results are excellent in the short term and tend to improve over time. Endodontic studies that categorize a decrease in size of apical rarefaction as an uncertain event will often show improved success rates during longer follow-up periods because some of these uncertain cases will become successful (Molven et al. 2002). On the other hand, implant studies evaluating survival as success might show an

opposite trend because some of the surviving, pathologically involved implants will be lost during longer follow-up periods (Iqbal and Kim 2008).

Effect of Coronal Restoration

Many practitioners consider root canal treatment incomplete without adequate coronal restoration. Nonrestored endodontically treated teeth are more prone to coronal leakage and fracture. Only 13 articles in endodontic literature reported the outcome of root canal–treated teeth with proper coronal restoration whereas the condition of the coronal restoration in the rest of the literature is unstated (Iqbal and Kim 2007). Radiographic examination of 1,010 endodontically treated teeth restored with a permanent restoration found that the quality of the coronal restoration was significantly more important than the quality of the endodontic treatment for the presence of apical periodontitis (Ray and Trope 1995). Based on several bacterial and endotoxin leakage studies, cases with root canal treatment that have been exposed to coronal leakage for more than 3 weeks should be retreated (Ray and Trope 1995; Alves et al. 1998; Khayat and Jahanbin 2005). It has been shown that teeth without adequate coronal restoration have four times greater incidence of extraction as compared with those that are properly restored (Lazarski et al. 2001).

Independent Comparison of Endodontic and Implant Literature

A recent review of 13,047 studies, including implant-supported crowns, fixed partial dentures, and root canal–treated teeth found that direct comparison of treatment was extremely rare. Review of 143 studies showed that the success rate of implant-supported single crowns were higher than root canal–treated teeth, but the success criteria differed greatly. Systematic review of endodontic and implant

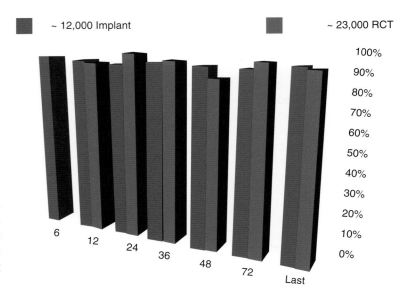

Figure 17.13 Derived from a meta-analysis comparison of the survival rates of the restored endodontically treated tooth and the restored single-tooth implant. No difference in the survival rates between the two treatment modalities over time. RCT, root canal treatment.

literature showed no difference in the survival rates between the two treatment modalities over time (Figure 17.13). In periodontally healthy teeth having pulpal and/or periradicular pathosis, root canal therapy resulted in outcomes (97%) equal to extraction and replacement of the missing tooth with an implant (Torabinejad et al. 2007). Studies on longevity of teeth and implants showed that teeth surrounded by healthy periodontal tissues yield a very high longevity, up to 99.5% over 50 years. In periodontally compromised, but treated and maintained teeth, the survival is still very high—92%–93%. Endodontically treated teeth had very high success rates. Survival of dental implants after 10 years varied between 82% and 94%. Teeth longevity is largely dependent on the periodontal health status of the pulp or periapical region and the extent of reconstructions. Dental implants did not surpass the longevity of even compromised and successfully treated natural teeth after 10 years (Holm-Pedersen et al. 2007). Other studies have shown that implants after restoration of function require more postoperative maintenance and tend to fail sooner than endodontically treated teeth over time (Doyle et al. 2006; Hannahan and Eleazer 2008). Independent studies on dental implants and surgical root canal treatment at a lower level of evidence (cohort and case series studies) show that both treatment modalities have comparable success rates. Both treatment modalities have improved over time, and their independent success rates have improved as well. One should keep in mind that modern dental implants as a treatment option should not be compared to surgical root canal treatment, specifically the modern microsurgical endodontic approach.

Treatment Decision

Priority in treatment planning should be given to tooth retention through root canal treatment or to replacement with an implant-supported single crown (Torabinejad et al. 2007). Iqbal and kim stated that the decision to treat a tooth endodontically or replace it with an implant must be based on factors other than the treatment outcomes of the procedures themselves, since both treatments have high success rate (Iqbal and Kim 2007). In order to formulate a proper treatment plan, an understanding of the difference between compromised and hopeless teeth is critical. Oftentimes, this difference is conspicuously missing from the literature. A uniform, objective, and precise definition must be given for each to allow for adequate treatment planning decisions to be made. Recently, Iqbal and Kim (2008) proposed these definitions:

Compromised tooth: Complex clinical syndrome that impairs the ability of a tooth to function properly. It requires removal of diseased tissue, and the optimal objective is restoration of removed tissue. Treatment strategies include placement of prosthetic restorations and various endodontic treatments.

End-stage tooth: Pathologic state or structural deficiency that cannot be successfully repaired with reconstructive therapies, including root canal treatment and retreatment, and continues to exhibit pathologic changes and clinical dysfunction of the tooth. Strategies for treatment include extractions and restoring function with placement of a fixed or removable prosthesis or an implant-supported restoration.

CONCLUSION

There is a common analogy that comparing various endodontic treatment procedures to dental implants is like comparing apples to oranges. These two treatment options each have their own indications and limitations. A dental implant is best seen as a replacement of a missing tooth, but not of an existing tooth. Since endodontic treatment on an end-stage tooth is unethical, extracting a restorable tooth and replacing it with a dental implant is just as unethical. Practitioners should not extract teeth requiring endodontic treatment based on the old understanding that endodontically treated teeth have low success rates. Endodontic therapy should be given priority in treatment planning for periodontally sound single teeth with pulpal and or periradicular pathology. Implants should be given priority in treatment planning for teeth that are planned for extraction. The most important factor in success of either one of the treatment modalities is case selection.

REFERENCES

Abedi HR, Van Mierlo BL, et al. 1995. Effects of ultrasonic root-end cavity preparation on the root apex. *Oral Surg Oral Med Oral Pathol Oral Radiol Endod*. 80(2):207–13.

Altonen M, Mattila K. 1976. Follow-up study of apicoectomized molars. *Int J Oral Surg*. 5(1):33–40.

Alves J, Walton R, et al. 1998. Coronal leakage: Endotoxin penetration from mixed bacterial communities through obturated, post-prepared root canals. *J Endod*. 24(9):587–91.

Andreasen JO, Rud J. 1972. Modes of healing histologically after endodontic surgery in 70 cases. *Int J Oral Surg*. 1(3):148–60.

August DS. 1996. Long-term, postsurgical results on teeth with periapical radiolucencies. *J Endod*. 22(7):380–83.

Beling KL, Marshall JG, et al. 1997. Evaluation for cracks associated with ultrasonic root-end preparation of gutta-percha filled canals. *J Endod*. 23(5):323–26.

Bogen G, Kuttler S. 2009. Mineral trioxide aggregate obturation: A review and case series. *J Endod*. 35(6):777–90.

Bondra DL, Hartwell GR, et al. 1989. Leakage in vitro with IRM, high copper amalgam, and EBA cement as retrofilling materials. *J Endod*. 15(4):157–60.

Boutsioukis C, Noula G, et al. 2008. Ex vivo study of the efficiency of two techniques for the removal of mineral trioxide aggregate used as a root canal filling material. *J Endod*. 34(10):1239–42.

Brocard D, Barthet P, et al. 2000. A multicenter report on 1,022 consecutively placed ITI implants: A 7-year longitudinal study. *Int J Oral Maxillofac Implants*. 15(5):691–700.

Brynolf I. 1967. A histological and roentgenological study of the periapical region of human upper incisors (Thesis). *Ondontol Revy*. 18(suppl. 11):1–176.

Carr G. 1992. Advanced techniques and visual enhancement for endodontic surgery. *Endod Rep*. 7(1):6–9.

Catuna M. 1953. Ultrasonic energy: A possible dental application. Preliminary report of an ultrasonic cutting method. *Ann Dent*. 12:256–60.

Chang M, Wennstrom JL, et al. 1999. Implant supported single-tooth replacements compared to contralateral natural teeth. Crown and soft tissue dimensions. *Clin Oral Implants Res*. 10(3):185–94.

Chong BS, Pitt Ford TR, et al. 2003. A prospective clinical study of Mineral Trioxide Aggregate and IRM when used as root-end filling materials in endodontic surgery. *Int Endod J*. 36(8):520–26.

Chong BS, Pitt Ford TR, et al. 2009. A prospective clinical study of Mineral Trioxide Aggregate and IRM when used as root-end filling materials in endodontic surgery. 2003. *Int Endod J*. 42(5):414–20.

Commission on Dental Accreditation of the American Dental Association. 2004. Standards for Advanced Specialty Education Programs in Endodontics, revised. http://www.ada.org/sections/educationAnd Careers/pdfs/endo.pdf

Danin J, Stromberg T, et al. 1996. Clinical management of nonhealing periradicular pathosis. Surgery versus endodontic retreatment. *Oral Surg Oral Med Oral Pathol Oral Radiol Endod*. 82(2):213–17.

Dorn SO, Gartner AH. 1990. Retrograde filling materials: A retrospective success-failure study of amalgam, EBA, and IRM. *J Endod*. 16(8):391–93.

Doyle SL, Hodges JS, et al. 2007. Factors affecting outcomes for single-tooth implants and endodontic restorations. *J Endod*. 33(4):399–402.

Doyle SL, Hodges JS, et al. 2006. Retrospective cross sectional comparison of initial nonsurgical endodontic treatment and single-tooth implants. *J Endod*. 32(9):822–27.

Dugas NN, Lawrence HP, et al. 2002. Quality of life and satisfaction outcomes of endodontic treatment. *J Endod*. 28(12):819–27.

Duggal M, Al Ansary M. 2006. Mineral trioxide aggregate in primary molar pulpotomies. *Evid Based Dent*. 7(2):35–36.

Estrela C, Bueno MR, et al. 2008. A new periapical index based on cone beam computed tomography. *J Endod*. 34(11):1325–31.

Frank AL, Glick DH, et al. 1992. Long-term evaluation of surgically placed amalgam fillings. *J Endod*. 18(8):391–98.

Gagliani MM, Gorni FG, et al. 2005. Periapical resurgery versus periapical surgery: A 5-year longitudinal comparison. *Int Endod J*. 38(5):320–27.

Gibbard LL, Zarb G. 2002. A 5-year prospective study of implant-supported single-tooth replacements. *J Can Dent Assoc*. 68(2):110–16.

Gilheany PA, Figdor D, et al. 1994. Apical dentin permeability and microleakage associated with root end resection and retrograde filling. *J Endod*. 20(1):22–26.

Goodacre CJ, Bernal G, et al. 2003. Clinical complications with implants and implant prostheses. *J Prosthet Dent*. 90(2):121–32.

Gorman MC, Steiman HR, et al. 1995. Scanning electron microscopic evaluation of root-end preparations. *J Endod*. 21(3):113–17.

Grung B, Molven O, et al. 1990. Periapical surgery in a Norwegian county hospital: Follow-up findings of 477 teeth. *J Endod*. 16(9):411–17.

Gutmann J. 1991. *Surgical Endodontics*. Boston: Blackwell Scientific. pp. 338–84.

Gutmann JL, Saunders WP, et al. 1994. Ultrasonic root-end preparation. Part 1. SEM analysis. *Int Endod J*. 27(6):318–24.

Hannahan JP, Eleazer PD. 2008. Comparison of success of implants versus endodontically treated teeth. *J Endod*. 34(11):1302–05.

Hargreaves CA. 2006. Periradicular Surgery. In: *Pathways of the Pulp*. St. Louis, MO: Mosby Elsevier.

Holland R, Otoboni Filho JA, et al. 1998. Effect of root canal filling material and level of surgical injury on periodontal healing in dogs. *Endod Dent Traumatol*. 14(5):199–205.

Holm-Pedersen P, Lang NP, et al. 2007. What are the longevities of teeth and oral implants? *Clin Oral Implants Res*. 18(Suppl)3:15–19.

Ingle J, Craig BL, Baumgartner J. 2007. Endodontic Surgery. In: *Ingle's Endodontics*. Hamilton, Ontario, Canada: BC Decker.

Iqbal MK, Kim S. 2007. For teeth requiring endodontic treatment, what are the differences in outcomes of restored endodontically treated teeth compared to implant-supported restorations? *Int J Oral Maxillofac Implants*. 22(Suppl):96–116.

Iqbal MK, Kim S. 2008. A review of factors influencing treatment planning decisions of single-tooth implants versus preserving natural teeth with nonsurgical endodontic therapy. *J Endod*. 34(5):519–29.

Jesslen P, Zetterqvist L, et al. 1995. Long-term results of amalgam versus glass ionomer cement as apical sealant after apicectomy. *Oral Surg Oral Med Oral Pathol Oral Radiol Endod*. 79(1):101–03.

Keller U. 1990. Aluminium oxide ceramic pins for retrograde root filling: experiences with a new system. *Oral Surg Oral Med Oral Pathol*. 69:737–42.

Kersten DD, Mines P, et al. 2008. Use of the microscope in endodontics: Results of a questionnaire. *J Endod*. 34(7):804–07.

Khayat A, Jahanbin A. 2005. The influence of smear layer on coronal leakage of Roth 801 and AH26 root canal sealers. *Aust Endod J*. 31(2):66–68.

Kim S. 1997. Principles of endodontic microsurgery. *Dent Clin North Am*. 41(3):481–97.

Kim S, Kratchman S. 2006. Modern endodontic surgery concepts and practice: A review. *J Endod*. 32(7):601–23.

Koh ET, Torabinejad M, et al. 1997. Mineral trioxide aggregate stimulates a biological response in human osteoblasts. *J Biomed Mater Res*. 37(3):432–39.

Lazarski MP, Walker WA, 3rd, et al. 2001. Epidemiological evaluation of the outcomes of nonsurgical root canal treatment in a large cohort of insured dental patients. *J Endod*. 27(12):791–96.

Ling J, Xu Q, et al. 2008. Microscopic management of teeth with open apices using mineral trioxide aggregate. *Pract Proced Aesthet Dent*. 20(1):49–51.

Lustmann J, Friedman S, et al. 1991. Relation of pre- and intraoperative factors to prognosis of posterior apical surgery. *J Endod*. 17(5):239–41.

Maddalone M, Gagliani M. 2003. Periapical endodontic surgery: A 3-year follow-up study. *Int Endod J*. 36(3):193–98.

Maroto M, Barberia E, et al. 2006. Dentin bridge formation after white mineral trioxide aggregate (white MTA) pulpotomies in primary molars. *Am J Dent*. 19(2):75–79.

Martin H. 1976. Ultrasonic disinfection of the root canal. *Oral Surg Oral Med Oral Pathol*. 42(1):92–99.

Martin H, Cunningham W. 1984. Endosonic endodontics: The ultrasonic synergistic system. *Int Dent J*. 34(3):198–203.

Martin H, Cunningham W. 1985. Endosonics—the ultrasonic synergistic system of endodontics. *Endod Dent Traumatol*. 1(6):201–06.

Martin H, Cunningham WT, et al. 1980a. A quantitative comparison of the ability of diamond and K-type files to remove dentin. *Oral Surg Oral Med Oral Pathol*. 50(6):566–68.

Martin H, Cunningham WT, et al. 1980d. Ultrasonic versus hand filing of dentin: A quantitative study. *Oral Surg Oral Med Oral Pathol*. 49(1):79–81.

Minnich SG, Hartwell GR, et al. 1989. Does cold burnishing gutta-percha create a better apical seal? *J Endod*. 15(5):204–09.

Moiseiwitsch J, Caplan D. 2001. A cost-benefit comparison between single tooth implant and endodontics. *J Endod*. 27:235.

Moiseiwitsch JR, Trope M. 1998. Nonsurgical root canal therapy treatment with apparent indications for root-end surgery. *Oral Surg Oral Med Oral Pathol Oral Radiol Endod*. 86(3):335–40.

Molven O, Halse A, et al. 2002. Periapical changes following root-canal treatment observed 20–27 years postoperatively. *Int Endod J*. 35(9):784–90.

Molven O, Halse A, et al. 1991. Surgical management of endodontic failures: Indications and treatment results. *Int Dent J*. 41(1):33–42.

Moradi DR, Moy PK, et al. 2006. Evidence-based research in alternative protocols to dental implantology: A closer look at publication bias. *J Calif Dent Assoc*. 34(11):877–86.

Naik S, Hegde AM. 2005. Mineral trioxide aggregate as a pulpotomy agent in primary molars: An in vivo study. *J Indian Soc Pedod Prev Dent*. 23(1):13–16.

Naoum HJ, Chandler NP, et al. 2003. Conventional versus storage phosphor-plate digital images to visualize the root canal system contrasted with a radiopaque medium. *J Endod*. 29(5):349–52.

Orstavik D. 1988. Reliability of the periapical index scoring system. *Scand J Dent Res*. 96(2):108–11.

Pannkuk TF. 1991. Endodontic surgery: Principles, objectives, and treatment of posterior teeth. Part 1. *Endod Rep*. 6(2):8–14.

Park JB, Lee JH. 2008. Use of mineral trioxide aggregate in the open apex of a maxillary first premolar. *J Oral Sci*. 50(3):355–58.

Penick E. 1961. Periapical repair by dense fibrous connective tissue following conservative endodontic therapy. *Oral Surg Oral Med Oral Pathol*. 14:239–42.

Percinoto C, de Castro AM, et al. 2006. Clinical and radiographic evaluation of pulpotomies employing calcium hydroxide and trioxide mineral aggregate. *Gen Dent*. 54(4):258–61.

Peterson J, Gutmann JL. 2001. The outcome of endodontic resurgery: A systematic review. *Int Endod J*. 34(3):169–75.

Pitt Ford TR, Roberts GJ. 1990. Tissue response to glass ionomer retrograde root fillings. *Int Endod J*. 23(5):233–38.

Plotino G, Pameijer CH, et al. 2007. Ultrasonics in endodontics: A review of the literature. *J Endod*. 33(2):81–95.

Rahbaran S, Gilthorpe MS, et al. 2001. Comparison of clinical outcome of periapical surgery in endodontic and oral surgery units of a teaching dental hospital: A retrospective study. *Oral Surg Oral Med Oral Pathol Oral Radiol Endod*. 91(6):700–09.

Rapp EL, Brown, CE Jr, et al. 1991. An analysis of success and failure of apicoectomies. *J Endod*. 17(10):508–12.

Ray HA, Trope M. 1995. Periapical status of endodontically treated teeth in relation to the technical quality of the root filling and the coronal restoration. *Int Endod J*. 28(1):12–18.

Reit C. 1987. Decision strategies in endodontics: On the design of a recall program. *Endod Dent Traumatol*. 3(5):233–39.

Richman R. 1957. The use of ultrasonics in root canal therapy and root resection. *Med Dent J*. 12:12–18.

Rubinstein RA, Kim S. 2002. Long-term follow-up of cases considered healed one year after apical microsurgery. *J Endod*. 28(5):378–83.

Rubinstein RK. 1999. Short-term observation of the results of endodontic surgery with the use of a surgical operation microscope and Super-EBA as root-end filling material. *J Endod*. 25(1):43–48.

Rud J, Rud V, et al. 1997. Effect of root canal contents on healing of teeth with dentin-bonded resin composite retrograde seal. *J Endod*. 23(8):535–41.

Rud J, Rud V, et al. 2001. Periapical healing of mandibular molars after root-end sealing with dentine-bonded composite. *Int Endod J*. 34(4): 285–92.

Salehrabi R, Rotstein I. 2004. Endodontic treatment outcomes in a large patient population in the USA: An epidemiological study. *J Endod*. 30(12):846–50.

Saunders W. 2008. A prospective clinical study of C surgery using mineral trioxide aggregate as a root-end filling. J *Endodont*. 34(6):660–65. doi:10.1016/j.joen.2008.03.002.

Saunders WP, Saunders EM. 1994. Coronal leakage as a cause of failure in root-canal therapy: A review. *Endod Dent Traumatol*. 10(3): 105–08.

Schwartz-Arad D, Yarom N, et al. 2003. A retrospective radiographic study of root-end surgery with amalgam and intermediate restorative material. *Oral Surg Oral Med Oral Pathol Oral Radiol Endod*. 96(4):472–77.

Silveira CM, Sanchez-Ayala A, et al. 2008. Repair of furcal perforation with mineral trioxide aggregate: Long-term follow-up of 2 cases. *J Can Dent Assoc*. 74(8):729–33.

Strindberg L. 1956. The dependence of the results of pulp therapy on certain factors. *Acta Odontologica Scandinavica*. 14(Suppl):21.

Taschieri S, Del Fabbro M, et al. 2007. Endodontic reoperation using an endoscope and microsurgical instruments: One year follow-up. *Br J Oral Maxillofac Surg*. 45(7):582–85.

Testori T, Capelli M, et al. 1999. Success and failure in periradicular surgery: A longitudinal retrospective analysis. *Oral Surg Oral Med Oral Pathol Oral Radiol Endod*. 87(4):493–98.

Tidmarsh BG, Arrowsmith MG. 1989. Dentinal tubules at the root ends of apicected teeth: A scanning electron microscopic study. *Int Endod J*. 22(4):184–89.

Torabinejad M, Anderson P, et al. 2007. Outcomes of root canal treatment and restoration, implant-supported single crowns, fixed partial dentures, and extraction without replacement: A systematic review. *J Prosthet Dent*. 98(4):285–11.

Torabinejad M, Chivian N. 1999. Clinical applications of mineral trioxide aggregate. *J Endod*. 25(3):197–205.

Torabinejad M, Pitt Ford TR. 1996. Root end filling materials: A review. *Endod Dent Traumatol*. 12(4):161–78.

Torabinejad M, Pitt Ford TR, et al. 1997. Histologic assessment of mineral trioxide aggregate as a root-end filling in monkeys. *J Endod*. 23(4):225–28.

Torabinejad M, Smith PW, et al. 1995. Comparative investigation of marginal adaptation of mineral trioxide aggregate and other commonly used root-end filling materials. *J Endod*. 21(6):295–99.

Tsesis I, Rosen E, et al. 2006. Retrospective evaluation of surgical endodontic treatment: Traditional versus modern technique. *J Endod*. 32(5):412–16.

von Arx T, Gerber C, et al. 2001. Periradicular surgery of molars: A prospective clinical study with a one-year follow-up. *Int Endod J*. 34(7):520–25.

von Arx T, Frei C, Bornstein MM. 2003. Periradicular surgery with and without endoscopy: A prospective clinical comparative study. *Schweiz Monatsschr Zahnmed*. 113(8):860–65.

Wang N, Knight K, et al. 2004. Treatment outcome in endodontics—The Toronto Study. Phases I and II: Apical surgery. *J Endod*. 30(11): 751–61.

Waplington M, Lumley PJ, et al. 1997. Incidence of root face alteration after ultrasonic retrograde cavity preparation. *Oral Surg Oral Med Oral Pathol Oral Radiol Endod*. 83(3):387–92.

Watts JD, Holt DM, et al. 2007. Effects of pH and mixing agents on the temporal setting of tooth-colored and gray mineral trioxide aggregate. *J Endod*. 33(8):970–73.

Wenzel A, Grondahl HG. 1995. Direct digital radiography in the dental office. *Int Dent J*. 45(1):27–34.

Wesson CM, Gale TM. 2003. Molar apicectomy with amalgam root-end filling: results of a prospective study in two district general hospitals. *Br Dent J*. 195(12):707–14; discussion p. 698.

Wuchenich G, Meadows D, et al. 1994. A comparison between two root end preparation techniques in human cadavers. *J Endod*. 20(6): 279–82.

Zuolo ML, Ferreira MO, et al. 2000. Prognosis in periradicular surgery: A clinical prospective study. *Int Endod J*. 33(2):91–98.

Section 6
Restoration of the Placed Implant

Chapter 18 What Every Surgeon Needs to Know About Implant-Supported Prosthodontics

Steven M. Morgano, DMD, Mohamad Koutrach, DDS, Fahad Al-Harbi, BDS, MSD, DScD

INTRODUCTION

Implant dentistry has allowed dentists to predictably replace missing teeth. The implant serves as an artificial root that supports and retains an artificial crown; therefore, implant dentistry is a branch of prosthodontics that has a prepros-thetic surgical component. To satisfy the patient's expectations related to aesthetics, phonetics, and function, the implant team—restorative dentist, surgeon, and dental laboratory technician—must work in concert with a clear understanding of the role or roles that each member of the team must play.

Patients request implant dentistry because of their desire for artificial teeth. Consequently, treatment planning should begin with the dentist who will fabricate the artificial tooth or teeth. Also, all members of the team should have a general understanding of the entire treatment process, including treatment planning, surgical procedures, clinical prosthodontic procedures, laboratory procedures, and follow-up care. This chapter reviews what every surgeon must know about implant-supported prosthodontics.

MANAGING THE SINGLE IMPLANT-SUPPORTED CROWN IN THE AESTHETIC ZONE

The conventional method of replacing a single missing tooth with an implant-supported crown involved surgical placement of the implant, covering of the implant with a soft tissue flap, surgical uncovering of the implant after osseointegration, and placement of a healing abutment. After sufficient healing of the soft tissue surrounding the healing abutment, an impression was made, a definitive abutment was placed, and the final crown was then delivered. This approach provided satisfactory results for tooth locations where aesthetic considerations were not paramount; however, when replacing teeth in the aesthetic zone, a more sophisticated approach has the

potential to improve the aesthetic outcome substantially (Wöhrle 1998; DeRouck et al. 2009).

Artificial crowns in the maxillary anterior region and the maxillary premolar region can be considered to be in the aesthetic zone, and favorable contours of the artificial crown and the soft tissues are critical to the success of the restorations. In addition, the location and angulation of the implant will influence the final result.

Soft Tissue Contours

When replacing a missing tooth in the aesthetic zone, an adequate thickness of soft tissue must be present to ensure the development of soft tissue contours that mimic natural gingival tissues. Figure 18.1 illustrates a patient who had a missing maxillary left central incisor. This patient was wearing, at the time, a maxillary provisional acrylic resin removable partial denture (RPD). To develop the soft tissue site to receive an implant, the pontic of the RPD was modified to an ovate style that indented the soft tissue and began the process of developing a pseudogingival margin and interdental papillae (Koutrach and Nimmo 2010; Figures 18.2, 18.3).

A surgical guide template was prepared that duplicated the position of the central incisor on the RPD, and the position and angulation of the implant was planned accordingly. A flapless surgical approach was used and the implant was immediately provisionalized. A 35-Ncm measurement of primary stability (final insertion torque measurement) of the implant is commonly recommended for immediate provisionalization; nevertheless, recommendations in the literature have ranged from as low as 30 Ncm (Drago and Lazzara 2006; Ostman, Hell, and Sennerby 2008) to as high as 40–45 Ncm (Hui et al. 2001; Nkenke and Fenner 2006). The provisional crown must be fabricated free of proximal contacts and occlusal contacts in maximal intercuspal position and in any eccentric positions (Nkenke and Fenner 2006). A

Practical Osseous Surgery in Periodontics and Implant Dentistry, First Edition. Edited by Serge Dibart, Jean-Pierre Dibart.
© 2011 John Wiley & Sons, Inc. Published 2011 by John Wiley & Sons, Inc.

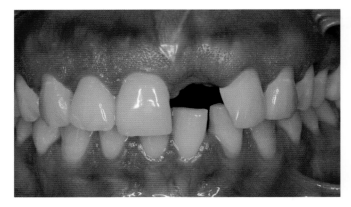

Figure 18.1 Patient with missing maxillary left central incisor. Site of missing tooth has adequate soft tissue. Soft tissue will be recontoured with a removable prosthesis prior to implant placement.

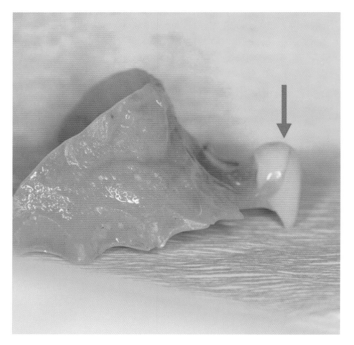

Figure 18.2 Removable partial denture (RPD) has been modified by adding tooth-colored acrylic resin to develop convex, ovate, pontic form (arrow).

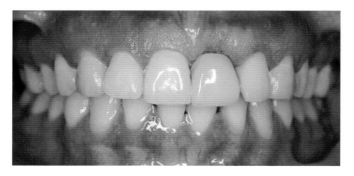

Figure 18.3 RPD in place.

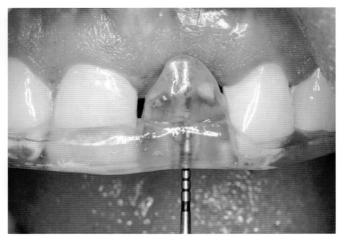

Figure 18.4 Flapless surgical procedure for implant placement. Initial drill is aligned and positioned with the aid of a surgical guide template.

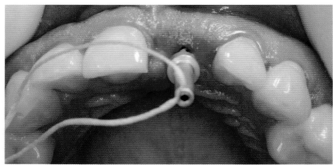

Figure 18.5 Occlusal view of angulation guide. Note optimal placement and angulation of initial osteotomy, as well as the indentation of soft tissue as a result of ovate pontic.

screw-retained provisional restoration is preferred to avoid the problem of cleaning excess cement in the presence of a surgical wound. Figures 18.4–18.9 illustrate the surgical and temporization procedures.

Fabrication and Delivery of the Definitive Crown

After osseointegration was achieved, a final impression was made. The provisional crown was removed, and an impression coping was placed. To ensure that the soft-tissue emergence profile was captured in the definitive cast, flowable composite resin was placed in the gap between the soft tissue and the impression coping (Figure 18.10). The impression was made, and an implant analog was attached to the impression coping (Figure 18.11).

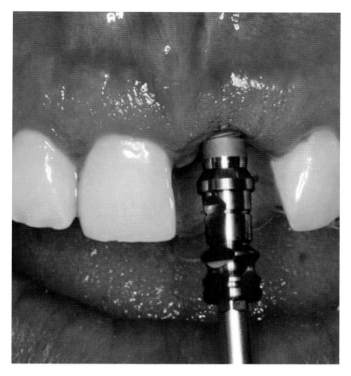

Figure 18.6 Implant placement.

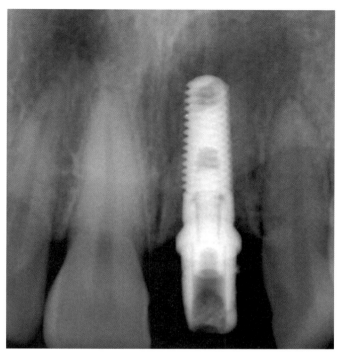

Figure 18.7 Radiograph displaying optimal placement of implant.

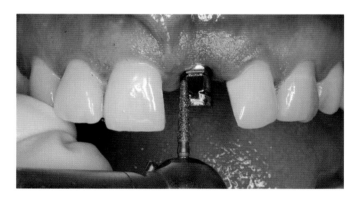

Figure 18.8 Surgical mount is cut back and recontoured in the laboratory to serve as provisional abutment for provisional crown. Contours of the abutment are finalized in the mouth with a coarse diamond rotary instrument and a high-speed hand-piece with copious water irrigation.

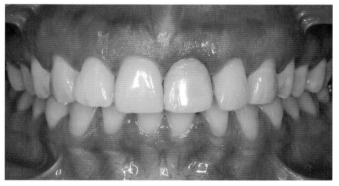

Figure 18.9 Contours of soft tissue around the provisional implant-supported crown after 8 weeks.

MULTIPLE IMPLANT-SUPPORTED CROWNS IN A PARTIALLY EDENTULOUS PATIENT

With multiple implant-supported crowns in series, there are limited landmarks to guide the technician in the fabrication of the custom abutments. After the definitive cast is fabricated (Figure 18.17), a diagnostic waxing is made of the planned final implant-supported crowns. The diagnostic waxing is duplicated in stone, and a clear plastic vacuum-formed template is fabricated (Figure 18.18). The clear plastic shell is used to assist the technician in developing the contours of the custom abutments (Figure 18.19).

A definitive cast was fabricated that included a silicone replica of the soft tissue (Figure 18.12). The final crown was waxed to complete the contour (Figure 18.13) and was then cut back to develop the wax pattern for the custom abutment (Figure 18.14). The custom abutment was cast (Figure 18.15). A definite crown was fabricated and delivered (Figure 18.16).

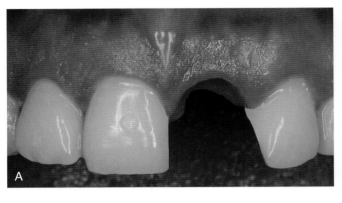

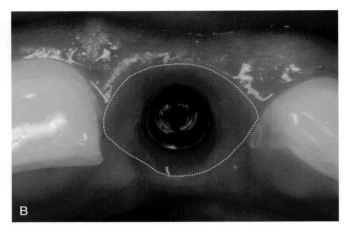

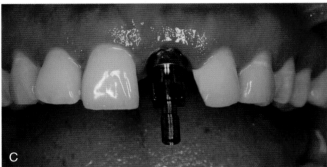

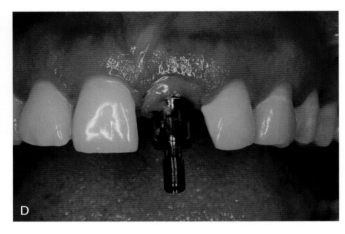

Figure 18.10 (A) Soft tissue contours with provisional crown removed (after 8 weeks). (B) Occlusal view of emergence profile of soft tissue. Note the classic triangular shape. (C) Implant impression coping in place. Note space between coping and soft tissue. (D) To prevent soft tissue from collapsing against impression coping, space is filled with flowable composite resin.

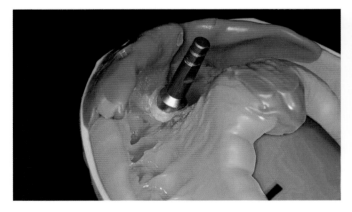

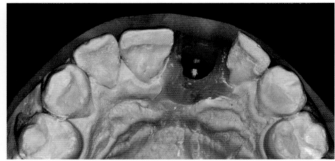

Figure 18.12 Definitive cast. Note silicone replica of soft tissue that preserves the emergence profile developed with the provisional crown.

Figure 18.11 Definitive impression with implant analog attached to the impression coping. Note flowable composite resin, which preserves emergence profile.

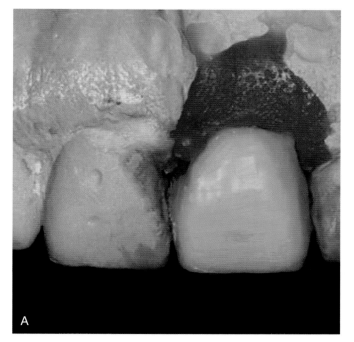

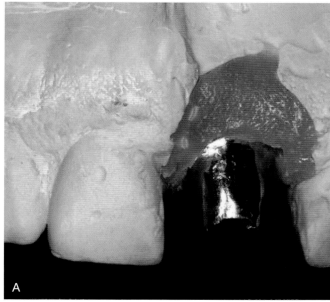

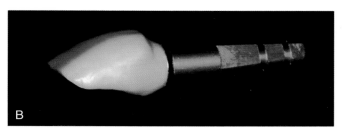

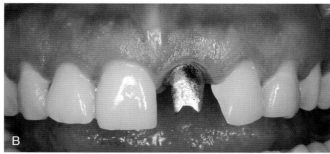

Figure 18.13 (A) Pattern for final crown waxed to complete contour. (B) Emergence profile contours.

Figure 18.15 Cast gold custom abutment on cast (A) and in the mouth (B).

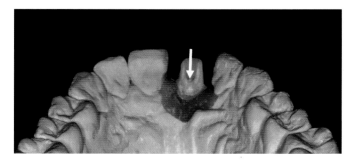

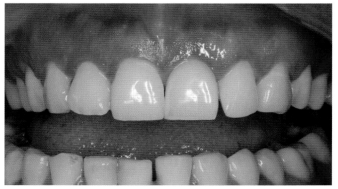

Figure 18.14 The wax pattern has been cut back to form the pattern for custom abutment, preserving emergence profile contours beneath the soft tissue replica. Note favorable location of screw access opening (at crest of cingulum; see arrow) because of controlled placement of implant by using the surgical guide template.

Figure 18.16 Final definitive crown. Note optimal soft tissue contours that mimic natural contours of contralateral incisor.

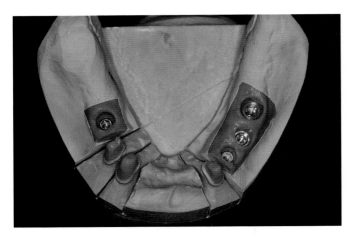

Figure 18.17 Definitive cast for implant-supported prosthodontics and conventional prosthodontics. Mandibular left first molar and premolars will be restored as splinted implant-supported crowns. Mandibular right first molar will be restored as a single implant-supported crown.

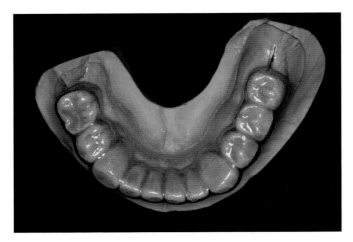

Figure 18.18 Clear plastic vacuum-formed template is fabricated.

Custom abutments are cast and milled to develop a common path of insertion for the definitive crowns (Figure 18.20). The custom abutments must have a common path of insertion because the crowns are commonly splinted to ensure favorable biomechanics. Castings are made for the splinted crowns and tried to verify their fit (Figure 18.21). The custom abutments are placed with a torque wrench at 30–35 Ncm of torque, and the definitive crowns are cemented (Figure 18.22).

SCREW-RETAINED VERSUS CEMENT-RETAINED FIXED RESTORATIONS

The original Branemark protocol for implant-supported fixed complete dentures incorporated screw retention for the prostheses, and Zarb and Schmitt (1991) continued with this protocol when designing their dentures. Because of initial uncertainty regarding the clinical outcomes of these restorations and their supporting implants, it was considered prudent to allow retrievability, whereby the prostheses were retained with screws. With the introduction of osseointegrated implants to restore partially edentulous patients, this screw-retained protocol was initially used with these restorations as well. It soon became apparent that the screw access openings could be located in very inconvenient places, often compromising aesthetics or the establishment of occlusal contacts (Hebel and Gajjar 1997).

Dentists began using prefabricated abutments, as well as custom abutments, cementing convention crowns and fixed partial dentures (FPDs) over these abutments, but results were variable. Abutment screw loosening beneath the crowns was a persistent problem. Often the crown covering an abutment with a loose screw was destroyed to gain entry into the screw access opening to retighten the screw.

With advances in the profession's knowledge and understanding of screw mechanics as well as changes in screw

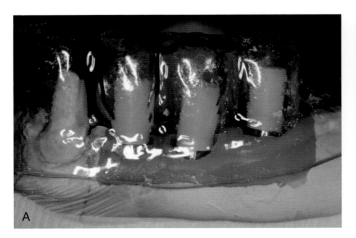

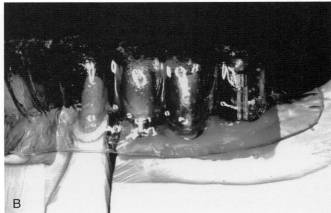

Figure 18.19 (A) UCLA-type abutments are reduced with the aid of the clear plastic template. (B) Wax patterns for custom abutments.

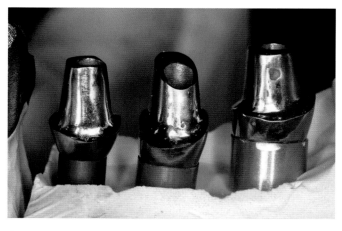

Figure 18.20 Custom abutments. Note that optimal placement of implants has resulted in screw access openings located at occlusal surfaces of abutments.

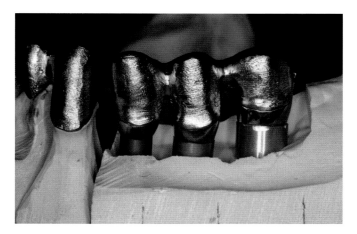

Figure 18.21 Casting for splinted crowns on custom abutments.

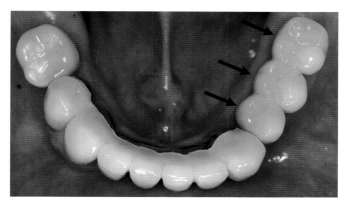

Figure 18.22 Definitive splinted implant-supported crowns in the mouth, occlusal view.

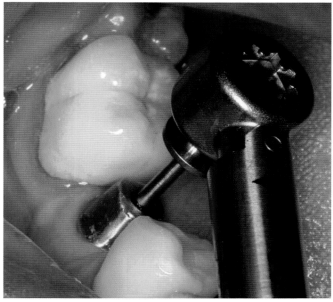

Figure 18.23 Torque wrench used to tighten abutment screw.

and connection designs, screw loosening became much less common. When a screw is tightened, the screw head places a clamping force against the screw threads, holding the abutment to the platform of the implant. This clamping force is called preload. The preload is related to the amount of torque placed on the screw, but the term "preload" is not synonymous with the term "torque" (Lang et al. 2003). Initially, screws were tightened by hand, producing inadequate preload. Special torque wrenches were designed to allow the dentist to place optimal torque on the abutment screw, which far exceeded the torque that could be developed by hand (Figure 18.23). Optimal torque ensures adequate, controlled development of preload without exceeding the tensile strength of the screw. If the tensile strength of the screw is exceeded, it will fracture within the implant.

After the screw is tightened, it can lose some of its preload. Because all surfaces have microroughness, when the screw

is tightened, the surfaces of the screw threads and the threads within the implant (mating thread surfaces) and the surfaces of the screw head and the abutment will lack precise uniform contact. Only the high points on the microroughened surfaces contact. Distortion of these high points with time, along with wear as a result of micromovement, produces a settling effect with the screw joint. The result is a reduction in the clamping force, and this process is called *embedment relaxation* (Aboyoussef, Weiner, and Ehrenberg 2000).

The initial process of embedment relaxation (loss of some of the preload) can be observed almost immediately after the screw has been tightened (Cantwell and Hobkirk 2004). If the dentist tightens the screw to a precise torque measurement using a torque wrench, and then retightens the screw to the same torque value 10 minutes later, the screw can usually be rotated further with the same torque value. In this short interval, the high points of contact on the mating surfaces have relaxed slightly, causing minor settling of the screw and some loss of preload. Further loss of preload occurs over the long term as a result of intraoral function.

Manufacturers have developed screws that are lubricated. With the same torquing force, a lubricated screw can become embedded further within the screw threads of the implant when compared with the embedment of an unlubricated screw. Further embedment within the screw threads of the implant will result in a higher preload or higher clamping force (Park et al. 2010).

The understanding of the connection of the abutment to the implant has also improved. The original Branemark-style implant possessed a hex on its platform that was 0.7 mm in height. This hex was designed to prevent rotation of the surgical implant mount when the surgeon was driving the implant into bone. Later, the hex was used to provide mechanical antirotation for an implant abutment; however, this hex was never designed for this purpose. Providing a more definitive antirotational effect with the mechanical connection could reduce stresses on the screw connection. Internal connections that extend deeply into the implant have been developed with the intention of reducing the potential for screw loosening by improving the antirotational stability of the joint. Nevertheless, internal connections are not a panacea. If there is mechanical overload of the prosthesis, something will eventually fail. With an internal connection, the internal implant connection itself may distort as a result of mechanical overload (Balfour and O'Brien 1995)

With advances in mechanics, screw loosening is less of a problem, although not entirely eliminated. As a result, most dentists have abandoned screw-retained, partial-arch fixed restorations in favor of cement-retained restorations.

OCCLUSION AND BIOMECHANICS

Fixed Implant-Supported Restorations

The mechanoreceptors within the periodontal ligaments of natural teeth are responsible for guiding the mandible through three-dimensional space during mastication. When a patient's anterior teeth prevent contact of the posterior teeth in eccentric positions (anterior guidance), the chewing stroke is guided by the tactile sensation and tactile memory of the anterior teeth. The mandibular anterior teeth pass by the maxillary anterior teeth without contact, except during the last millimeter of the chewing stroke, where there are gliding contacts on the anterior teeth. However, these gliding contacts are of short duration and low magnitude when compared with contacts in the maximal intercuspal position (Gibbs and Lundeen 1982).

Osseointegrated implants lack a periodontal ligament; therefore, the sensation generated from occlusal contacts is completely different from the sensation experienced with natural teeth. The passive tactile sensation threshold of an implant-supported prosthesis has been reported to be up to 50 times greater when compared with the passive threshold for unrestored natural teeth; that is, an implant-supported prosthesis can be subjected to a force 50 times greater than a force directed to a natural tooth before the patient can sense the force (Jacobs and van Steenberghe 1993). This marked difference in sensation suggests that a patient could easily, and without awareness, overload an implant-supported restoration.

An understanding of the biomechanics of implant-supported artificial occlusion is essential for all members of the implant team. Unfavorable implant placement can result in mechanical overload. Occlusal interferences can also lead to biomechanical overload. Mechanical overload can produce problems manifested in the implant, the prosthesis, the implant-abutment connection or the bone. Problems can include chronic screw loosening, screw fracture (Figure 18.24), implant fracture, or loss of osseointegration (Miyata et al. 2000). A retrospective study by Eckert et al. (2000) of fractured implants reported that screw loosening preceded implant fracture for the majority of the implants, suggesting that screw loosening can be a first sign of biomechanical overload that can eventually lead to more serious complications.

The method of implant support will also influence the biomechanics. A mandibular single molar supported by a 5-mm-diameter implant will result in approximately 50% reduction in abutment strain and micromotion of the crown when compared with a 3.75-mm-diameter implant (Soeng, Korioth, and Hodges 2000; Geramy and Morgano 2004). Micromotion of the artificial crown is an important consideration in implant prosthodontics. Micromotion has been reported to produce various clinical problems for implant-supported crowns, including soft tissue complications (Dixon et al. 1995), bone loss (Hermann et al. 2001), and mechanical problems, including fracture and loosening of screws (Gratton, Aquilino, and Stanford 2001). Ensuring favorable implant placement, angulation, and distribution can ensure favorable biomechanics. Biomechanics can also be improved by splinting implants in series (Guichet, Yoshinobu, and Caputo 2002).

Implant-Supported Overdentures

Occlusion and biomechanics are also important considerations with implant-supported overdentures. Enhanced denture retention and stability, when compared with conven-

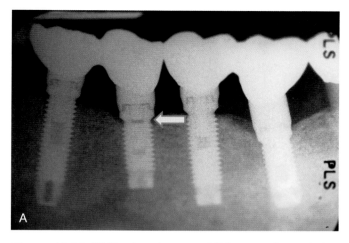

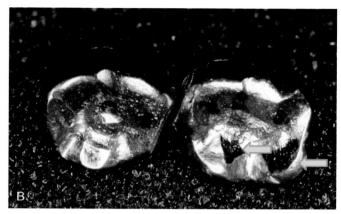

Figure 18.24 (A) Fractured screw visible on radiograph (arrow). (B) Note obvious signs of working occlusal interference on the crown (arrows).

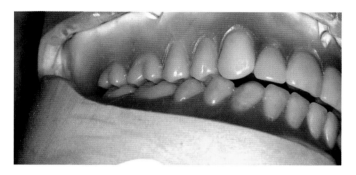

Figure 18.25 Anatomical teeth with sharp, pointed cusps reduce the amount of force required to penetrate food (wax trial dentures). Reduction in force results in improved biomechanics and better stress control.

tional complete dentures, allows patients to function better, with improved neuromuscular activity (Heckmann et al. 2009). This improvement in retention and stability also allows patients to generate considerably more force with implant-supported overdentures (Rismanchian et al. 2009). It is important for the dentist to control stresses generated from these higher-force magnitudes.

The use of teeth with sharp, pointed cusps can improve masticatory performance by reducing the amount of force required to penetrate food, therefore reducing the forces directed to the supporting implants and edentulous ridges (Figure 18.25) (Ohguri et al. 1999). Because mastication involves lateral, protrusive, and retrusive three-dimensional movements, arranging the artificial teeth of complete dentures to allow simultaneous contact of the teeth in eccentric

positions (balanced articulation) can enhance denture stability, uniformly distribute the forces directed to the edentulous ridges and implants, and enhance patient comfort (Figure 18.26; Ohguri et al. 1999; Khamis, Zaki, and Rudy 1988; Sutton and McCord 2007).

A modified form of balanced articulation involves the arrangement of the artificial teeth with cross-arch balance but not cross-tooth balance (Figure 18.27). The term "lingualized occlusion" was later used to describe this method of developing an artificial occlusion (Pound 1970). This occlusal concept has become popular and is commonly advocated for implant-supported removable prosthodontics. Clinical and in vitro studies have shown that balanced lingualized occlusion can be as effective at controlling stresses and enhancing masticatory function as classical balanced articulation (Ohguri et al. 1999; Khamis, Zaki, and Rudy 1988; Sutton and McCord 2007).

PLANNING OVERDENTURES AND SCREW-RETAINED FIXED COMPLETE DENTURES

Patient Assessment

Overdenture restorations and screw-retained fixed complete dentures require careful planning to ensure predictable results. Treatment planning begins with the dentist who will be responsible for the fabrication of the prosthesis. The clinical procedures for screw-retained fixed complete dentures are similar to those used for implant-supported overdentures; therefore, these procedures will be discussed simultaneously in this section.

When planning these types of prostheses, the dentist must ensure adequate space for the implant components and the

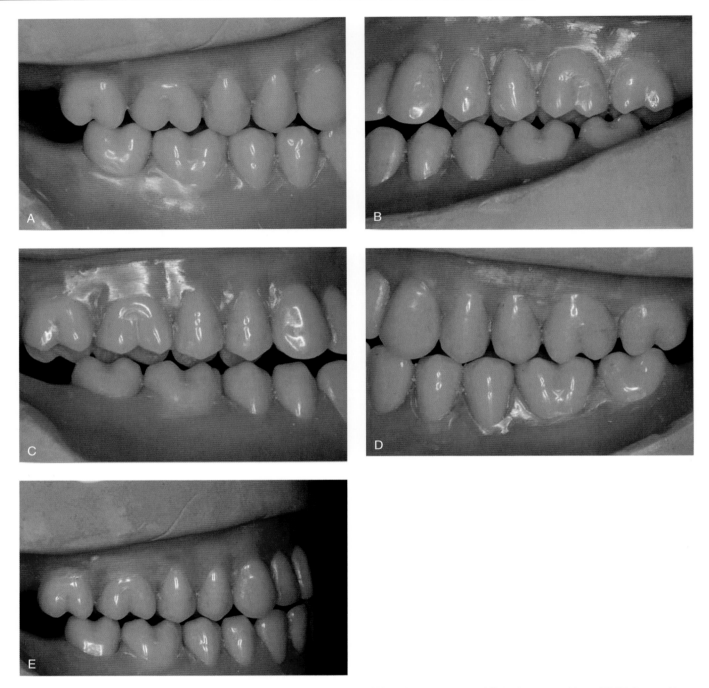

Figure 18.26 Classical balanced articulation. (A) Right working. (B) Left nonworking. (C) Left nonworking. (D) Right working. (E) Protrusion.

prosthetic components. This space assessment is accomplished by fabricating a wax trial denture, similar to that used in a conventional complete denture technique. After the wax trial denture is evaluated for aesthetics, phonetics, and the vertical dimension of occlusion, the mounting is verified with a new centric relation record. This new record must match the mounting on the articulator.

Once it has been determined that tooth positioning is correct, the technician can make an index of the occlusal surfaces and incisal edges of the artificial teeth. The artificial teeth are then removed from the wax, seated into the index, and attached with sticky wax. The relationship of the ridgelaps of the artificial teeth to the residual alveolar ridge can now be assessed to ensure adequate space. A similar index is used

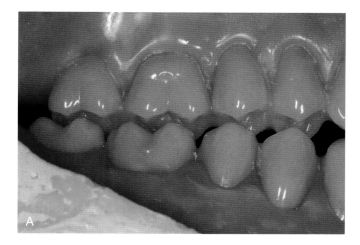

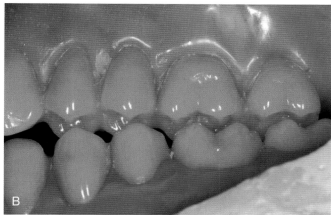

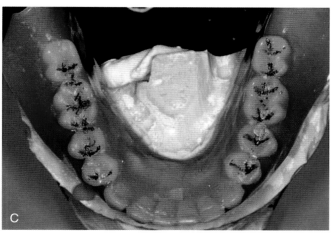

Figure 18.27 (A, B) Lingualized occlusion (wax trial dentures). Compare with occlusal arrangement in Figure 18.25. (C) Clinical remount of final denture and final occlusal equilibration. Note paths traveled by maxillary palatal cusps in eccentric movements.

during the fabrication process itself when a bar is fabricated for an overdenture or a framework is fabricated for a screw-retained fixed complete denture to permit the technician to design the bar or framework in the correct relationship to the planned positions of the teeth (Figure 18.28).

Implant Placement

There are many options for the design of an implant-supported overdenture. The simplest design in the mandible is the placement of two implants with retention derived from two stud attachments. The optimal position of the implants is immediately behind the cingula of the canines. A well made surgical guide template can ensure the desired position and avoid errors in placement (Figure 18.29). If a bar is planned for retention when two conventional-diameter implants are placed, the distance between the two implants from center to center should be 20 mm to permit the placement of two clips (Figure 18.30). This distance will usually place the

implants behind the cingula of the canines. For a mandibular implant-supported overdenture that will be retained with a bar supported by four implants, the center-to-center distance between the two anterior implants should be 20 mm, and the center-to-center distance between the anterior implant and the posterior implant on each side should be 13 mm to allow placement of one posterior clip on each side between the two implants.

With maxillary overdentures, four implants are recommended, and bar retention is commonly preferred over retention by individual stud attachments because of angulation problems (Figure 18.31). The two anterior implants should be placed behind the cingula of the canines, and the two posterior implants should be placed as far distally as the maxillary sinuses will permit (Figure 18.32).

With a screw-retained implant-supported complete denture, implants should be placed to ensure optimal position of the

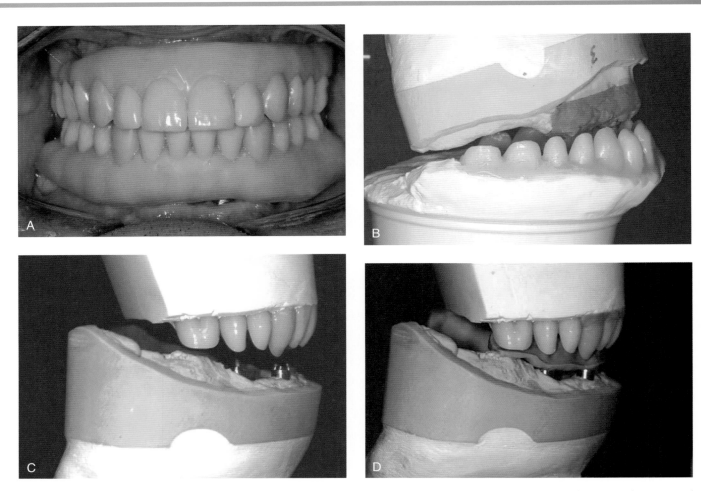

Figure 18.28 (A) Wax trial dentures for patient who will receive bar-retained implant-supported maxillary overdenture and screw-retained implant-supported mandibular complete denture. (B) Maxillary tooth index indicates available space for bar. (C) Mandibular tooth index indicates available space for framework. (D) Pattern for mandibular framework and its relationship to ridgelaps of artificial teeth.

Figure 18.29 Mandibular overdenture retained with stud attachments. Implants have been placed too far posteriorly. Optimal position is immediately behind the cingula of the canines. A surgical guide template would have avoided this error.

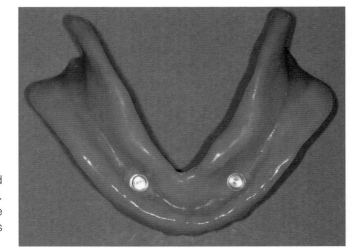

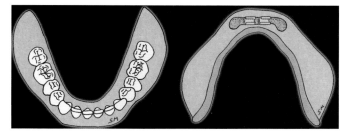

Figure 18.30 Mandibular implant-supported overdenture retained by a bar and two clips. Distance from center to center of conventional-diameter implants should be 20 mm.

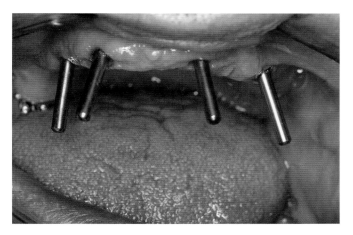

Figure 18.31 Because of the shape of the maxillary alveolar process, maxillary implants for overdenture retention are frequently divergent. Placement of a bar can correct this divergence.

screw-access openings in the final prosthesis. A surgical guide template can assist in the placement of the implants. The two most posterior implants should be placed as far distally as vital structures will permit. There is commonly an anterior loop of the inferior alveolar nerve of about 2 mm before it exits the mental foramen. A cone beam CT scan can assist in locating the loop. The distal surface of the most posterior implant on either side should be located 2 mm anterior to the loop.

AUTHORS' VIEWS AND COMMENTS

The final result of any implant-supported prosthesis depends on the treatment-planning process and a team approach. With the introduction of implant-supported prosthodontics, the revolutionary ability to retain a mandibular complete denture with screws and implants improved the quality of life for many edentulous patients. With these restorations, aesthetics were not of overriding importance, and planning was less critical. Today, patients are expecting highly aesthetic results along with comfort and function. It is essential that all members of the implant team have a clear understating of all steps involved in the treatment process—treatment planning, implant surgery (including grafting procedures), clinical and laboratory prosthetic treatment, and follow-up care. Treatment planning must start with the dentist who will provide the restorative treatment. It is no longer acceptable for a surgeon to place implants without any input from the restorative dentist. This chapter gives a brief summary of what every surgeon must know not only about what occurs after the implants are placed but also what should occur before the they are placed.

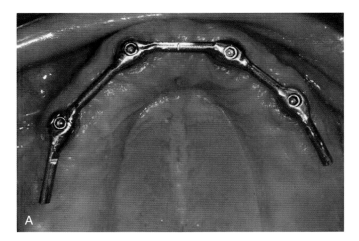

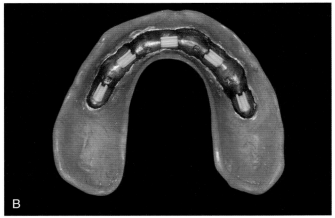

Figure 18.32 (A) Maxillary bar for overdenture retention. Note cantilevers distal to the most distal implants to support occlusal table. Posterior implants were placed as far distally as sinuses would permit. (B) Intaglio of U-shaped denture with clips.

REFERENCES

Aboyoussef H, Weiner S, Ehrenberg D. 2000. Effect of an antirotation resistance form on screw loosening for single implant-supported crowns. *J Prosthet Dent.* 83:450–55.

Balfour A, O'Brien GR. 1995. Comparative study of antirotational single tooth abutments. *J Prosthet Dent.* 73:36–43.

Cannizzaro G, Leone M, Consolo U, et al. 2008. Immediate functional loading of implants placed with flapless surgery versus conventional implants in partially edentulous patients: A 3-year randomized controlled clinical trial. *Int J Oral Maxillofac Implants.* 23:867–75.

Cantwell A, Hobkirk JA. 2004. Preload loss in gold prosthesis-retaining screws as a function of time. *Int J Oral Maxillofac Implants.* 19:124–32.

De Rouck T, Collys K, Wyn I, et al. 2009. Instant provisionalization of immediate single-tooth implants is essential to optimize esthetic treatment outcome. *Clin Oral Implants Res.* 20:566–70.

Dixon DL, Breeding LC, Sadler JP, et al. 1995. Comparison of screw loosening, rotation, and deflection among three implant designs. *J Prosthet Dent.* 74:270–78.

Drago CJ, Lazzara RJ. 2006. Immediate occlusal loading of osseotite implants in mandibular edentulous patients: A prospective observational report with 18-month data. *J Prosthodont.* 15:187–94.

Eckert SE, Meraw SJ, Cal E, et al. 2000. Analysis of incidence and associated factors with fractured implants: A retrospective study. *Int J Oral Maxillofac Implants.* 15:662–67.

Geramy A, Morgano SM. 2004 Finite element analysis of three designs of an implant-supported molar crown. *J Prosthet Dent.* 92:434–40.

Gibbs CH, Lundeen HL. 1982. Jaw movements and forces during chewing and swallowing and their clinical significance. In Gibbs CH, Lundeen HL. *Advances in Occlusion.* John Wright PSG, Boston. pp. 2–50.

Gratton DG, Aquilino SA, Stanford CM. 2001. Micromotion and dynamic fatigue properties of the dental-implant interface. *J Prosthet Dent.* 85:47–52.

Guichet DL, Yoshinobu D, Caputo AA. 2002. Effect of splinting and interproximal contact tightness on load transfer by implant restorations. *J Prosthet Dent.* 87:528–35.

Hebel KS, Gajjar RC. 1997. Cement-retained versus screw-retained implant restorations: Achieving optimal occlusion and esthetics in implant dentistry. *J Prosthet Dent.* 77:28–35.

Heckmann SM, Heussinger S, Linke JJ, et al. 2009. Improvement and long-term stability of neuromuscular adaptation in implant-supported overdentures. *Clin Oral Implants Res.* 20:1200–05.

Hermann JS, Schoolfield JD, Schenk RK, et al. 2001. Influence of the size of the microgap on crestal bone changes around titanium implants. A histometric evaluation of unloaded non-submerged implants in the canine mandible. *J Periodontol.* 72:1372–83.

Hui E, Chow J, Li D, et al. 2001. Immediate provisional for single-tooth implant replacement with Branemark system: Preliminary report. *Clin Implant Dent Relat Res.* 3:79–86.

Jacobs R, van Steenberghe D. 1993. Comparison between implant-supported prostheses and teeth regarding passive threshold level. *Int J Oral Maxillofac Implants.* 8:549–54.

Khamis MM, Zaki HS, Rudy TE. 1998. A comparison of the effect of different occlusal forms in mandibular implant overdentures. *J Prosthet Dent.* 79:422–29.

Koutrach M, Nimmo A. 2010. Preservation of existing soft-tissue contours in the transition from a tooth to an implant restoration in the esthetic zone using a flapless approach: A clinical report. *J Prosthodont.* 19:391–96.

Lang LA, Kang B, Wang R-F, et al. 2003. Finite element analysis to determine implant preload. *J Prosthet Dent.* 90:539–46.

Miyata T, Kobayashi Y, Araki H, et al. 2000. The influence of controlled occlusal overload on peri-implant tissue. Part 3: A histologic study in monkeys. *Int J Oral Maxillofac Implants.* 15:425–31.

Nkenke E, Fenner M. 2006. Indications for immediate loading of implants and implant success. *Clin Oral Implants Res.* 17(Suppl 2):19–34.

Ohguri T, Kawano F, Ichikawa T, et al. 1999. Influence of occlusal scheme on the pressure distribution under a complete denture. *Int J Prosthodont.* 12:353–58.

Ostman PO, Hellman M, Sennerby L. 2008. Immediate occlusal loading of implants in the partially edentate mandible: A prospective 1-year radiographic and 4-year clinical study. *Int J Oral Maxillofac Implants.* 23:315–22.

Park J-K, Choi J-U, Jeon Y-C, et al. 2010. Effects of abutment screw coating on implant preload. *J Prosthodont.* 19:458–64.

Rismanchian M, Bajoghli F, Mostajeran Z, et al. 2009. Effect of implants on maximum bite force in edentulous patients. *J Oral Implantol.* 35:196–200.

Seong WJ, Korioth TW, Hodges JS. 2000 Experimentally induced abutment strains in three types of single-molar implant restorations. *J Prosthet Dent.* 84:318–26.

Sutton AF, McCord JF. 2007. A randomized clinical trial comparing anatomic, lingualized, and zero-degree posterior occlusal forms for complete dentures. *J Prosthet Dent.* 97:292–98.

Wöhrle PS. 1998. Single-tooth replacement in the aesthetic zone with immediate provisionalization: Fourteen consecutive case reports. *Pract Periodontics Aesthet Dent.* 10:1107–14.

Zarb GA, Schmitt A. 1991. Osseointegration and the edentulous predicament. The 10-year-old Toronto Study. *Br Dent J.* 170:439–44.

Index

Practical Osseous Surgery in Periodontics and Implant Dentistry, First Edition. Edited by Serge Dibart, Jean-Pierre Dibart.
© 2011 John Wiley & Sons, Inc. Published 2011 by John Wiley & Sons, Inc.

root-, ratio, 228–29
single implant-supported, 249–51
splinted, 255f
CT. *See* Computer tomography
CTX1. *See* Carboxyterminal telopeptide
of type 1 collagen
Cunningham, W., 232–33
Cuspid
angle to alveolar bone, 115f
CBCT, 86f
eminence, 112f, 113f
endodontic abscess on right, 104f
Cusps pointed, 257, 257f
Cylindrical implants, 176
Cytokine, 3, 4, 5. *See also specific
cytokines*
inflammation markers and, 21
inflammatory, 21–22
proinflammatory, 51–52

Daughaday, W. H., 55
Deep probing pockets, 4, 7
Definitive cast, 252f, 253f, 254f
Definitive crown, 250–51, 251f, 252f,
253f
Definitive impression, 252f
Definitive therapy, 42
Deformation, 79f, 80f
Demineralized freeze-dried bone allograft
(DFDBA), 216
Dentures, 254
bar-retained implant supported, 260f
mandibular, 69
modified prosthetic design, 71f
retention by maxillary implant, 261f
screw-retained fixed complete, 70f,
257–58
like templates, 217f
u-shaped with clips, 261f
wax trial, 258, 259f, 260f
DFDBA. *See* Demineralized freeze-dried
bone allograft
Diabetes, 3
clinical parameters, 14
emergencies, 12
patient management, 11–12
periodontitis and, 11–15
surgery and, 12
uncontrolled, 11
Diabetes mellitus type 1, 11
periodontal treatment and, 14–15
Diabetes mellitus type 2, 11
periodontal treatment and, 12–14
Diabetic microangiopathy, 11
DICOM. *See* Digital Imaging and
Communication in
Medicine
Diet, 4, 6
Digital Imaging and Communication in
Medicine (DICOM), 208

Diseased teeth, 236
Disease-modifying antirheumatic drugs
(DMARDS), 27
Docosahexaenoic acid, 31
Double parabola, 43, 48f
Dynamic surgical guides, 210
Dyslipidemia, 20

Edentulous mandible treatment, 69
Edentulous maxillae treatment, 69
Edentulous patients, 24
implant treatment for partially, 69,
71
partially, 251, 254, 254f, 255f
Edentulous ridge expansion (ERE),
159–66
mandible, 171f
Edentulous sites, biomechanical
stabilization in, 107
Eicosapentaenoic acid, 31
Elasticity calculation models, 79f
Elevated antibody titer, 23
Endocrine, 51
Endodontic abscess, 104f
Endodontic literature
case selection, 240
follow-up period, 241
implant literature compared to,
239–42
indices in, 236, 239
publication bias, 241
resurgery - outcomes assessment
studies, 239
success *versus* survival, 240
summary of selected, 237–38t
surgery - outcomes assessment
studies, 239
Endodontic microsurgery, 227–39
anatomical considerations in, 229f
considerations concerning, 228–30
indications, 227–28, 229f
instruments, 231–32
objectives, 227
outcome assessment, 236, 239
surgical procedure, 230, 231f
traditional *versus* modern techniques
in, 230–31, 232t
ultrasonics used in, 232–33
Endodontic treatment, 242–43
implant treatment compared to, 228f,
240, 241tf, 242–43
Endosseous implants, 75
protocol for placement and loading,
107
Endothelial dysfunction, 20
pathogenesis, 24–25
End-stage tooth, 242
ERE. *See* Edentulous ridge
expansion
Erythrocyte sedimentation rate, 21

Extension crest device, for ridge splitting,
161

FGF. *See* Fibroblast growth factor
Fibrinogen, 21
Fibroblast growth factor (FGF), 51, 52t,
55
Fish oil, 5, 31
Fissure bur, 183
5s rule, 182–83
Fixed implant-supported restoration,
256–57
Fixed partial dentures (FPD), 254
Flap
abbreviated trapezoidal, 213
elevation and piezosurgery, 195
full-thickness mucoperiosteal, 162
mucoperiosteal, 230, 231f
osteoperiosteal, 162
partial-thickness, 39f, 40f, 162
passive adaptation of, 187f
u-shaped peninsula, 213
Flapless surgery, 213–14
for implant placement, 250f
indications, 213–14
Flap surgery, 48
flapless compared to, 213–14
ridge expansion technique and,
162
FPD. *See* Fixed partial dentures
Fractured tooth, 118f
Free radicals, 5–6
Friedman, N., 37
Frost, H. M., 195
Full-thickness mucoperiosteal flap, 162
Fusobacterium-stimulated
polymorphonucleocytes, 6

Garlic, 7
GBR. *See* Guided bone regeneration
Generalized aggressive periodontitis,
215f
Gingival crevicular fluid, 6
Gingival recession, 142f, 197f
piezocision and, 199f
Gingivitis, 22
Glucose monitoring, 12
Glycated hemoglobin, 13–14
Glycemic control, 11
Glycosylated hemoglobin (HbA1c), 11
Gold custom abutment, 253f
Graft. *See also* Bone graft
biomaterial, 139f
connective tissue, 198f
hard tissue, 195
onlay, 179
protection, 187f
soft tissue, 189f, 195
Gram-negative bacteria, 20
Green tea, 7

Jaw
  osteonecrosis of, 17–18
  osteoporosis, 32
Juvenile idiopathic arthritis, 31

Keratinized tissue, 212–13
Kim, S., 242
Kramer, Gerald M., 48
Kronfield R., 37
Kurrek, A., 148

Lateral incisor site, 107, 110
Lateral window approach, 145–46,
      146t
  complication possibilities, 146–47
Lazarra, R., 107
Leukocytes, 21
Ligament, 76f
  supported teeth, 75
  vascular net of space, 75
Limiting canals, 97
Lindhe, J., 37
Lingualized occlusion, 257, 259f
Lipopolysaccharide, 23
Lipoprotein parameters, 24
Loaf slicer, 89f
Long-term studies, 241
Lubricated screw, 256
Luc, H., 145
Lycopene, 5–6

Macrovascular pathology, 11
Magnification
  power of, 235–36
  recommended, for different
      procedures, 235t
Major histocompatibility complex, 27–28
Malar process, 112f
Malnutrition, 6
Mandible
  anterior, 197f
  axial CT original, parallel to base of,
      94f
  axial CT reformats when using base
      of, 95f
  cortical bone location in, 95, 97
  edentulous, 69
  ERE, 171f
  lower posterior, 170f
  membrane exposure in, 174
  one-stage ridge splitting of, 169,
      173–74
  three-dimensional view of lower, 200f
  two-stage ridge splitting of, 169
  virtual implant planning in, 218f
Mandibula
  incisors-sockets, 109f
  intraoral view of incisor area, 58f
  resorption, 101f
  three-dimensional CT scan of, 59f

Mandibular
  canal, 99f
  chin grafts and, 180
  dentures, 69
  framework, 260f
  implant placement, 222f, 223f
  molars, 40
    first, 111f
    socket, 109f
  osteoporosis, 31
  overdentures, 260f
    implant supported, 261f
  ramus block graft, 180
Mandibular bicuspids
  alveolar housing projection midline,
      112f
  first, 111f
  sockets, 109f
MAPK. See Mitogen activated protein
      kinase
MAP system tips, 232f
Marginal bone, 42, 45f
Martin, H., 232–33
Matrix Metalloproteinases (MMP), 30, 51
Maxilla, 220f, 221f
  cortical bone location in, 95
  edentulous, 69
  implant placement in, 220f, 221f
  interproximal incisions completed in,
      197f
  intraoral view of incisor area, 58f
  overdenture, 72f
  physical models of, 209f
  three-dimensional CT scan of, 59f
  virtual implant planning in, 219f
Maxillary
  bar, 261f
  implant for denture retention, 261f
  overdentures, 259
    implant-supported, bar-retained, 72f
  posterior, 99f
  reconstruction and chin grafts, 180
  right second premolar CBCT scan, 73f
Maxillary bicuspid
  alveolar housing projection midline,
      112f
  extraction sites, 114f, 115f
  first, 111f
Maxillary molars
  extraction sites, 114f
  first, 111f, 112
  sockets, 109f
Maxillary sinus, 97, 99f
  bleeding, 146
  buccal wall of, 100f
  cyst, 103f
  extension, 113f
  floor augmentation using rhBMP-2/
      ACS, 56–57, 57f
  incisive foramen variations, 102f

leakage seen in CAT scan, 104f
  minimally invasive surgery, 145–58
  Underwood's septa in, 100f
Mental foramen, 99f
Mesenchymal stem cells, 53
Metabolic disorder, 11
Metabolic syndrome, 4–5, 6
Metal plate, 175f
MIAMBE. See Minimally invasive antral
      membrane balloon elevation
Microbial antigens, cross-reactivity
      between self-antigens and, 20
Microbial dental plaque, 19
Microbial infection, 20
Microbial pathogenesis, of rheumatoid
      arthritis, 30
Microvascular circulation, 29
Microvascular pathology, 11
Mineral trioxide aggregate (MTA), 233,
      234–35
  gray and white, 235f
Minimally invasive antral membrane
      balloon elevation (MIAMBE), 156
Minimally invasive maxillary sinus
      surgery, 145–58
Mitogen activated protein kinase (MAPK),
      55
MMP. See Matrix Metalloproteinases
Moghaddas, H., 41
Molecular mimicry, 20
MTA. See Mineral trioxide aggregate
Mucoperiosteal flap, 230, 231f
Mylohyoid attachment, 100f

Navigation systems, 210
  Image-guided bur tracking, 211
Negative architecture, 42
Neurosensory disturbances, 189
Nitrogen-containing bisphosphonates, 18
Nondefinitive therapy, 42
Non-nitrogen-containing
      bisphosphonates, 18
Nonsmokers, 3
Normal architecture, 42
Noxious stimulus, 185
Nutrition, 5–8
Nutritional status, 6
Nyman, S., 37, 43

Obesity, 3–5
Oblique images, 101f
  occlusal plane and, 97f, 98f
  posterior, 96f
  reference slice, 94f
  reformatted, 85f, 91–95, 102f, 113f
Oblique slice, 90f
  cleared, 93f
  reformatted, 93f
Obstructed tooth extraction, 140f,
      141f

Occlusal
interference on crown, 257f
loads, 79f
fracture related to, 81f
view, 77f
Occlusal plane, 75
implant at right angle to, 108f
reference plane for axials parallel to, 96f
reference plane used for reformat as parallel to, 97f
reformats with plane reference parallel to, 98f
transfer of forces from, 83
Occlusion
biomechanics and, 256–57
implant placement and, 75–106
lingualized, 257, 259f
Ochsenbein, C., 38, 40
O'Connor, T. W., 40
Olive loaf
loaf slicer with, 89f
reformatting, 90f
Olsen, C., 41
Omega-3
fatty acids, 31
Polyunsaturated Fatty Acids, 5
Oncology treatment, for osteonecrosis cases, 17–18
One-stage ridge splitting, 159, 162, 165–66, 172f
of mandible, 169, 173–74
preoperative CT scan prior to, 164f, 168f, 169f
Onion, 7
Onlay grafting, 179
Oral maxillofacial procedures, growth factor BMP-2 use in, 56
Orban, B., 37
Orstavik, D., 236
Orthodontic appliances, 196, 196f
Orthodontic tooth movement. See Periodontally accelerated orthodontic tooth movement
Orthodontist, 199–200
Orthograde treatment, 229
Oscillating saws, for ridge splitting, 161, 161f
Osseointegrated implant, 75, 256
Osseous defects, 46
techniques to eliminate, 38–40
Osseous surgery, 43f, 44f, 45f, 46f, 47f, 48f
bone loss after, 40–41
clinical steps for, 42
comparisons table, 41f
completion of, 46
limitations, 42–43, 46
long-term healing after, 40–41
piezoelectric instruments used for, 41f

postsurgical management, 46
regenerative, 51–64
resective, 37, 39f, 40f
sequence, 42
Ostectomy, 38
Osteoblasts, 3
Osteo-integrated implant, 138f, 139f
OsteoMed kit, 185
Osteonecrosis of jaw, 17–18
Osteoperiosteal flap, 162
Osteoplasty, 37–38
Osteoporosis
jaw, 32
periodontitis and, 31–32
treatment, 17–18
Osteotomy, 132, 135
crestal, 172f
with diameter 2.8–3 mm, 152f
Overdentures
implant-supported, 256–57, 259, 261f
mandibular, 260f
implant-supported, 261f
maxillary, 259
implant-supported, bar-retained, 72f
planning, 257–58
retention, 261f
Oxidative stress, 5

P. gingivalis, 5
elevated antibody titer and, 23
PAI. See Periapical index
Palatal, 76f
Panoramic radiographs, 206
Panoramic reformat, 85f, 86, 91, 101f, 104f
Panoramic slice
cleared, 93f
reformatted, 86, 91
Panorex film, 83, 83f, 104f
PAOO. See Periodontally accelerated osteogenic orthodontics
Paracrine, 51
Paroxysmal positional vertigo, 174, 176
Partial-thickness flap, 39f, 40f, 162
Pathogenesis
arthritis, 27–28
cardiovascular disease, 19–20
endothelial dysfunction, 24–25
of rheumatoid arthritis, microbial, 30
Pathophysiology, 29
PDGF. See Platelet-derived growth factor
PDI. See Prosthetic-driven implantology
Periapical index (PAI), 236
Periapical radiograph, 206
conventional compared to digital, 83, 83f
Peri-implant disease, 5–6

Periodontally accelerated orthodontic tooth movement, 195–201
Periodontally accelerated osteogenic orthodontics (PAOO), 195
Periodontal treatment, 15
diabetes and, 12
diabetes mellitus type 1 and, 14–15
diabetes mellitus type 2 and, 12–14
rheumatoid arthritis and, 30–31
Peroxyl radicals, 5
Persistent periapical lesion, 229f
Physical activity, 4
Physical models, 209
of maxilla, 209f
Physiologic adaption, 75
bite collapse with, 77f
Piezocision, 195–201, 197f
after, 200f
advantages, 198–99
complete, 198f
effect on bone, 196
equipment, 196
gingival recession and, 199f
indications for use of, 196
interproximal incisions, 196, 196f, 197f
possible complications, 198
postoperative care, 198
prior to, 200f
surgical sheet, 199f
technique, 196–98
Piezoelectric
corticotomy, 197f
method to remove implant, 135
Piezoelectrical tips, 127–28, 128f, 129f, 130f, 131f, 132f
Piezoelectric instruments
access and, 135, 144
osseous surgery use of, 41f
Piezoelectric surgery (PS), 179
Piezosurgery
atraumatic extractions, 127–44
chin graft incision with, 182f
flap elevation and, 195
implant removal and, 135
indications, 128, 132
osteotomy and, 132, 135
postoperative treatment and healing period, 174, 176
for ridge expansion, 166, 168–69, 169f, 170f, 171f, 172f, 173–74, 173f, 176
for ridge splitting, 161, 161f
standard technique compared with, 127–28, 129f, 130f, 131f, 132f
Piezotome, 197f
BS1 tip, 196
Pikos Bur Kit, 188f
Platelet activation, 20, 25
Platelet-derived growth factor (PDGF), 51, 52, 52t, 54–56